Anesthesia
for Veterinary Technicians

Anesthesia
for Veterinary Technicians

Susan Bryant, CVT, VTS (Anesthesia)

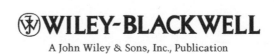

WILEY-BLACKWELL

A John Wiley & Sons, Inc., Publication

Edition first published 2010
© 2010 Blackwell Publishing

Blackwell Publishing was acquired by John Wiley & Sons in February 2007. Blackwell's publishing program has been merged with Wiley's global Scientific, Technical, and Medical business to form Wiley-Blackwell.

Editorial Office
2121 State Avenue, Ames, Iowa 50014-8300, USA

For details of our global editorial offices, for customer services, and for information about how to apply for permission to reuse the copyright material in this book, please see our website at www.wiley.com/wiley-blackwell.

Library of Congress Cataloging-in-Publication Data

Anesthesia for veterinary technicians / [edited by] Susan Bryant.
       p. ; cm.
   Includes bibliographical references and index.
   ISBN 978-0-8138-0586-3 (pbk. : alk. paper)   1. Veterinary anesthesia.   2. Animal health technicians.   I. Bryant, Susan, 1963-.   [DNLM: 1. Anesthesia—veterinary.   2. Anesthesia—methods. SF 914 A579 2010]
   SF914.A54   2010
   636.089'796—dc22

                                                                           2009031849

A catalog record for this book is available from the U.S. Library of Congress.

Set in 10 on 12 Sabon by Toppan Best-set Premedia Limited
Printed in Singapore

1   2010

Contents

On the Web: www.wiley.com/go/bryant

Contributors

Courtney Beiter, RVT, VTS (Anesthesia)
Ohio State University Veterinary School
Columbus, Ohio

Susan Bryant, CVT, VTS (Anesthesia)
Tufts Cummings School of Veterinary
Medicine
North Grafton, Massachusetts

Heather Carter, CVT, VTS (Anesthesia)
Southpaws
Fairfax, Virginia

Michelle Cheyne, CVT, VTS (Anesthesia)
Pet Emergency Center
Veterinary Hospitals
Fort Lauderdale, Florida

Deb Coleman, RVT, VTS (Anesthesia)
VetAMac, Inc.
Ames, Iowa

Kristen Cooley, CVT, VTS (Anesthesia)
Veterinary Medical Teaching Hospital
UW-Madison School of Veterinary Medicine
Madison, Wisconsin

Wendy Curtis-Uhle, CVT, VTS (Anesthesia)
Matthew J. Ryan Veterinary Hospital
University of Pennsylvania
Philadelphia, Pennsylvania

Lynette DeGouff, CVT, VTS (Anesthesia)
Cornell University College of Veterinary
Medicine
Ithaca, New York

Heather Dulong, CVT, VTS (Anesthesia)
New England Medical Center
West Bridgewater, Massachusetts

Jennifer Dupre, CVT, VTS (Anesthesia)
Ross University School of Veterinary Medicine
St. Kitts, West Indies

Trish Farry CVN, VTS (Anesthesia, ECC)
Veterinary Teaching Hospital
School of Veterinary Science
The University of Queensland, Australia

Sharon Fornes, RVT, VTS (Anesthesia)
Western Career College
San Leandro, California

Lori Fuehrer CVT, VTS (Anesthesia)
Rocky Mountain Veterinary Neurology
Veterinary Referral Center of Colorado
3550 S. Jason St.
Englewood, CO

James Gaynor, DVM, MS, DACVS, DAAPM
Peak Performance Veterinary Group
Colorado Springs, Colorado

Ami Gilkey, LVT, VTS (Anesthesia)
VMR-CVM VTH
Blacksburg, Virginia

Susan Holland, LVT, VTS (Anesthesia)
Animal Cancer and Imaging Center
Canton, Michigan

Sharon Johnston, CVT, VTS (Anesthesia)
Simpsonville, North Carolina

Sharon Kaiser-Klinger, RVT, VTS
(Anesthesia)
Premier Equine Veterinary Services
Whitesboro, TX

Jennifer Keefe, CVT, VTS (Anesthesia, ECC)
Dover Veterinary Hospital
Dover, New Hampshire

Harry Latshaw, CVT, VTS (Anesthesia)
VetAMac, Inc.
Ames, Iowa

Amy Levensaler, CVT, VTS (Anesthesia)
Port City Veterinary Referral Hospital
Portsmouth, New Hampshire

Kim Lockhead, CVT, VTS (Anesthesia)
Tufts Cummings School of Veterinary
Medicine
North Grafton, Massachusetts

Ellen LoMastro, CVT, VTS (Anesthesia)
Matthew J. Ryan Veterinary Hospital
University of Pennsylvania
Philadelphia, Pennsylvania

Samantha McMillan, VTS (Anesthesia),
DipAVN (Medical), RVN
Davies Veterinary Specialists,
United Kingdom

Lawrence E. Nann, CVT, VTS (Anesthesia)
University of Pennsylvania
Veterinary Teaching Hospital
New Bolton Center
Kennett Sq., Pennsylvania

Christopher L. Norkus, BS, CVT, VTS
(Anesthesia, ECC)
Ross University School of Veterinary
Medicine
St Kitts, West Indies

Darci Palmer, LVT, VTS (Anesthesia)
VSPN and VSPN CE Member Services,
CE Instructor
Veterinary Support Personnel Network
a division of the Veterinary Information
Network
Davis CA

Heidi L. Reuss-Lamky, LVT, VTS (Anesthesia)
Oakland Veterinary Referral Services
Bloomfield Hills, Michigan

Sandra Robbins, CVT, VTS (Anesthesia)
Tufts Cummings School of Veterinary
Medicine
North Grafton, Massachusetts

Christine Slowiak, CVT, VTS (Anesthesia)
Arlington Veterinary Surgery Specialists
Arlington Heights, Illinois

Kim Spelts, CVT, VTS (Anesthesia), CCRP,
CCMT
Peak Performance Veterinary Group
Colorado Springs, Colorado

Jennifer Stowell, CVT, VTS (Anesthesia)
Tufts Cummings School of Veterinary
Medicine
North Grafton, Massachusetts

Shawn Takada, CVT, VTS (Anesthesia)
The Bobst Hospital
Animal Medical Center
New York, New York

Katy W. Waddell, RVT, VTS (ECC,
Anesthesia)
College of Veterinary Medicine
Texas A & M University
College Station, Texas

Connie Warren, CVT, VTS (Anesthesia)
Tufts Cummings School of Veterinary
Medicine
North Grafton, Massachusetts

Preface

Anesthesia for Veterinary Technicians is intended to act as a reference guide for the aspiring or accomplished veterinary anesthetist. It is intended to be a resource for technicians of varying levels of skill and knowledge, but it also contains advanced material and is suitable as a study guide for those preparing to sit for the Veterinary Technician Specialty in Anesthesia exam.

The book's purpose is to provide veterinary anesthetists with the skills and knowledge to develop safe and effective anesthesia protocols and to be able to avoid or at least proactively anticipate and plan for the treatment of potential complications. The ultimate goal, of course, is to collaborate with our supervising veterinarians to improve the lives of our veterinary patients through informed, compassionate anesthesia and pain management.

Acknowledgments

I believe that behind every successful anesthetist stands a mentor who has inspired enthusiasm for excellent patient care in the field of veterinary anesthesia. For most of the contributors in this book our mentors have been members of the American (or Australian or British) College of Veterinary Anesthesiologists (ACVA). To them we owe a world of thanks and gratitude. We dedicate this book to their endless patience, guidance, and selfless sharing of their vast experience and knowledge. Thank you for believing in us.

I would like to acknowledge veterinary anesthesiologists Dr. Lois Wetmore, Dr. Alicia Karas, Dr. Cheryl Blaze, and Dr. Emily McCobb who, along with our past and present anesthesia residents, Dr. Amanda Abelson, Dr. Elizabeth Armitage-Chan, and Dr. Alex Hawley, have inspired in me an endless quest for the perfect anesthesia protocol; smooth, uncomplicated recoveries; and a passion for pain management. They have discussed and debated complicated workups with me, shared the latest anesthesia drug information, encouraged and allowed me to try new protocols or improve upon old ones, and patiently followed me to the wards for many, many pain consults. In doing all this, they have inspired me to become a better teacher and to share with others what they gave to me. I am forever grateful for their mentorship.

I also want to acknowledge my colleagues in the Academy of Veterinary Technician Anesthetists (AVTA), many of whom contributed chapters to this book. Your dedication and devotion to excellence in veterinary anesthesia and pain management are inspirations to many and gifts to your animal patients. It is a pleasure to work alongside so many talented individuals with the common goal of improving the lives of their patients.

I want to thank Erica Judisch at Wiley-Blackwell for walking me through this experience. Her patience, support, and guidance through this whole process has been amazing. I could not have accomplished this without her.

Finally, I would like to express my sincere gratitude to my family for their support and encouragement during this process. To my fiancé, Leo, who became a "book widow" throughout the writing of this book, yet was ever supportive, I give a heartfelt thank you for putting up with me and my whims. For my dad, Dan Bryant, the man who is my hero, who has always encouraged me to be the best I can possibly be, I say "this one's for you, Bear Bryant."

Susan Bryant, CVT, VTS (Anesthesia)

Anesthesia
for Veterinary Technicians

Review of Cardiovascular and Respiratory Physiology

Susan Bryant

Most anesthetic drugs affect the cardiovascular and/or pulmonary systems in some way. It is important for the anesthetist to have at least a basic understanding of how these systems function and what impact anesthetic drugs are likely to have on them. This chapter reviews the basic physiology of the cardiovascular and respiratory systems, and some of the terminology related to them, as they relate to anesthesia.

The Cardiovascular System

Anatomy and physiology of the heart

The cardiovascular system consists of the heart, which is a muscular pumping device, and a closed system of vessels: the arteries, veins, and capillaries. The heart is responsible for pumping blood around the body, carrying nutrients to all parts of the body, and carrying waste away for removal. The heart consists of four chambers: the right atrium, the right ventricle, the left atrium, and the left ventricle. Arteries are the vessels that carry blood from the heart, and veins carry blood to the heart. Sodium, chloride, potassium, and calcium are the electrolytes that are most important for normal cardiac function. Depolarization of the cell occurs when sodium channels in the cell membrane open increasing sodium permeability. Resting membrane potential becomes less negative due to an influx of positive sodium ions. Cells begin repolarizing when the sodium gates close and negatively charged chloride ions begin to move into the cell. This causes calcium channels to open, allowing an influx of these ions. Final repolarization occurs when the calcium channels close and potassium permeability increases. Any alterations of normal plasma concentrations of these electrolytes can affect cardiac muscle function.

The *sino-atrial (SA) node* in the wall of the right atrium initiates the heartbeat. Impulses from this node transmit to the *atrioventricular (AV) node*. Other impulses in the heart are transmitted by the bundle of HIS, the bundle branches, and the purkinje fibers. Any damage to the cardiac muscle can result in unsynchronized impulse transmission, irregular heart contractions, and reduced cardiac output. The SA node acts as an intrinsic pacemaker and controls the rate of contractions. Both parasympathetic and sympathetic nervous systems innervate the SA node. Acetylcholine and noradrenaline are nervous system mediators that affect sodium,

3

calcium, and potassium channels and can increase or decrease depolarization. Many drugs used for anesthesia purposes can affect heart rate, and therefore monitoring is strongly indicated.

Cardiac cycle

The *cardiac cycle* is the complete series of events that happens in the heart during one heartbeat. Blood flows into the atria from the vena cava and pulmonary veins. The cycle starts with depolarization at the SA node leading to atrial contraction. The atrioventricular valves, called the *mitral* and *tricuspid* valves, open when atrial pressure exceeds ventricular pressure. While the atria contract, blood flows into the relaxed ventricles. This is *diastole*, when the ventricles are relaxed and filling. Next, the atria relax and the ventricles contract (*systole*) pushing blood out the aortic and pulmonary valves. Ventricular systole causes closure of the atrioventricular valves and this action is the first heart sound heard on auscultation. The second heart sound is generated when ventricular relaxation occurs and the pulmonic and aortic valves close. *Murmurs* are abnormal cardiac sounds and usually result from malfunction of the valves (Reece 1997).

Electrical activity

As the heart undergoes depolarization and repolarization, the electrical currents that are generated (as described above) spread not only within the heart, but also throughout the body. This electrical activity generated by the heart can be measured by electrodes placed on the body surface. The recorded tracing of this activity is called an *electrocardiogram* (ECG or EKG). The different waves that comprise the ECG represent the sequence of depolarization and repolarization of the atria and ventricles. The complete cardiac cycle that is portrayed on the ECG is represented by waves that are identified as P wave, QRS complex, T wave.

The *P wave* represents the wave of depolarization that spreads from the SA node throughout the atria. The brief isoelectric period after the P wave represents the time in which the impulse is traveling within the AV node and the bundle of HIS. The period of time from the onset of the P wave to the beginning of the QRS complex is termed the *P-R interval*. This represents the time between the onset of atrial depolarization and the onset of ventricular depolarization. If the interval is prolonged or no QRS complex follows (the impulse is unable to be conducted to the ventricles), there is an *AV conduction block* (1st, 2nd, or 3rd degree AV block).

The *QRS complex* represents the ventricular depolarization. The duration of the QRS complex is normally of relatively short duration, which indicates that ventricular depolarization occurs very rapidly. If the QRS complex is prolonged, conduction is impaired within the ventricles. This can occur with bundle branch blocks or whenever an abnormal pacemaker site becomes the pacemaker driving the ventricle. Changes in the height and width of the QRS complex can indicate left heart enlargement. The shape of the QRS complex can also change depending on placement of the electrodes. The isoelectric period following the QRS (ST segment) is the time at which the entire ventricle is depolarized. The ST segment is important in the diagnosis of ventricular ischemia or hypoxia because under those conditions, the ST segment can become either depressed or elevated.

The *T wave* represents ventricular repolarization and is longer in duration than depolarization. The *Q-T interval* represents the time for both ventricular depolarization and repolarization to occur and therefore roughly estimates the duration of an average ventricular action potential. At high heart rates, ventricular action potentials shorten in duration, which increases the Q-T interval. Prolonged Q-T intervals can be diagnostic for susceptibility to certain types of tachyarrhythmias.

Determining heart rate from an ECG strip

Heart rate can be determined by examining an ECG rhythm strip. The ventricular rate can be determined by measuring the time intervals between the QRS complexes, which is done by looking at the R-R intervals. Assuming a recording speed of 25 mm/sec and a lead II ECG, one method is to divide 1500 by the number of small squares on the recording paper between two R waves. Or one can divide 300 by the number of large squares between waves (Blaze and Glowaski 2004). If the heart rate is irregular, it is important to determine a time-averaged rate over a longer interval. Changes in heart rate can affect the function of the heart. Very fast heart rates can reduce cardiac output by not allowing the ventricles to fill adequately (Clark 2003). Bradycardia can also affect cardiac output. Troubleshooting heart rate abnormalities should include identifying and correcting the underlying cause if possible. Treatment with fluid therapy and/or additional analgesics may be necessary for tachycardic patients. Lightening anesthetic depth and/or treatment with an anticholinergic may be necessary for bradycardic patients. Arrhythmias should be identified and their effect on cardiovascular function should be determined before treatment therapy is decided on.

Contractility is the intrinsic ability of cardiac muscle to develop force for a given muscle length. It is also referred to as *inotropism*. *Preload* is the force acting on a muscle just before contraction, and it is dependent on ventricular filling (or end diastolic volume). Preload is related to right atrial pressure. The most important determining factor for preload is venous return. Hypovolemia, vasodilation, and venous occlusion decrease preload.

Afterload is the tension (or the arterial pressure) against which the ventricle must contract. If arterial pressure increases, afterload also increases. Afterload for the left ventricle is determined by aortic pressure; afterload for the right ventricle is determined by pulmonary artery pressure.

Blood pressure is the driving force for blood flow (perfusion) through capillaries that supply oxygen to organs and tissue beds of the body. Blood pressure is needed to propel blood through high-resistance vascular beds, including those of the brain, heart, lungs, and kidneys. Blood pressure variations are detected by baroreceptors that are present throughout the cardiovascular system. These baroreceptors are capable of stimulating the autonomic nervous system in response to increases and decreases in blood pressure. If blood pressure falls, the sympathetic nervous system is stimulated and outflow will be increased, causing an increase in heart rate and blood pressure. If blood pressure increases, the parasympathetic system works to slow the heart rate and decrease pressure (Fraser 2003).

Blood pressure values are expressed in millimeters of mercury (mm Hg) and as three measurements: *systolic, mean,* and *diastolic*. Remember that the systolic pressure is the pressure generated when the left ventricle is fully contracted. Diastolic pressure is the pressure measured when the left ventricle relaxes. Pulse pressure felt on peripheral arteries is the difference between the two numbers. Mean arterial pressure (MAP) is calculated as diastolic pressure + 1/3 systolic pressure (systolic pressure − diastolic pressure) (Smith 2002). Mean blood pressure determines the average rate at which blood flows through the systemic vessels. It is closer to diastolic than to systolic because, during each pressure cycle, the pressure usually remains at systolic levels for a shorter time than at diastolic levels. Most times, under anesthesia, a patient's mean pressure is what the anesthetist focuses on. A mean arterial pressure of at least 60 mm Hg (70 in horses) is needed to properly perfuse the heart, brain, and kidneys. Mean arterial blood pressures consistently below 60 mm Hg can lead to renal failure, decreased hepatic metabolism of drugs, worsening of hypoxemia, delayed recovery from anesthesia, neuromuscular complications, and central nervous system abnormalities, including blindness after anesthesia (Smith 2002). Prolonged hypotension (> than 15–30 minutes) can lead to nephron damage. Although the effects may not be immediately apparent because 65–75% of nephrons need to be damaged before renal disease becomes clinically observable, the effects may play a role in the onset of renal disease later in a pet's life. Severe untreated hypotension can lead to cardiac and respiratory arrest. Hypertension, or excessively high blood pressure, can lead to problems as well. Ideally, any animal under anesthesia should have should have regular blood pressure monitoring because most anesthetic drugs affect blood pressure in some way.

Mean arterial blood pressure (MAP) = cardiac output (CO) × systemic vascular resistance (SVR). *Cardiac output* is defined as the amount of blood pumped by the heart in a unit period of time. Cardiac output is a term that is often used in anesthesia because it is extremely important in the overall function of the cardiovascular system. In general, the term applies to how well the cardiovascular pump (heart) is working. Many factors affect CO, directly or indirectly, including some anesthesia drugs. CO = heart rate (HR) × stroke volume (SV). *Contractility* is the amount of force and velocity that the ventricles can exert to eject the volume within them (Hamlin 2000). *Systemic vascular resistance* is the amount of resistance to flow through the vessels. Some vessels may be dilated and therefore allow more flow at less resistance. Constriction of vessels may limit blood flow and require more pressure to get blood through. It's important to know that many of the drugs used for anesthesia affect one or more of these systems in some way.

Normal systolic blood pressures in the conscious awake patient are 100–160 mm Hg, normal diastolic pressures are 60–100 mm Hg, and normal mean arterial blood pressure ranges are 80–120 mm Hg. Hypotension is classified as MAP of less than 60 mm Hg. It is important to be able to identify the cause of a blood pressure abnormality to know how to begin treatment for it. There are generally three things to consider when looking for causes of hypotension. Look for drugs or physiological/pathological factors that may reduce systemic vascular resistance (SVR), look at heart rate, and look for things that affect stroke volume (preload/contractility) (Smith 2002). As mentioned earlier, many of the drugs used in anesthesia cause some degree of hypotension, and less often, hypertension. Knowing the side effects of these drugs and how they work will help in determining treatment. Drugs that decrease SVR (and cause vasodilation) in a dose-dependent manner include acepromazine, thiobarbiturates, propofol, and the inhalants. Other physiologic factors that may cause a decrease in blood volume or vascular tone

include hemorrhage, inadequate volume administration or replacement, dehydration, shock, sepsis, anaphylaxis, or severe hypercapnia (high CO_2) (Smith 2002). Patients with acid/base abnormalities should be stabilized prior to anesthesia if possible to help reduce the possibility of hypotension. Drugs that can decrease heart rate include opioids, alpha 2 agonists, and the inhalant drugs isoflurane and sevoflurane. Patients with intracranial disease, hypothermic patients, and extremely fit pets may have low heart rates (bradycardia). Anesthetic drugs affecting the contractility of the heart include the inhalants, thiobarbiturates, propofol, and alpha-2 agonists. The inhalant drugs are potent vasodilators, with up to a 50% reduction in cardiac contractility at surgical planes of anesthesia as well. The other drugs' effects on contractility are more transient and less profound. Alpha-2 agonists and phenylephrine cause vasoconstriction of blood vessels, which results in hypertension. The effects of hypertension from the alpha-2 agonists are transient, lasting only a few minutes before the vessels relax and hypotension can result. The dissociative drugs, ketamine and Telazol, have indirect positive effects on the cardiovascular system and thus increase heart rate, but this can cause a reduction in stroke volume depending on how severely heart rate is affected. Patient positioning can affect blood pressure. Obese or bloated patients or patients with large abdominal masses placed in dorsal recumbency may be hypotensive due to excessive pressure on the caudal vena cava. This pressure may compromise venous return and result in hypotension. The same can happen when positive pressure ventilation is used.

Certain disease states can cause hypertension, including renal disease, pheochromocytomas, pulmonic stenosis, heartworm disease, and hyperthyroidism. Ideally, these patients will have their hypertension well controlled before surgery. The exception may be the pheochromocytoma patient whose hypertension may spike up during surgery when the tumor is manipulated. A nitroprusside CRI may be indicated for these patients if systolic pressure exceeds 200 mm Hg. If a patient develops hypertension under anesthesia that is not related to a disease state, the cause is most likely related to inadequate anesthetic depth and/or inadequate analgesic administration. Adjusting anesthetic depth and providing additional pain medications should result in normotension.

Changes in blood volume affect arterial blood pressure by changing cardiac output. During general anesthesia, the rate of normal ongoing losses of fluid from the body is increased by high oxygen flow rates. The oxygen dries the respiratory system and causes rapid evaporation from mucous membranes. To offset this loss, intravenous fluid administration of crystalloids at a rate of 10 mL/kg/hr is recommended to help "fill the space" caused by vasodilation and to replace normal ongoing losses that occur in patients (with normal cardiovascular and renal function; patients with certain cardiac diseases may not be able to "handle" excessive fluid overload) under anesthesia. Fluid therapy is best begun before hypotension exists. For suspected hypovolemia a fluid bolus of "1 hour's worth" of the patient's maintenance rate may be given (i.e., 35 kg pet = 350 mL bolus, along with maintenance fluids). Reassess following the bolus. If the patient is instrumented with a Doppler monitor you may be able to hear the improvement and "stronger" flow. Blood loss should be replaced with 2–3 times the suspected amount of loss. One mL of blood loss should be replaced with 2–3 mL of crystalloid. Excessive hemorrhage will require replacement with colloids and blood products. The best way to prevent hypotension is to detect changes in blood pressure as soon as they begin and start treatment to restore it as soon as possible.

Volume status

Central venous pressure is the blood pressure within the intrathoracic portion of the caudal or cranial vena cava. It can be measured to gain information about intravascular blood volume and cardiac function. CVP correlates with the volume reaching the right atrium during diastole. A single measurement of CVP yields little information, but serial measurements are useful. Measuring CVP can be helpful in determining hypovolemia or fluid overload. Normal CVP should be 2–7 cm H_2O in anesthetized patients (Muir et al. 2000).

Urine output can also be measured to determine volume status. Normal urine output should be 1–2 mL/kg/hr.

Respiratory Physiology

Every cell in the body needs a constant supply of oxygen to produce energy to grow, repair, or replace itself and to maintain normal vital functions. The respiratory system is the body's link to its supply of oxygen. It includes the diaphragm and chest muscles, the nose and mouth, the pharynx and trachea, the bronchial tree and the lungs. The bloodstream, heart, and brain are also involved. The bloodstream takes oxygen from the lungs to the rest of the body and returns carbon dioxide to them to be removed. The heart creates the force to move the blood at the right speed and pressure throughout the body. The smooth functioning of the entire system is directed by the brain and the autonomic nervous system.

Anatomy of the respiratory system

The main function of the lungs is to provide continuous gas exchange between the inspired air and the blood in the pulmonary circulation. The lungs supply oxygen during inspiration and remove carbon dioxide (CO_2) during expiration. During inspiration air containing oxygen (at sea level, atmospheric air contains 21% oxygen) enters the body through the nose and mouth. From there it passes through the pharynx on its way to the trachea. The trachea divides into two main *bronchi* upon reaching the lungs. One bronchus serves the right lung and the other serves the left lung. The bronchi subdivide several times into smaller bronchi, which then divide into smaller and smaller branches called *bronchioles*. After many subdivisions, the bronchioles end at the alveolar ducts. At the end of each alveolar duct are clusters of *alveoli*. The oxygen transferred through the system is finally

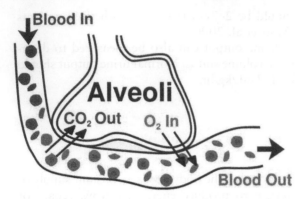

Figure 1.1.   Illustration of perfusion. (Drawing by Melanie Tong.)

transferred to the bloodstream at the alveoli. Blood vessels from the pulmonary arterial system accompany the bronchi and bronchioles. These blood vessels also branch into smaller and smaller units ending with *capillaries*, which are in direct contact with each alveolus. Gas exchange occurs through this *alveolar-capillary membrane* as oxygen moves into and carbon dioxide moves out of the bloodstream (perfusion) (Fig. 1.1).

In the blood, oxygen is transported in two forms: dissolved in plasma (which is measured by PO_2) and bound to hemoglobin (measured by SpO_2). The amount of oxygen bound to hemoglobin is much larger than the amount dissolved in plasma (Fig. 1.2).

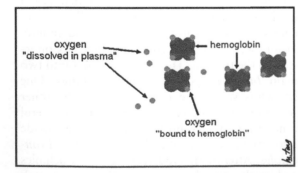

Figure 1.2.   The amount of oxygen bound to hemoglobin is much larger than the amount dissolved in plasma. (Drawing by Melanie Tong.)

The "matching" of ventilation and perfusion is important to proper lung function. It does no good to ventilate an alveolus that is not being perfused (*alveolar dead space*) or to perfuse an alveolus that is not being ventilated because of *atelectasis* (collapse of alveoli). In the normal lung, ventilation (V) and perfusion (Q) are not evenly matched (known as *V/Q mismatch*), and this worsens with lung disease and dorsal or lateral recumbencies. Both ventilation and perfusion increase toward the dependent regions of the lung, but since blood is heavier than lung parenchyma, perfusion increases at a faster rate than ventilation. Vasodilation or vasoconstriction, caused by disease or anesthetic drugs, enhances V/Q mismatching and hypoxemia. From an anesthetic point of view, *alveolar ventilation* is very important because it will control the amount of volatile or gaseous anesthetic agent that can diffuse into the bloodstream. Any increase in alveolar ventilation will increase anesthetic uptake into the pulmonary blood (Fraser 2003).

The movement of air into and out of the lungs is called *ventilation*. The contraction of the inspiratory muscles, mainly the diaphragm, causes the chest cavity to expand, creating negative pressure. This is inspiration. During maximal inspiration, the diaphragm forces the abdominal contents ventrally and caudally. The external intercostal muscles are also involved. These muscles contract and raise the ribs during inspiration, increasing the diameter and volume of the chest cavity. Ventilation is the process by which gas in closed spaces is renewed or exchanged. As it applies to the lungs, it is a process of exchanging the gas in the airways and alveoli with gas from the environment. Breathing provides for ventilation and oxygenation.

Normal expiration is a passive process resulting from the natural recoil or elasticity of the expanded lung and chest wall. However, when breathing is rapid, the internal intercostal muscles and the abdominal muscles contract to help force air out of the lungs more fully and quickly. At the end of inspiration, the elasticity of the lung causes it to return to its smaller, unexpanded size. The ability to do this is called *elastic recoil*. The volume of air remaining in the lung at the end of a normal breath (the end expiratory lung volume) is called the *functional residual capacity* (FRC). FRC is composed of the expiratory reserve volume and the residual volume. On expiration, there is still air left in the lungs; if there weren't, all of the alveoli would collapse. FRC decreases slightly in supine and lateral recumbency compared to prone. Certain conditions such as pregnancy, obesity, and abdominal distention due to gas-filled organs or masses can exacerbate decreases in FRC. FRC is diminished with small airway diseases. At FRC the alveoli in the nondependent lung sections are larger than those in the dependent regions because of gravity and the weight of the lung. Alveoli in the dependent regions are squashed and compressed by the weight of the overlying lung tissue. In lateral or dorsal positions the dependent alveoli are also compressed by the weight of the mediastinal structures and by the weight of the abdominal contents pressing against the diaphragm. In patients with large abdominal masses or excessive bloating (such as gastric dilatation volvulus GDV or obstructive colic in horses), the problem becomes especially significant.

In spite of many protective mechanisms in place in the lungs, including FRC, small airway and alveolar collapse (atelectasis) still occurs in the normal animal. Atelectasis is especially prominent in the dependent lung regions when an animal is recumbent. Intermittent deep positive pressure breaths in the anesthetized patient can help minimize small airway and alveolar collapse. The use of *positive end expiratory pressure* (PEEP) is known to help as well. PEEP increases airway pressure and FRC to help keep small airways and alveoli open during expiration (Battaglia 2001). PEEP valves are commercially available (in 5, 10, and 15 cm H_2O) and can be added to the anesthesia machine for this purpose. Unfortunately, once atelectasis has occurred, it is very difficult to open the closed alveoli. Applying excessive pressure in an attempt to open alveoli (as in the case of attempting to reinflate a packed-off lung during a thoracotomy) tends only to damage the already working tissue (barotrauma) before reinflation takes place. Reinflation is a slow, delicate process and will happen on its own in healthy tissue over time or once recumbency or insult changes.

The degree of stiffness or *compliance* of the lung tissue affects the amount of pressure needed to increase or decrease the volume of the lung. With increasing stiffness, the lung becomes less able to return to its normal size during expiration. Virtually all diseases cause the compliance of the lungs to decrease to some extent.

The amount of airflow resistance can also affect lung volumes. *Resistance* is the degree of ease in which air can pass through the airways. It is determined by the number, length, and diameter of the airways. An animal with a high degree of resistance may not be able to exhale fully, thus some air becomes trapped in the lungs.

Tidal volume is the volume of gas passing into and out of the lungs in one normal respiratory cycle. Normal tidal volume for mammals is 10–20 mL/kg. *Minute volume* is used to describe the amount of gas moved per minute and is approximately 150–250 mL/kg/minute. *Minute volume = tidal volume × respiratory rate*. It is *alveolar ventilation* that is important for gas exchange, however. Alveolar ventilation is the portion of ventilation that contributes to gas exchange (McDonnell and Kerr 2007). Tidal volume is used to ventilate not only the alveoli, but also the airways leading to the alveoli. Because there is little or no diffusion of oxygen and carbon dioxide through the membranes of the airways, they comprise what is known as *dead space ventilation* (Fig. 1.3).

The other part of dead space is made up of alveoli with diminished capillary perfusion. Ventilating these alveoli is ineffective and will do nothing to improve blood gases. The nonperfused alveoli and the airways are known as *anatomic dead spaces*. Therefore tidal volume has a dead space component and an alveolar component. Dead space ventilation is about 30–40% of tidal volume and minute volume in a normal patient breathing a normal tidal volume. Dead space ventilation has a purpose. It assists in humidifying and tempering inhaled air, and it cools the body, as in panting. Panting is predominantly dead space ventilation. During panting, the respiratory frequency increases and the tidal volume decreases so that alveolar ventilation remains approximately constant. This is the reason that when animals under anesthesia

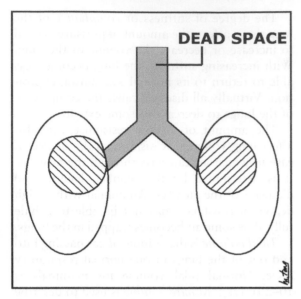

Figure 1.3. Anatomical dead space where no gas exchange takes place. (Drawing by Melanie Tong.)

pant, they very often wake up. They are not effectively ventilating their alveoli and exchanging gas well. Often times these patients will be hypercarbic because they are not able to effectively reduce their carbon dioxide levels. Slower, deeper breaths are usually more efficient. Certain pieces of anesthesia equipment can add to the anatomical dead space of a patient by "extending" its airway. This is called *mechanical dead space*. Endotracheal tubes that are too long and extend far beyond the patient's nose would be an example. Adding this dead space presents a further challenge to patients trying to effectively ventilate.

Monitoring ventilation on patients under anesthesia can be done a number of ways. Ventilation is assessed in terms of rate, rhythm, and tidal volume. First of all, a good look at the patient's chest excursions should be done to evaluate for quality and effort. Auscultation of the lungs should be performed prior to sedating or anesthetizing any patient. Normal lung sounds should be heard on both sides of the chest. Any abnormal sounds should be investigated prior to moving forward with anesthesia because anesthetic drugs can depress respiration and ventilation and may worsen existing problems.

Mucous membrane color should be assessed regularly. The tongue and gums should be pink. Any change in color, especially blue or purple tingeing, can indicate hypoxemia.

Spirometers or ventilometers can be used to measure tidal volume and minute volume. Apnea or respiratory monitors detect the movement of gas through the proximal end of the endotracheal tube. They sound an alarm when no gas movement is detected. They provide no information on tidal volume or the physiologic state of the patient. They can be falsely activated by pressure on the chest or abdomen of the patient or by cardiac oscillations that cause gas movement in the trachea.

Positive pressure ventilation (PPV) is indicated when an animal cannot ventilate adequately on its own. This indication may be defined as one or more of the following: *hypercarbia* (increased CO_2 > 60 mmHg), *desaturation* (SpO_2 < 95%) in spite of oxygen therapy, *hypoxemia* (PaO_2 of less than 100 mmHg on oxygen), or a low observed or measured minute volume. PPV is always indicated in any surgery requiring an open chest, whenever paralytic neuromuscular blocking drugs are to be used, neuromuscular diseases, chest wall problems, abdominal enlargements, or pulmonary parenchymal disease. Any patient that is to be anesthetized with potentially increased intracranial pressure should be mechanically ventilated. Positive pressure ventilation is of great benefit to many patients, but it is not without potential complications. These can be avoided with careful monitoring, attention to detail, and a good understanding of the underlying physiological processes. A major contraindication for positive pressure ventilation is a closed pneumothorax, because positive pressure ventilation will make it worse. Positive pressure ventilation can decrease arterial blood pressure and reduce cardiac output, especially if airway pressures are consistently more than 10 mmHg or if circulating blood volume is low. Artificial ventilation decreases pulmonary blood flow and therefore may lead to ventilation-perfusion abnormalities. These depressant effects can be seen on the arterial wave form during direct blood pressure measurement and on the waveform when measuring oxygen saturation. It is seen as a dampening of the wave form following an artificial breath. The changes in circulatory flow during IPPV are caused by prolonged increases in mean airway pressures and decreases in CO_2 (Muir, et al., 2000). Hypovolemia worsens these effects.

References

Abbott, JA. 2000. Small Animal Cardiology Secrets. Philadelphia: Hanley & Belfus, Inc.

Battaglia, AM. 2001. Small Animal Emergency and Critical Care. Ithaca, NY: WB Saunders Co.

Blaze, C, Glowaski, M. 2004. Veterinary Anesthesia Drug Quick Reference. St. Louis: Elsevier Inc., p.175.

Clark, L. 2003. Monitoring the anaesthetised patient. In Anaesthesia for Veterinary Nurses, edited by Welsh, E. Ames, IA: Blackwell Publishing, pp.227–233.

Fraser, M. 2003. Physiology relevant to anaesthesia. In Anaesthesia for Veterinary Nurses, edited by Welsh, E. Ames, IA: Blackwell Publishing, p.20.

Hamlin, R. 2000. Cardiovascular physiology. In Small Animal Cardiology Secrets, edited by Abbott, J. Philadelphia: Hanley and Belfus, Inc., pp.1–9.

McDonnell, W, Kerr, C. 2007. Respiratory system. In Lumb and Jones' Veterinary Anesthesia and Analgesia, edited by Tranquilli, WJ, Thurmon, JC, Grimm, KA. Ames, IA: Blackwell Publishing, p.121.

Muir, WW, Hubbell, J, Skarda, R, Bednarski, R. 2000. Handbook of Veterinary Anesthesia, 3rd ed. St. Louis: Mosby, Inc., pp.236–257, 295–269.

Reece, WO. 1997. Physiology of Domestic Animals, 2nd ed. Philadelphia: Lippincott Williams & Wilkins, p.179.

Smith, L. 2002. Hypotension. In Veterinary Anesthesia and Pain Management Secrets, edited by Greene, S. Philadelphia: Hanley & Belfus, Inc., pp.135–140.

The Preanesthetic Workup

2

Jennifer Dupre

Failing to plan is planning to fail.

Allen Lakelin

The anesthesia workup is essential for successful anesthesia management. Potential complications that can develop during the preanesthetic, perianesthetic, and postanesthetic phases are projected in this planning period. A preanesthetic workup will be of great assistance in developing the best anesthetic plan possible for each patient. Failure to collect the information is very likely to have a negative impact on the patient outcome of the anesthetic event. Each patient will have its own itinerary that will include signalment; physical exam; diagnostics; ASA status or risk status; and choice of drugs, dosages, and route of administration. The plan also will determine choice of monitors and monitoring techniques as well as special techniques needed, such as local anesthesia, controlled ventilation, arterial catheter placement, and so forth. Being familiar with the procedure to be performed as well as the use of the anesthetic drugs, including their advantages and disadvantages, will keep the anesthetist alerted to potential complications such as hypotension, hypothermia, hypoventilation, arrhythmias, and so forth. Begin charting the preanesthetic workup by referring to Figure 2.1.

Influencing Factors

Signalment is the first step in planning the anesthesia. It consists of general information pertaining to the patient including age, breed, species, and sex.

Information about the client is important, especially phone numbers in the event of an emergency.

Different species have special considerations; feline species show a tendency to develop laryngospasm during intubation (Hall et al. 2001). On the contrary, this complication is unlikely in the dog. Metabolic requirements vary among species and have a direct influence on dosaging of anesthetic drugs.

Within the same species, breeds can display specific characteristics that might be relevant to the anesthetist. For example in dogs, sight hounds (Greyhound, Whippet, Saluki, Borzoi, and so forth) have little to no body fat and an alteration of liver enzymes. Both features can impact metabolism and redistribution of drugs such as the thiobarbiturates; this results in prolonged recovery. Brachycephalic dogs and cats (Persian and Himalayan) (Blocker and van der Woerdt 2001) may suffer from upper airway obstruction syndrome, which could be aggravated by

13

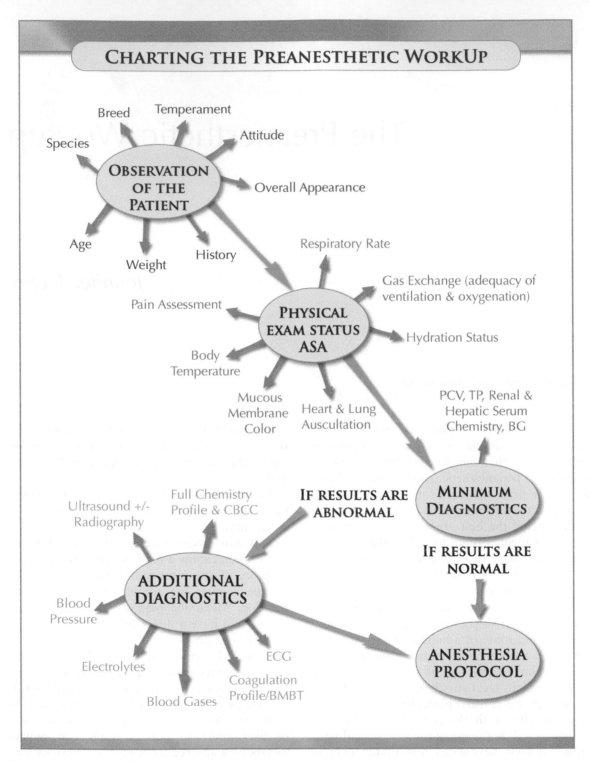

Figure 2.1. Flow chart of preanesthetic workup.

premedication and/or anesthesia. Although endotracheal intubation is advised for most species to protect the airways, it is mandatory with this group of dogs and cats.

Boxers seem to be sensitive to acepromazine (boxer-ace syndrome) (Hall et al. 2001). Its administration might cause hypotension and fainting in that breed. The presence of a higher vagal tone and slower heart rate in the breed is believed to be the cause of this syndrome. The drug has to be used with caution in boxers, and its administration must be followed by a very close monitoring of the blood pressure. Anticholinergics such as atropine and intravenous fluids need to be available.

Miniature Schnauzers may develop sick sinus syndrome. The abnormal cardiac rhythm may worsen with anesthesia, leading to decreased cardiac output potentially severe enough to cause a cardiovascular collapse. A preanesthetic electrocardiogram (ECG) may be indicated if the patient has a questionable history (Seymour and Duke-Novakovski 2007).

Doberman Pinschers can develop von Willebrand's disease, a coagulation disorder. Any carrier of the disease should ideally be identified prior to any surgical procedure with a bleeding potential. Preferably, von Willebrand's factor can be checked or a buccal mucosal bleeding time (BMBT) can be assessed before surgery (Seymour and Duke-Novakovski 2007).

Different genders bring different considerations. A female patient might be pregnant, and physiological as well as pharmacological characteristics in both the mother and fetus will have to be considered.

Immature (neonate or pediatric) patients have undeveloped organ function and have specialized needs. For instance, their small body mass will make them very prone to hypothermia, and temperature support should be maintained throughout the anesthesia and into the postoperative period. Hypoglycemia is another complication observed in neonates because they have a higher metabolic rate than do adult patients. A mature (geriatric) patient is more prone to age-related changes in organ function. These changes are progressive and unalterable.

The behavior of the animal can impact the choice of drugs dramatically. This is a subjective evaluation. The animal should be observed with and without the owner. Some owners might make their animal more nervous; others might be very useful in helping to keep the patient calm during the initial exam as well as answering any questions related to patient history.

The choice of drug and dose for anesthesia sedation, tranquilization, or immobilization is largely dependent on the temperament of the species/breed. Catecholamines (hormones from the adrenal glands) are increased in stressed patients. This can cause arrhythmias, hypotension, and even cardiac arrest.

The existence of a preexisting condition may require additional diagnostics. A patient with a history of increased thirst and urination may indicate a renal or endocrine disorder, and organ function will have to be investigated because behavioral problems could also cause similar symptoms. Excessive fatigue might be the sign of a cardiopulmonary disease or might result from arthritis or other conditions and should be checked. In ferrets, a loss of fur may indicate a change in hormones, which could be due to a recent ovariohysterectomy or could indicate adrenal associated endocrinopathy (AAE).

It is important in all cases that pertinent information is obtained. The following questions can be asked routinely of all clients (Alef et al. 2007):

1. Is the animal intact?
2. What is the food/water intake? (Get actual measurement in cups, mL, and so forth.)
3. What is the frequency of urination/ defecation?
4. Is there any coughing, sneezing, wheezing, and so forth?
5. Were there any previous illnesses?
6. Is there any exercise intolerance?
7. Have there been any recent treatments/ medications (organophosphates, cardiovascular meds, analgesics, herbal therapies?
8. Are there allergies or adverse reactions to certain drugs?
9. What is the vaccination and heartworm history?

10. Has there been any fainting, seizure-like activity, or signs of CNS depression?
11. What is the activity level (couch potato or marathon runner)?
12. Has the owner noticed any pain or discomfort in the animal?

Current medication

Good knowledge of the patient's current medication and the possible interaction with commonly used anesthesia drugs will help influence decisions made when planning the anesthetic protocol. This includes choice of drugs as well as route of administration (oral versus injectable).

Minimize oral intake of medication during the fasting period and change to injectable, if possible. If there is concurrent drug use, take precaution. Organ system function should be evaluated via diagnostic testing.

Antibiotics (AB)

The aminoglycocides (gentamycin) can be nephrotoxic and might also interfere with normal neuromuscular function. Check renal function before using such ABs and ensure good kidney perfusion through fluid therapy and arterial blood pressure monitoring during the procedure. Avoid using aminoglycocides if neuromuscular blockade is necessary.

Analgesics

Nonsteroidal antiinflammatory drugs (NSAIDs). NSAIDs (meloxicam, carprofen, deracoxib) are analgesics that inhibit prostaglandin formation in the inflammatory pathway. Side effects from the use of NSAIDs come from the fact that some prostaglandins are also important in renal, clotting, GI, and liver function. Monitor blood pressure closely, provide fluids, and evaluate chemistry serum profiling prior to anesthesia.

Adjunctive analgesic drugs (AADs). These drugs have varying pharmacodynamic interactions when used with traditional analgesics (opioids, NSAIDs, local anesthetics). The effects will involve some of the same receptors and could potentiate or enhance analgesic action, whether a patient is in acute or chronic pain. Choose the anesthetic regime carefully if a patient is currently on one of the AADs (oral, injectable, or topical) because organ function may already be compromised (liver, kidney, heart, and so forth).

Cardiovascular drugs

The anesthetist should be familiar with the physiological effect, as well as the pharmacology, of each of these drugs (positive inotropes, vasodilators, beta-2 blockers) because they will alter the CV function, such as the heart rate, blood pressure, stroke volume, and overall cardiac output.

Phenylpropanolamine HCL

A sympathomimetic agent, which releases norepinephrine by stimulation of both the alpha and beta-adrenergic receptors, phenylpropanolamine HCL is used primarily to treat incontinence. Patients treated with this drug are prone to vasoconstriction, increased heart rate and blood flow, increased blood pressure, and mild CNS stimulation. Be cautious when adding drugs in the anesthesia regime that may potentiate these effects (α_2 agonists, anticholinergics, positive inotropes, and so forth).

Chemotherapy drugs

It is important to evaluate the possible pharmacokinetic/pharmacodynamics (PK/PD) interaction of each drug individually with commonly used anesthesia agents as well as the pharmacologic effects on each patient. Cancer patients might have various systemic disorders, and caution is necessary when designing an anesthetic protocol.

Phenobarbital

Phenobarbital is a barbiturate drug used to control seizures. This drug might potentiate the effect of some anesthetic agents, and dosage needs to be modified accordingly. Any drugs that might potentiate seizure activity will have to be avoided. Attempt to eliminate any factor that might trigger a seizure (stress, pain, and so forth).

Organophosphates

These are insecticides used to treat endo/ecto-parasites. They inhibit plasma cholinesterases and might prolong activity of certain local anesthetics and potentiate neuromuscular blocking drugs (atricurium, pancuronium).

Insulin

Diabetic patients have special needs during anesthesia. A modified fasting protocol, as well as frequent monitoring of blood glucose, should be part of the anesthesia plan for these patients.

Physical Exam

A preanesthetic physical exam is required for every patient. Be consistent in the approach. This may be a head-to-tail or a body systems approach. All the systems are interesting to the anesthetist, but the cardiovascular, respiratory, renal, and hepatic are most important. Recognizing abnormal changes of the body systems during a physical exam will be difficult unless you are familiar with normal physiological vital signs of individual species and breeds (Ettinger and Feldman 2006).

Cardiovascular system

When evaluating the cardiovascular system during physical examination, look for signs of adequate tissue perfusion (Perkowski 2000). The capillary refill time (CRT) indicates adequacy of perfusion but is not the most accurate method because many things can affect it. Blood pressure monitoring is more ideal. By looking and touching the mucous membranes, a patient

is assessed for hydration; normal is moist and pink.

Auscultate heart sounds while trying to identify abnormal sounds (murmurs) and palpate peripheral pulses. The heart rate should be auscultated while palpating the pulse and these should match, one heart beat for every pulse. Below are common pulse locations on the dog and cat:

- **DOG.** Femoral, tibial, dorsopedal, palmar digital, lingual, caudal arteries
- **CAT.** Femoral, tibial, dorsopedal, caudal

Pulse pressure (PP) is the difference between systolic arterial pressure (SAP) and diastolic arterial pressure (DAP). A strong pulse equals a large PP; a weak pulse equals a small PP. Pulse quality may be similar for two different blood pressure measurements. The pulse will feel the same; however, the tonicity of the artery will be different (vasoconstricted, vasodilated, and so forth).

Cardiovascular disease should be controlled prior to anesthesia. A diagnosis should be made and a further workup may be indicated to assess the risk associated with anesthesia. Tools used to diagnose cardiovascular disturbances include auscultation (murmurs and arrhythmias), complete blood count (anemia and thrombocytopenia), diagnostic imaging (ultrasound and radiography). ECG is a measurement of electrical function of the heart. This test should be performed if there is a notion of an arrhythmia or a disease potentially causing electrical changes in the heart. Situations that might trigger arrhythmias would be trauma, pain, electrolyte alterations, catecholamine release, hypoxemia, hypercapnia, certain anesthetics, and myocardial disease.

Cardiac murmurs are classified on a scale of 1–6. A murmur intensity greater than 3/6 may warrant a workup, which would involve measurement of the valve function through cardiac ultrasound, echocardiogram, or possibly radiography (if ultrasound or echo is not available).

Any patient with cardiovascular disease should be identified, treated if necessary, and monitored constantly. Intravenous fluid therapy will be unique to each patient dependent on the type and severity of disease. The heart is the "fluid pump." If the pump does not function well, it will not pump fluid around the body as it should, and it may not be able to process additional fluid efficiently. Fluid volume as well as type should be carefully administered.

Dehydration and hypovolemia should ideally be treated prior to anesthesia. Both might reduce tissue perfusion and ultimately reduce drug clearance. *REHYDRATE* anesthesia patients prior to anesthesia.

Respiratory system

The main function of the respiratory system is to allow gas exchange (oxygenation and CO_2 elimination). The respiratory system is composed of an upper and lower tract. The upper part of the tract consists of the nasal cavity, pharynx, larynx, and trachea. Symptoms of diseases associated with the upper respiratory tract may include sneezing or snorting. There may be facial swelling or rubbing, nasal discharge, and/or dyspnea (difficulty breathing). Parts of the lower tract include bronchi, bronchioles, and alveoli. Open mouth breathing, tachypnea, dyspnea, or orthopnea (difficulty breathing unless sitting or standing up), as well as cyanosis, tachycardia, and collapse, can be symptoms of lower respiratory tract disease. If these symptoms are found on exam, there is potential for a decreased ability for the lungs to exchange CO_2 for oxygen at the level of the alveoli. If patients are severely dyspneic during physical examination, oxygen therapy can be beneficial as long as it does not stress the patient.

Normal function of the respiratory system is examined through auscultation of all lung fields as well as observing the quality (depth and rhythm) and rate of ventilation. Wheezes, crackles, and stridor sounds heard with or without a stethoscope are problematic and can reveal respiratory tract disease. Moist, pink mucous membranes (MM) with a CRT of <2 seconds indicate adequate oxygenation/perfusion. Pale MM can be an indication of hypotension, hypothermia,

hypoxemia, vasoconstriction (from α_2 agonists), and low packed cell volume. A red brick coloring can point to venodilation, blood sludging, hypercarbia, or endotoxemia.

Arterial blood gases, which include oxygen arterial tension (PaO_2) and carbon dioxide arterial tension ($PaCO_2$), can be beneficial in determining the oxygen CO_2 exchange. Radiography and/or ultrasound can also be helpful in recognizing abnormalities within the thorax. It is important to remember that pain, stress, discomfort, and central nervous system depression (CNS) can alter the function of the respiratory system and should be considered if there are abnormalities noted. Almost all anesthetics are respiratory depressants; therefore, a patient with a respiratory disorder may need ventilation support during the anesthetic period.

Renal system

Palpation of the kidneys should be performed for size and symmetry. Record history and clinical findings such as polyuria/polydipsia (PU/PD) or vomiting and lethargy. Owners may recognize a strange smell to either the patient's breath or urine. Renal serum chemistry, urine specific gravity (USG), and full urinalysis will help diagnose renal disorders. An azotemic or uremic (retaining nitrogenous wastes in blood can indicate poor kidney function) patient is more sensitive to anesthetics and must be stabilized prior to anesthesia. A postrenal azotemia is severe in nature and usually associated with a urethral obstruction (blocked cat). Decreased renal perfusion under anesthesia may worsen preexisting disease. In chronic renal failure, there is a multisystemic compromise (anemia, hypertension) on top of renal dysfunction. Maintenance of adequate perfusion is essential.

Fluids may be required to stabilize the patient prior to anesthetic drug administration. Also, metabolism and excretion of anesthetics may be prolonged; therefore, use drugs that are eliminated quickly (e.g., Propofol) as well as lower dosages.

Hepatic system

A thorough evaluation of the hepatic system is essential because it determines how well the patient can metabolize and excrete anesthetic drugs. On physical exam, record history of lethargy, jaundice (hyperbilirubinemia), increased thirst, or dark-colored urine. In certain patients, the abdomen may appear enlarged. Hepatic diseases that may affect function include infection, toxicity, portosystemic shunts (PSS), overdose of medication, cancer, and hereditary disease. Progressed disease may lead to seizure, coma, and death.

Plasma proteins, alkaline phosphatase (ALK Phos), and alanine aminotransferase (ALT) are diagnostic tests that will help identify the severity of disease. Animals with PSS will often have increased bilirubin, bile acids, white blood cell count, and clotting times as well. It is common with the PSS or patients with hepatic disease to see decreased blood glucose, albumin, total plasma proteins, and packed cell volume as well. Diagnostic imaging (DI) can be useful to diagnose obvious abnormalities. Anesthesia may be required to take fine needle aspirates (FNAs) of the liver for tissue sampling during ultrasound examination.

Many anesthetics will have prolonged action in patients with hepatic disease. Highly protein bound drugs with prolonged metabolism (thiobarbiturates, benzodiazepines) should be used cautiously in liver dysfunction patients. If there is profound CNS depression as well as lethargy, dosages can be decreased dramatically. Use short-acting/metabolizing anesthetic drugs for which recovery does not rely heavily on liver metabolism (e.g., propofol, inhalants).

Nervous system

The nervous system plays an essential role in anesthesia management. If there is an indication of a disorder, such as head trauma or paralysis, a full neurologic exam must be performed. Some diagnostic testing available for neurology may require general anesthesia (EEG, computed

tomography or CAT Scan, MRI); therefore, plan the anesthesia regime accordingly.

Evaluate the mental status of each patient because all anesthetics will cause some degree of CNS depression; drug requirement may be decreased if there is evidence of such depression. Some nervous system disorders may require respiratory support (cervical spinal injuries interfering with the phrenic nerve will alter normal diaphragm movement). Intracranial trauma or lesions will require close monitoring of CO_2, which, when elevated, can cause intracranial pressure to increase. Neuromuscular blocking drugs, dissociative agents, some antibiotics, and local anesthetic techniques may be contraindicated in certain neuropathies.

Gastrointestinal system (GI)

A thorough history from the owner is vital when evaluating the GI system. Diet, behavior, and duration and consistency of vomiting ± diarrhea should be noted. Electrolytes will be altered with any substantial losses—particularly a decrease in potassium. Evaluate hydration status on physical exam. Abnormalities, such as tumors and foreign bodies can be detected during abdominal palpation. A full CBC and chemistry profile including electrolytes should be evaluated. Diagnostic imaging can be beneficial for further assessment of the GI organs. Pain management is an important part of the protocol because many GI abnormalities that require anesthesia are likely to be painful. There may be the potential of a reduction in venous return due to the distension of abdominal organs. Measurement of arterial blood pressure is essential as well as ventilation; abdominal pressure may increase pressure to the thoracic cavity causing hypoventilation.

Integument system

Common abnormalities found on the skin include ectoparasites, infection or abscess, masses or swelling, petechiation or bruising (can be an indication of a clotting problem), alopecia (may be endocrine dysfunction), and fungus. Skin scrapings/slides can be prepared to help identify certain fungi, parasites, and bacteria; histological examination of abnormal cells can indicate types of cancer (melanoma, sarcoma). It is important to identify the cause of the abnormality, although identification may not alter anesthetic protocol. The approach to disinfection may be altered. Sterile saline may be used in place of rubbing alcohol, intravenous catheters should be placed in nondiseased skin (if possible), and local anesthetic techniques may be contraindicated (epidural, infiltrative line block, and so forth). The use of gloves can be beneficial to both you and the patient.

Endocrine system (ES)

Suspicion of endocrine disease should be investigated with a full physical exam as well as CBC, chemistry (including BG and electrolytes), urinalysis, ECG, radiographs, and ultrasound. The endocrine system influences many of the body systems as a whole, and management of a patient with an ES disorder is multifactorial. Any metabolic disturbance should be corrected or stabilized prior to anesthesia. Diseases of this system may include one or more of the following: diabetes mellitus, insulinoma, Cushing's disease, Addison's disease, thyroid disorder (hypo/hyperthyroidism), hypo/hyperadrenocortism, adrenalassociated endocrinopathy (ferrets), and hypo/hyperglycemia.

Overall body condition

Evaluate overall body condition. This includes body weight, temperature, age, gender, and possibility of pregnancy. It also includes hydration status and pain assessment.

A dehydrated patient must be stabilized prior to anesthesia as this can increase drug uptake, metabolism, and clearance. Hypovolemia can affect cardiovascular function. Use skin turgor, eyeball position, moisture of mucous membranes, the simple lab tests, packed cell volume, total solids, and azo stick to determine hydration status. Body temperature can indicate disease and/or stress. Overall body condition can be

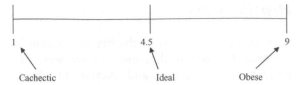

Figure 2.2.   Scale used to assess body scoring.

altered by age. Although age is not a disease, the risk status increases as certain disease processes are expected in older patients.

Pain and discomfort should be assessed before, during, and after anesthesia whether an animal is in pain or not. This will provide baseline values. Body conditioning should also be noted. Extremely fit patients may have very low resting heart rates. Body scoring can provide information on overall system function due to weight changes such as obesity and cachexia. If an animal has a chronic disease, body scoring will reveal how severe the disease is. Obese animals will have more cardiopulmonary stress (potential difficulty with ventilation and tissue perfusion) due to the excessive weight on system organs, while the cachectic patient will have minimal reserves and are at risk for overdosage, hypoglycemia, and hypothermia. The scoring is based on a number scale of 1–9 (Fig. 2.2). Normally, drug dosages and ventilation tidal volumes should be based on lean body weight.

ASA—American Society of Anesthesiologists

After obtaining all pertinent exam information on your patient, an anesthetic plan can be developed based on an ASA status (Fig. 2.3). This status is designed to help the anesthetist determine a risk category for each patient undergoing general anesthesia.

ASA status—examples

CLASS   I—castration,   ovariohysterectomy, diagnostic orthopedic radiographs, dental prophylaxis

ASA STATUS

I-   Minimal risk of a healthy patient

II-   Slight risk w/ slight to mild systemic change

III-   Moderate risk w/ systemic change & some clinical alterations

IV-   High risk w/ preexisting disease; surgical intervention may preserve life.

V-   Extreme risk where patient has little chance of survival w/ or w/o surgery

E-   Attached to an individual class if an emergency

Figure 2.3.   Scale used to assess ASA status.

CLASS II—pediatric or otherwise healthy geriatric patients, cruciate repair

CLASS III—blocked cat or goat; some cardiac diseases; fracture with pulmonary contusions; a depressed, anemic dog OHE with a pyometra

CLASS IV—cat that is in liver failure, shocky patients, hemoabdomen, uncompensated heart disease

CLASS V—severe shock, massive hemorrhage, massive trauma, ruptured colon in a colic case

An "E" denotes an emergency. The "E" should be placed next to the ASA class if the procedure requires anesthesia immediately (e.g., ASA IV E).

Preanesthetic Diagnostics

Preanesthetic laboratory tests should be performed on patients suspected to be at an increased risk status. This may decrease or eliminate unexpected complications. If stabilizing is necessary, diagnostics can guide therapeutic techniques. These tests are usually dictated based on availability, cost, environment, and patient-related factors (breed, age). There is evidence that in animals under 6 years of age, diagnostic tests may not be necessary (Alef et al. 2007). To minimize anesthetic risk, the following sections present recommendations for a basic minimum database and advanced diagnostic testing.

Basic minimum database (BMD)

■   <6yrs of age: PCV, TP, BUN, creatinine, ALT, Alk Phos, blood glucose (*These 7 tests can detect many diseases.*)

Advanced diagnostic testing (ADT)

■   >6yrs of age or systemically compromised: Full CBC, chemistry profile as well as other diagnostic tests may be required. *If any disease is suspected or the BMD is abnormal, further testing may be indicated.*

PCV (packed cell volume)—whole blood

This is an indicator of hydration. It will give you information on the patient's oxygen-carrying capacity. Minimum PCV for preop is 27–30%. The minimum intraop is 20%. The maximum is 60% (patient's cardiac output is reduced in half when blood viscosity doubles). The delivery of crystalloid fluids can hemo-dilute an already low PCV and so should be used judiciously. A whole blood transfusion may be necessary for patients with a PCV less than 20%.

TP or TPP (total plasma protein)

The TPP will affect the patient protein binding ability. A patient with a low TPP (hypopro-teinemia) will have fewer protein molecules for the drug to bind to, thus increasing the amount of free drug and its potency. An increase in TPP may indicate dehydration in a patient.

CBC (complete blood count)—whole blood

This will include PCV, TPP, and hemoglobin but also will provide information about the red and white blood cell counts. An alteration in white cell count may indicate stress or infection. CBC should also include a count of platelets, which will reveal information about clotting ability.

USG (urine specific gravity) centrifuged urine

The USG is used to assess tubular function of the renal system.

BUN and creatinine

These serum tests are used to help diagnose renal insufficiencies.

Aminotransferases: alanine aminotransferase (ALT), aspartate aminotransferase (AST) serum, alkaline phosphatase (alk phos) serum

These serum tests are used as sensitive indicators of liver disease.

Blood glucose

Blood glucose is an inexpensive, quick test that can be used on patients having anesthesia or patients suspected to have disorders of the glucose homeostasis (diabetes mellitus, insulin-oma). Neonates, pediatric patients, and patients with disease (sepsis, PSS) should be screened as well. Be sure to obtain the blood sample from veins that do not contain substances such as glucose-containing fluids and/or any other medication.

Full chemistry profile—serum

There are a variety of tests that assess organ function and disease. A full chemistry profile includes renal, hepatic, and endocrine tests as well as blood glucose, and it may include electrolytes.

Additional Diagnostics

Additional tests are available for further evaluation of specific disorders.

Coagulation profile

Any animal that may be suspected of having a bleeding abnormality (a Doberman or an animal with liver disease, coagulation disorder, and so forth) should be tested with coagulation profiling. Patients undergoing elective procedures may need to be rescheduled until more stable. If the procedure is an emergency, blood products (plasma, cryoprecipitate) can be made available to treat coagulation disorders prior to anesthesia.

Buccal mucosal bleeding time (BMBT)

A bleeding disorder is most likely due to inadequate platelet numbers or improperly functioning platelets. These do not involve the coagulation factors. Coagulation factor deficiencies will not cause a prolonged bleeding time. In small animals, a small incision is made with an "automated incision" (devices available on the market for purchase) on the inside of the upper buccal mucosa. The small wound begins bleeding and is timed. Filter paper is used to blot the blood. When the bleeding has ceased and a clot is formed, the time is stopped. The time from beginning of bleeding until clot forms is the BMBT. This test is a crude evaluation of the ability of the platelets to form an initial plug in a wound. A normal BMBT is < 3 minutes. If the patient is sedated or under general anesthesia, the BMBT is expected to be <4 minutes. Abnormalities that may cause a prolonged BMBT include acquired platelet function defect and disseminated intravascular coagulation (DIC).

Platelet or thrombocytopenic count

A platelet count is usually part of the CBC but can be done individually if the full CBC is not performed. If there is any indication of a clotting disorder, the platelets should be counted. Normal platelet count in a dog is about 150,000 to 450,000 platelets per microliter ($\times 10^{-6}$/L) of blood. If platelet levels fall below 100,000 per microliter, spontaneous bleeding can occur and is considered a life-threatening risk. Bone marrow disease such as leukemia or another cancer in the bone marrow, as well as certain ectoparasites, can cause thrombocytopenia. These patients will often experience excessive bleeding. Whole blood products are considered when stabilizing these patients prior to anesthesia.

Full urinalysis

This can reveal diseases that are not uncovered by other tests because the patient does not have signs or symptoms. Examples include diabetes mellitus, glomerulonephritis, and chronic urinary tract infections (UTI).

Electrolytes

The following serum tests provide information on the essential electrolytes in the body.

Potassium (K⁺)

This positively charged electrolyte will generate electricity, contract muscles, and move water and fluids within the body. Intracellular osmolality is controlled through K^+. The kidneys will filter and excrete potassium. If a patient retains K^+, they can become hyperkalemic (when glomerular filtration rate slows down in renal disease, a patient may not be able to excrete potassium properly).

Sodium (Na⁺)

Sodium is a positive ion that is responsible for generating electricity, contracting muscles, and moving water and fluids within the body. Na^+ influences the maintenance of osmotic pressure of extracellular fluid. Any type of fluid loss will cause an increase in Na^+ (hypernatremia), such as vomiting, diarrhea, burns, peritonitis, and fever.

Calcium (Ca⁺)

Calcium is a positive electrolyte that affects neuromuscular performance and contributes to skeletal growth and blood coagulation. A hypocalcemic patient may have a cardiac contraction deficiency.

Magnesium (Mg⁺⁺)

Magnesium is a positive electrolyte that influences muscle contractions and intracellular activity.

Chloride (Cl⁻)

Chloride is a negative electrolyte that helps regulate blood pressure.

Phosphate (HPO4⁻)

Phosphate is a negative electrolyte that impacts how the body metabolizes and regulates acid-base balance and calcium levels.

Bicarbonate (HCO3⁻)

Bicarbonate is a negatively charged electrolyte that keeps the acid-base status of the body in balance and assists in the regulation of blood pH levels. Bicarbonate insufficiencies and elevations cause acid-base disorders.

Diagnostic imaging

Radiography

Radiography is the most popular method of obtaining information through imaging. It is used to assess size and shape of the internal organs; any fluid, air, tumor, or misshapen organ (mass, GDV, genetic disorder); and bone formation/fractures.

Ultrasound (US)

If there is evidence of disease on radiographs, US (echo, sonography, ultrasonography) can be beneficial because it is a safe diagnostic imaging technique used to visualize internal organs for size, structure, and any pathological change. Internal images and organ sections are visualized. Oxygenated and deoxygenated blood flow of each internal structure can be evaluated as well. US is often used in place of radiography to determine diagnosis of abnormalities.

Arterial blood gases

This is a test to assess respiratory function, and it will provide information on the patient's oxygenation and ventilation status. It will give body pH as well as provide some information on metabolic function.

Electrocardiogram (ECG)

The heart's electrical system controls timing of the heartbeat by regulating heart rate and rhythm. An ECG will measure the electrical function of the heart but not the mechanical function. Anything interfering with the normal rhythm of each patient's heart should be evaluated with an ECG prior to anesthesia.

Endocrine testing

Any animal revealing thyroid dysfunction may require additional workup including thyroid function tests. Hypothyroidism is associated with a decreased metabolism and is seen commonly in dogs. Anesthetic drug dosages will be altered (decreased) dramatically if this condition is not stabilized in the patient prior to anesthesia. A patient may be seen with low heart rates, low blood pressure, and prolonged recoveries. An overactive thyroid (hyperthyroidism) is common in cats and they will have an increased metabolic state. Risks associated with this condition are increased workload on the heart and patients may be cachectic or underweight. Hypertrophic cardiomyopathy can develop if not treated.

Conclusion

After completing a history, physical exam, and diagnostic testing, develop an anesthesia protocol based on the findings specific to that patient. Refer to the organ systems chart in Figure 2.4. Use all information available and keep a good record of each patient. Provide evidence of your plan on a preanesthetic workup document. The acronym "SOAP" is used for a preanesthetic evaluation short form; see below for definition. The author recommends using a form similar to Figure 2.5 to chart your findings.

SOAP

Subjective: Behavior, pain assessment
Objective: Physical exam and diagnostic findings
Assessment: ASA status (I–V) + E
Plan: Anesthetic protocol

Organ System	Cardiovascular	Respiratory	Renal	Hepatic	Nervous	GI	Integument	Endocrine
Common Disorders	Murmurs, Arrhythmias Hypovolemia Hyper/hypo-tension Myocardial disease Dehydration Heart failure	Pneumonia, Asthma, Diaphragmatic Hernia, Neoplasia FB, Bronchitis Pulmonary edema Tracheal collapse	ARF, CRF Endocrine DZ Nephrotoxin Diabetes Glomerulo-nephitis Urethral Obstruction	Infection Viral Toxin, Drug Overdosage Hereditary PSS	Seizures Infection Tumor Hydro-cephalus Trauma Pain	Vomiting Diarrhea FB Tumor IBD Perio-dontal disease	Parasites Infection Viral, Fungal Cancer Alopecia	Diabetes Insulinoma Cushing's Adison's Thyroid & Adrenal DZ
Diagnostics Available	CBC, Chem Blood Gases, Electrolytes, DI, Blood Pressure	Blood Gases, CBC, Chem DI, Pulse Oximetry	CBC, Chem Urinalysis w/ USG, Electrolytes,	CBC, Chem TP, Albumin coagulation profile, Platelets, BMBT, DI Electrolytes	CBC, Chem ECG, DI Blood Gases Neuro Exam Pain Scoring	CBC, Chem, DI Electro-lytes	CBC, Chem Skin scraping Ultraviolet light Histology Bacterial culture	CBC, Chem, Specific endocrine testing, DI Electrolytes
Concerns Pertaining to Anesthesia	Use drugs w/ minimal CV depression such as Benzodiaze-penes, Opioids, Etomidate, Hypotension, Arrhythmias, Anemia	Hypoxemia, Hypercarbia, Acidosis, Use short acting drugs w/ minimal sedation, Reduce stress, Provide O_2 as needed, May need to provide IPPV	↓ perfusion, Electrolyte imbalance Hyperkalemia	Use short acting drugs Delayed metabolism, Caution w/ protein binding drugs; Bleeding, Slow recovery	CNS Depression, Seizures, Coma, Exaggerated response to drugs	Hypo-volemia, Special fluid therapy, Risk of aspiration, Impaired motility	Wear gloves, Caution using local anesthetics, May use alternative disinfection techniques	Electrolyte imbalances, Arrhythmias ARF, CRF, CV instability Slow recovery

Figure 2.4. Organ system chart describing common disorders, diagnostics, and concerns pertaining to anesthesia. FB: foreign body; ARF: acute renal failure; CRF: chronic renal failure; DZ: disease; PSS: porto-systemic shunt; IBD: inflammatory bowl disease; CBC: complete blood count; Chem: chemistry; DI: diagnostic imaging; USG: urine specific gravity; TP: total protein; BMBT: buccal mucosal bleeding time; ECG: electrocardiogram; CV: cardiovascular; O_2: oxygen; CNS: central nervous system.

ANESTHESIA "SOAP" FORM

DATE:	SIGNALMENT

DATE:

ANESTHETIST _____
SURGEON/ASSIST _____
PROCEDURE _____
BODY WEIGHT (Kg) _____

SIGNALMENT

NAME _____
SPECIES _____
BREED _____
SEX _____
AGE _____

COLOR/MARKINGS _____

SUBJECTIVE FINDINGS (Behavior) _____

OBJECTIVE FINDINGS

Temp _____ Pulse _____ Resp _____
Cardiac Ascultation _____
Pulse Quality _____
Mucous Membrane Color _____
Capillary Refill Time _____
Respiratory Ascultation _____

LABWORK

PCV _____   TP _____

OTHER _____

ASSESSMENT ASA STATUS   I   II   III   IV   V   E

History/ Current Meds

PRIOR ANESTHESIA
Dates:
Complications:

PLAN ANESTHESIA REGIME

	Drug	Route	Dosage	mg	ml
Premeds					
Induction					
Maintenance					
Analgesia					

Advantages/Disadvantages

COMPLICATIONS ANTICIPATED: (pre-op, intra-op, post-op: consider age, body wt., breed, position, surgical procedure, physical status)

ADMINISTRATION SET

10 drops/ml ☐   20 drops/ml ☐   60 drops/ml ☐

IV FLUID TYPE

Dose ml/hr _____ Drops per minute/second _____

APPROVED: _____

Drugs Received _____ / _____

MONITORING
(circle)

Doppler	Arterial Line
ECG	Capnograph
Esoph Stethoscope	Pulse Oximeter
Temp. Probe	IPPV
Blood Gas	Other _____

Drugs Wasted _____ / _____

Figure 2.5. Preanesthetic document used at Ross University School of Veterinary Medicine, St Kitts.

References

Alef, M, von Praun, F, Oechtering, G. 2007. Is routine pre-anesthetic haematological and biochemical screening justified in dogs? Vet Anaesth Analges 35:132–140.

Blocker, T, van der Woerdt, A. 2001, A comparison of corneal sensitivity between brachycephalic and domestic short-haired cats. Vet Opthalmol 4(2):127–130.

Ettinger, SJ, Feldman, EC. 2006. Textbook of Veterinary Internal Medicine, 6th ed. Volume 1, Physical Exam. St Louis: Elsevier Saunders.

Hall, LW, Clarke, KW, Trim, CM. 2001. Veterinary Anaesthesia, 10th ed. London, UK: WB Saunders, pp. 77, 393, 511.

Perkowski, SZ. 2000. Anesthesia for the emergency patient. Emergency Surgical Procedures, VCNA: SAP, Volume 30, Number 3, May.

Seymour, C, Duke-Novakovski, T. 2007. BSAVA Canine and Feline Anaesthesia and Analgesia, 2nd ed. Gloucester: BSAVA, p.9.

Mathematics and Calculations for the Veterinary Anesthetist

3

Sharon Johnston

Anesthetic agents are dose-dependent. To administer an effective dose, the anesthetist must be able to perform basic mathematical calculations.

The most common error in drug administration is using the wrong medication or a medication with the incorrect concentration. To ensure patient safety, it is essential that the veterinary anesthetist develop the knowledge and skill to accurately write, read, interpret, and carry out drug orders (Bill 2000). The following are the seven rights of medication administration (Booth and Whaley 2007):

1. Right Patient
2. Right Agent
3. Right Dose
4. Right Route
5. Right Time
6. Right Technique
7. Right Documentation

The Basics: Metric System

Conversion of units requires the use of a "conversion factor," which is any equivalent equation in which the known and the unknown units are involved (Tables 3.1–3.4) (Bill 2000). You must set up a proportion of values on either side of the equation.

$$\frac{\text{Unknown unit}}{\text{Known value unit}} = \frac{\text{Conversion factor with same units as unknown}}{\text{Conversion factor with same units as known}}$$

50 pounds = X kg

Cross-multiply and divide.

$$\frac{X\,kg}{50\ \text{pounds}} \qquad \frac{1\ kg}{2.2\ \text{pounds}} \qquad = 50 = 2.2\ X$$

Solve for **X**

50 = 2.2 **X** $\qquad \frac{50}{2.2} \quad \frac{2.2}{2.2} = 22.7$ kg

50 pounds = 22.7 kg

Table 3.1. Weight.

Unit	Fraction	Symbol
Kilogram	1000 grams	kg
Gram	1000 milligrams	g
Milligram	1/1000 of a gram	mg
Microgram	1/1,000,000 of a gram	μcg or μg

Table 3.2. Weight.

Unit	Fraction	Decimal	Symbol
Kilo	1000		k
Deci	10	0.1	d
Centi	1/100	0.01	c
Milli	1/1000	0.001	m
Micro	1/1,000,000	0.000001	μ

Table 3.3. Volume.

Unit		Amount	Symbol
Liter	=	1000 mL	L
Milliliter	=	0.001 L	mL
Microliter	=	0.000001 L	mcL or μL

Table 3.4. Common unit conversions.

1 kilogram	=	2.2 pounds
1 teaspoon	=	5 mL
1 tablespoon	=	15 mL
1 grain	=	60 mg

Percentages

Percent can be expressed as "out of 100" or "for every 100." For example: 25% can be written as

$$\frac{25}{100} = 0.25$$

The decimal point can be moved two places to the left to achieve the same calculation.

$$25\% = 25.0 = 2\ 5\ .0 = 0.25$$

Agent strength as percent solution

Agents with the dose listed as a concentration percent represent grams in 100 mL.

Lasix as a 5% solution has a concentration of 50 mg/mL.

$$5\% \text{ means } \frac{5 \text{ grams}}{100 \text{ mL}} = \frac{5000 \text{ mg}}{100 \text{ mL}} = \frac{5000 \text{ mg}}{100 \text{ mL}}$$
$$= \frac{50 \text{ mg}}{1 \text{ mL}}$$

Lidocaine as a 2% solution has a concentration of 20 mg/mL.

$$2\% \text{ means } \frac{2 \text{ grams}}{100 \text{ mL}} = \frac{2000 \text{ mg}}{100 \text{ mL}} = \frac{2000 \text{ mg}}{100 \text{ mL}}$$
$$= \frac{20 \text{ mg}}{1 \text{ mL}}$$

The decimal point can be moved one place to the right in any percent solution to discern the mg/mL concentration.

$$5\% = 5.00 = 5.0\ 0 = 50.0 = 50 \text{ mg/ml}$$

Agent Dose Calculation

The dose is the amount of the drug administered. It is generally calculated using the animal's lean body weight.

Concentration is listed on the drug package or in the package insert.

Agents should be recorded using the generic name where possible, such as in the following examples:

carprofen (generic)   bupivicaine (generic)
Rimadyl (Brand)   Marcaine (Brand)

To calculate a dose of an agent you can use the following:

$$\frac{\text{Patient weight (kg)} \times \text{dose of agent (mg/kg)}}{\text{Concentration of agent (mg/mL)}} = \text{mL of agent}$$

Example: To administer 2 mg/kg of an agent with the concentration of 10 mg/mL to a 22.7 kg dog:

$$\frac{22.7 \text{ kg} \times 2 \text{ mg/kg}}{10 \text{ mg/mL}} = \frac{45.4 \text{ mg}}{10 \text{ mg/mL}} = 4.54 \text{ mL}$$

Using an Excel Worksheet for Drug Calculations

An Excel worksheet can be set up as in Table 3.5 to calculate basic agent doses. The *formulas* displayed should be entered in the D2 cell and E2 cell.

Use the following website for anesthesia agent calculations:

vet-medicine.net/vetmednet/index.
php?pageid=5011

Calculating fluid drip rates

IV administration sets are calibrated to a set number of drips equal to 1 mL:

Macrodrip   10 drops/mL
Macrodrip   15 drops/mL
Microdrip   60 drops/mL

To administer a set amount of fluid over a set amount of time:

$$\frac{\text{Volume to be infused} \times \text{dripset rate}}{\text{Time of infusion in minutes}} = \text{drops/minute}$$

Example: To administer 150 mL using a 10 drops/mL dripset:

$$\frac{150 \text{ mL} \times 10}{60 \text{ minutes}} = \frac{1500 \text{ mL}}{60 \text{ minutes}} = 25 \text{ drops/minute}$$

To calculate the milliliters per minute rate, divide the drops per minute by the dripset rate:

$$\frac{25 \text{ drops/minute}}{10 \text{ drops/mL}} = 2.5 \text{ mL/minute}$$
(Dripset rate)

Example: To administer 150 mL using a 15 drop/mL dripset

$$\frac{150 \text{ mL} \times 15}{60 \text{ minutes}} = \frac{2250 \text{ mL}}{60 \text{ minutes}} = 37.5 \text{ drops/minute}$$

Table 3.5. Worksheet for calculating doses.

	A	B	C	D	E
1	Patient weight (kg)	Agent dose (mg/kg)	Agent concentration (mg/mL)	Agent to be administered (mg)	Agent to administer (mL)
2	22.7	2.0	10.0	45.4	4.5
				= SUM(A2*B2)	= SUM(D2/C2)

Table 3.6. Worksheet for fluid calculations.

	A	B	C	D	E
1	Fluids to be administered (mL)	Dripset rate drops/mL	Time to administer (minutes)	Drops/minute	mL/minute
2	150	10	60	25	2.5
	⬆			=SUM(A2*B2)/C2	=SUM(D2/B2)

$$\frac{37.5 \text{ drops/minute}}{15 \text{ drops/mL}} = 2.5 \text{ mL/minute}$$
$$\text{(Dripset rate)}$$

Example: To administer 150 mL using a 60 drop/mL dripset

$$\frac{150 \text{ mL} \times 60}{60 \text{ minutes}} = \frac{9000 \text{ mL}}{60 \text{ minutes}} = 150 \text{ drops/minute}$$

$$\frac{150 \text{ drops/minute}}{60 \text{ drops/mL}} = 2.5 \text{ mL/minute}$$
$$\text{(Dripset rate)}$$

Using an Excel Worksheet for Fluid Calculations

An Excel worksheet can be set up as in Table 3.6. The *formulas* displayed should be entered in the D2 cell and E2 cell.

Preparing a % Solution

A proportion equation can be used to prepare solutions with a designated percent of an agent.

Example: Your orders state to deliver a 5% dextrose solution to the patient. You have a 1 L bag of NaCl and a bottle of dextrose with a 50% concentration.

First calculate that a 5% solution requires 50 mg/mL of dextrose. You have a 1000 mL bag. **X** represents the unknown amount of mg needed in 1000 mL to deliver 50 mg in 1 mL:

$$\frac{50 \text{ mg}}{1 \text{ mL}} = \frac{X \text{ mg}}{1000 \text{ mL}}$$

Cross-multiply and divide:

$$X = 50,000 \text{ mg}$$

If the dextrose solution on hand is a 50% solution, it contains 500 mg/mL. You need to add 50,000 mg to the 1000 mL fluid bag. By dividing the amount needed by the concentration of the agent, you will find you need 100 mL of 50% dextrose.

You must remove 100 mL of the NaCl from the fluid bag and then add the 100 mL of 50% dextrose, which will give you 50 mg of dextrose in 1 mL.

Example: Your orders state to deliver a 5% dextrose solution to the patient. You have a 1 L bag of fluids that currently is a 2.5% solution of dextrose and a bottle of dextrose with a 50% concentration.

Your proportion equation would look like the following:

$$\frac{50 \text{ mg}}{1 \text{ mL}} = \frac{X \text{ mg}}{1000 \text{ mL}}$$

Constant Rate Infusion—CRI

CRI is used to administer an agent over a period of time in order to ensure that the medication achieves and sustains therapeutic concentrations while avoiding unnecessarily high peak concentrations and their subsequent toxic reactions or side effects (Bill 2000).

Administering an Agent by Adding the Agent to IV Fluids

To calculate the amount of agent to add to a bag of fluids for a CRI the following formula may be used:

$$\underset{\substack{\text{Amount (ml) of} \\ \text{agent to add}}}{X} = \frac{\frac{\text{(CRI rate)}}{\text{mg/kg/hr}}}{\frac{\text{ml/kg/hr}}{\text{(fluid rate)}}} \times \underset{\text{(mls)}}{\text{Diluent volume}}$$

To set up a 1000 mL fluid bag with MLK (post op dose) for a patient using the above formula:

Morphine

$$X = \frac{0.1 \text{ mg/kg/hr}}{2 \text{ mL/kg/hr}} \times 1000 \text{ mL bag of fluids}$$

$$X = 0.05 \times 1000$$

$$X = 50 \text{ mg of morphine}$$

$$X = 50 \text{ mg/15 mg/mL} = \textbf{3.3 mL}$$

Ketamine

$$X = \frac{0.18 \text{ mg/kg/hr}}{2 \text{ mL/kg/hr}} \times 1000 \text{ mL bag of fluids}$$

$$X = 0.09 \times 1000$$

$$X = 90 \text{ mg of ketamine}$$

$$X = 90 \text{ mg/100 mg/mL} = \textbf{0.9 mL}$$

Lidocaine

$$X = \frac{3 \text{ mg/kg/hr}}{2 \text{ mL/kg/hr}} \times 1000 \text{ mL bag of fluids}$$

$$X = 1.5 \times 1000$$

$$X = 1500 \text{ mg of lidocaine}$$

$$X = 1500 \text{ mg/20 mg/mL} = \textbf{75 mL}$$

To assemble the CRI in a 1000 mL bag of fluids:

Morphine 3.3 mL = 0.05 mg of morphine/mL

Ketamine 0.9 mL = 0.09 mg of ketamine/mL

Lidocaine 75 mL = 1.5 mg of lidocaine/mL

Total   79.2 mL

Remove 79.2 mL of fluid from the 1000 mL bag and add the three agents in doses calculated. Administer the combined fluid/agent combination at the fluid rate of 2 mL/kg/hr.

Example: Administering the above assembled bag of fluids with agents added will administer the following agent amounts at the fluid rate of 2 mL/kg/hr to a 22.7 kg dog:

$$22.7 \text{ kg} \times 2 \text{ mL/kg/hr} = 45.4 \text{ mL/hr}$$

$$\text{Morphine} = 0.05 \text{ mg of morphine/mL} \times 45.4 \text{ mL}$$
$$= 2.27 \text{ mg/hr}$$

$$\text{Ketamine} = 0.09 \text{ mg of ketamine/mL} \times 45.4 \text{ mL}$$
$$= 4.08 \text{ mg/hr}$$

$$\text{Lidocaine} = 1.5 \text{ mg of lidocaine/mL} \times 45.4 \text{ mL}$$
$$= 68.1 \text{ mg/hr}$$

Remember! To increase the patient's fluid rate, DO NOT increase the CRI; a secondary set of fluids should be used.

References

Bill, R. 2000. Medical Mathematics and Dosage Calculations for Veterinary Professionals. Ames, IA: Blackwell Publishing.

Booth, K, Whaley, J. 2007. Math and Dosage Calculations for Medical Careers. New York: McGraw-Hill.

Web Resources—CRI Calculators

The Veterinary Anesthesia Support Group has a wide variety of calculators at www.vasg.org/resources_&_support_material.htm#item3

Barber Vet has a pop-up calculator on their website at www.barberveterinary.co.uk/CRICalculation.htm

Records and Record Keeping

4

Heather Dulong

The veterinary medical record is comprised of many forms and logs that account for the management and care given to our veterinary patients. Among these is the anesthetic log or record. Having moved out of the Stone Age where monitoring consisted of someone's foot tapping to the beat of the heart and the anesthetic record reflecting this simplicity, today's advancements in veterinary medicine have greatly increased the amount of information available to us during the anesthetic period. Not only is it important in the support of patient care, but the anesthetic record also serves as a legal document. The value that we place on our beloved pets today has prompted these advancements as well as the legal issues that may be lurking in wait.

The Anesthetic Record

The anesthetic record serves as a literal witness to significant events and physiological changes that occur during the anesthetic period. It acts as a reminder of the parameters that need to be assessed and prompts the anesthetist to continuously stay vigilant in evaluating the patient. The level of information recorded is dictated by the complexity or simplicity of the case. The amount of information documented should increase as the level of monitoring increases.

Information that should be included in the anesthetic record:

1. Patient and client identification
2. Date and procedure
3. Preoperative physical evaluation and ASA status
4. Previous and current medications
5. Previous anesthetic episodes
6. Laboratory results (BUN, PCV, TS, ALT, Glucose, and so forth)
7. Drugs administered (dose, time, and route)
8. Parameters monitored (HR, RR, BP, temp, and so forth)
9. Significant events (Example: estimated blood loss, fluid bolus, complication, treatment, response)
10. Supportive therapy (dobutamine, fluids)
11. Endotracheal tube size and anesthetic circuit used

The anesthetic record is probably the most involved and complex form found within the patient's medical file. It is generally found in a grid format with a 5-minute interval timeline going across the top and a left, downward column used to record the patient's data, inhalants administered (oxygen, anesthetic gas, nitrous oxide), fluids given, and drugs used. Although no symbol or symbols are standardized, the right-side-up and upside-down letter Vs are commonly used to represent systolic and diastolic blood pressure. Other symbols such as Xs, dots, and circles can be used to indicate heart rate, end tidal carbon dioxide, temperature, and pulse oximetry (Fig. 4.1). Graphing of symbols allows the anesthetist to quickly recognize trends and adjust anesthesia accordingly. Recording the patient's vitals in a graph format also allows other personnel to quickly evaluate and continue proper anesthetic management of the patient.

The anesthetic record should extend to include a recovery form to ensure that continued monitoring is provided during transfer of care. Like the anesthetic log, the recovery form should mirror the complexity or simplicity of each case (McCurnin, Bassert 2002).

The automated anesthetic record

The very important job of recording and graphing information can, admittedly, be a tedious task. It can also be difficult to decipher such a large amount of information in the confining typical grid format. In the human medical field this has been resolved with the automated anesthesia record (AAR). This automated system uses a computer to collect data obtained directly through monitoring equipment attached to the patient, creating a hands-free recording of the patient's vital signs. During an uneventful anesthetic period, documenting vital signs manually can be done easily. However, during an emergency situation it is almost impossible to manually record every event without neglecting the patient. The AAR system allows greater attention to be given to the patient while maintaining an accurate record.

The legal document

Whether electronically or handwritten, human or veterinary, the anesthetic record serves as a legal document subjected to subpoena. Every year, countless numbers of disciplinary actions are brought against veterinary professionals for failing to maintain complete and accurate records. For example, between the years of 2001 and 2003, 53% of the disciplinary actions taken by the Florida Board of Veterinary Medicine involved inappropriately maintained medical records (Lacroix 2006).

Proper documentation can make the difference in potential malpractice litigation. When something unexpectedly goes wrong, the grieved or angry client will sometimes look for someone to blame. Although not required by law, the signed anesthesia/surgery consent form documents the clients understanding of the anesthetic and surgical risks.

The value of the anesthetic record can often be underestimated. It's this blasé attitude that can lead to a more time-consuming legal battle when an appropriately documented record could have prevented the issue from the start. It is important that the anesthetic record is legible and is accurately stated. There should be no whiteout or scribbling out of any mistakes made. Instead a single or double line should be drawn through any mistakes and initialed. Pencil should not be used and although there is no legal standard on the color of pen, black is typically the color of choice. Depending on the state, records should be kept for a minimum of 3 to 5 years (Pettit 1994).

Recording every single event during the anesthetic period can prove to be impossible, especially during a time of crisis when the patient should have priority over record keeping. It is important though to write down the chain of events as soon as possible. It is far better to document retrospectively than it is to not document at all. Any court of law would understand the position of a patient's needs taking priority over record keeping in a time of crisis (Powers 1994).

Record Keeping of Controlled Substances

All controlled drugs are regulated by the Drug Enforcement Agency (DEA), which is responsi-

ANESTHETIC RECORD

DATE:	SURGEON:	ANESTHETIST:	CLIENT #:

PROCEDURE:	POSITION:	ASA STATUS	PATIENT NAME:

BODY WT:	TEMP:	PULSE:	RESP:	PCV:	TPP:	MM/CRT:	SPECIES:	BREED:

OTHER PE or LAB:	FACILITY:

PRE-ANESTHETIC AGENT(s)

AGENT	DOSE(MG)	ROUTE	TIME

INDUCTION AGENT(s)

AGENT	DOSE(MG)	ROUTE	TIME

	TIME:	:15	:30	:45	:15	:30	:45	:15	:30	:45	:15	:30	:45	TOTALS
IV 1:TYPE: RATE:														
IV 2:TYPE: RATE:														

Bair Hugger ☐ TEMP
Circ. Water Blanket ☐

OXYGEN L/min

VAPORIZER SETTING × %

8
7
6
5
4
3
2.5
2
1.5
1
0.5

AGENT:
☐ DESFLURANE
☐ ISOFLURANE
☐ SEVOFLURANE
☐ HALOTHANE

SYMBOLS
PULSE ● RESP O
ET CO2 ▲ SP O2 ■
BLOOD PRESSURE
SYSTOLIC V
MEAN ↑
DIASTOLIC ^
DIRECT ☐
INDIRECT ☐
DOPPLER ☐

TIMES:
TOTAL ANES:
PROCEDURE:
EXTUBATION:
STERNAL:
STANDING:

AIRWAY MAINTENANCE
☐ ET TUBE ☐ MASK
SIZE:

SYSTEM:
☐ CIRCLE
☐ NON-REBREATHING
☐ MECH VENT

CATHETER:
SIZE:
TYPE:
LOCATION:
SIZE:
TYPE:
LOCATION:

POST-OP AGENTS:

REMARKS

TEMP

180
160
140
120
110
100
90
80
70
60
50
40
30
20
10

Post-Op
TPR	TIME

Figure 4.1. The handwritten anesthesia monitoring grid. (Courtesy of Sharon Johnston, VTS, Anesthesia, AVTA webmaster.)

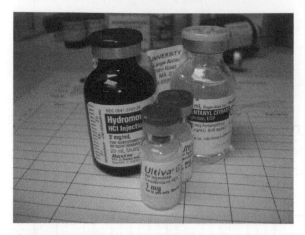

Figure 4.2. Controlled drugs and log.

ble for enforcing the 1970 Controlled Substances Act. This Act states that all controlled substances be properly documented when ordered, received, and used within any and all veterinary facilities (Bill 2006; McCurnin and Bassert 2002; Pettit 1994).

When dispensing controlled drugs to a patient in the hospital, it's important to include the following information in the drug logbook (Fig. 4.2):

1. Patient's full name and identification number
2. Date and name of drug, including dose in mL and mg
3. Initials of the individual drawing up the drug as well as the doctor overseeing the case

The logbook should be maintained with bound pages containing sequentially printed page numbers. This type of system, unlike that of a three-ring binder, makes it hard to alter any information that would render the record an untrustworthy document.

Computer systems with software that allows minimal editing of entries and uneditable notes of any changes made to preexisting entries can also be used to legally document controlled substances. These systems should not allow any deletions or alterations of records without the traceable fingerprint of such acts.

Records of dispensing, ordering, and receiving controlled drugs are required by law to be kept for a minimum of 2 years and should be easily accessible. Be aware that certain states may impose their own regulations in addition to those already established by the Act. Some states require a paper document or hard copy when a computer system is used. To find out more about what your state requires you can contact the American Veterinary Medical Associations (AVMA) as well as your local DEA office.

Summary

The anesthetic record is crucial to the successful management of the anesthetic patient. Whether manually or electronically written, its medical and legal value is directly related to the accuracy and thoroughness in which it is compiled. Much like the anesthetic record, the controlled drug log should represent the same diligence in documentation. All medical records are viewed as an integral part of the veterinary field and, as such, their value should never be underestimated.

References

Bill, RL. 2006. Clinical Pharmacology and Therapeutics for the Veterinary Technician, 3d ed. St. Louis: Mosby, Inc., an affiliate of Elsevier, Inc.

Lacroix, CA. 2006. Legally Sound Medical Record Keeping. NAVC Clinician's Brief (Vol. unk)12–14.

McCurnin, DM, Bassert, JM. 2002. Clinical Textbook for Veterinary Technicians, 5th ed. Philadelphia: WB Saunders Company.

McKelvey, D, Hollingshead, KW. 1994. Mosby's Fundamentals of Veterinary Technology. Small Animal Anesthesia: Canine and Feline Practice, 1st in 3 series. St. Louis: Mosby-Year Book, Inc.

Pettit, TH. 1994. Hospital Administration for Veterinary Staff. Goleta: American Publication Company, Inc.

Powers, MJ. 1994. Record-keeping in anesthesia: What the law requires. Brit J Anaesth 73:22–24.

Web Addresses

http://www.aana.com/resources.aspx?ucMenu_TSMenuTargetID=51&ucNAVMENU_T Documenting the Standard Care: The Anesthetic Record.

http://www.apsf.org/resource_center/newsletter/2000/winter/09CriticalIncidents.htm Cooper JB, 2008. Critical Incidents, Anesthesia Safety and Record Keeping.

http://www.clinicalwindow.net/cw_issue_08_index.htm Comparison of automated and manual anesthesia record keeping.

Preanesthetic Preparation 5

Connie Warren

After the patient has been worked up and a protocol has been chosen and approved by the clinician in charge, the next step is to prepare for anesthesia. The importance of preparation cannot be overemphasized. A thorough patient workup will help to make sure all of the possible complications have been anticipated. It is vital to have the appropriate supplies close at hand because it may be impossible to retrieve forgotten items when the patient requires immediate attention.

First, make sure all of the anesthesia equipment and monitors are set up properly and are in good working condition. Anesthetizing a patient without first checking the equipment is like starting on a trip across the country in your car without checking the oil—it might be possible to make the whole trip without incident, or the engine may blow before you finish. Make sure the anesthesia machine is in good working condition. Confirm that it does not have any leaks by performing a pressure check. It is very difficult to maintain a steady plane of anesthesia if some of the gas is leaking out of the machine, and this also poses a safety issue because personnel may be exposed to waste gas. In addition, a leak will also make it extremely difficult to

mechanically ventilate a patient because positive pressure will not be maintained.

To perform a pressure check of an anesthesia machine, close the pop-off valve, place a thumb or another rebreathing bag over the end of the "y" rebreathing tube, and fill the system with oxygen by either using the oxygen flush valve or by turning the oxygen flow meter up until the pressure reads 30 cm H_2O (Fig. 5.1). Turn off the oxygen, and watch the pressure meter. The pressure should hold steady and not decrease for at least 10 seconds (Hartsfield 2007).

After establishing that there is no leak, open the pop-off valve and squeeze the rebreathing bag empty before unblocking the end of the Y-piece (Fig. 5.2).

The high pressure in the system can create a vacuum, of sorts, and if the thumb is removed before releasing the pressure in the system, it can cause some of the carbon dioxide (CO_2) absorbent to be sucked up into the Y-piece, which could end up in the patient's lungs. Empty the rebreathing bag before unblocking the Y-piece to reduce the exposure to anesthetic gases left in the Y-piece from previous use and also to ensure that the pop-off valve does not inadvertently get left closed.

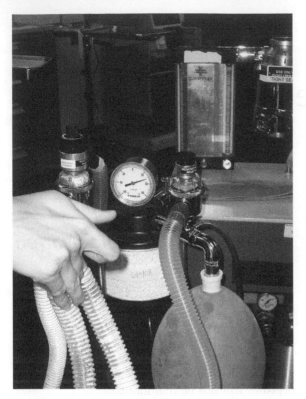

Figure 5.1.   Pressure-checking the machine prior to use.

After successfully pressure checking the anesthesia machine, check the vaporizer to make sure it has enough liquid inhalant. Next check to make sure the CO_2 absorbent is fresh. The absorbent granules should be soft and crumble easily if they are fresh. Exhausted absorbent is hard and will not crumble. Absorbent granules are designed to change to a violet color as they are exhausted. A canister should be completely changed when two-thirds of the canister turns violet during use. The absorbent will change back to white when not in use, so it is necessary to make note of the color change during a procedure. Active absorbent will produce heat as it is being used. The violet-colored exhausted absorbent will not produce heat because no chemical reaction is taking place within it. When filling the canister the contents should be shaken gently to settle them so that channeling of gases does not occur and the gas flows evenly throughout the canister. The machine should be pressure-checked after the canister is replaced to

make sure it has sealed. Absorbent that is too old and exhausted will not absorb CO_2 and could result in elevated inspired CO_2. If oxygen tanks are being used, check to make sure that the tanks are not depleted. The last step in preparing the anesthesia machine is to connect the appropriate size of Y-piece and rebreathing bag or nonrebreathing system.

Monitoring equipment should be set up prior to induction and should be checked to make sure that it is working properly. EKG, pulse oximetry, blood pressure (oscillimetric or Doppler instrument), and end-tidal carbon dioxide ($ETCO_2$) are some of the common parameters to monitor. Not every clinic has the same monitoring equip-

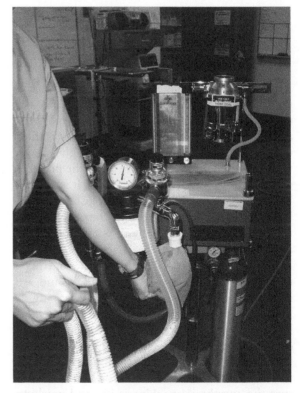

Figure 5.2.   After the pressure check is complete, open the APL or pop-off valve and squeeze the bag empty while the Y-piece is still occluded. This sends waste gas from the system out through the scavenge system instead of releasing it into the room air (although only oxygen is used to pressure check the machine, residual anesthetic gases can still be in the system from last use). This method also ensures that the APL valve does not inadvertently remain closed following the pressure check.

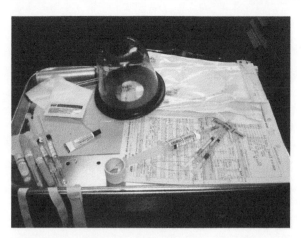

Figure 5.3. The individualized preanesthetic tray setup with all anticipated supplies needed for premed, catheterization, and induction processes.

ment, but whatever equipment is present should be checked prior to starting a procedure. Turn on the monitor(s), and confirm that the battery is charged or that it is plugged into an outlet. If it is a multifunction monitor, make sure the screen turns on and has every needed function turned on. A Doppler monitor can be checked by placing the probe on a staff member and confirming that it will produce sound with the pulse without static.

Once all of the equipment is checked out, the next step is to prepare for induction. A good method is to dedicate a tray, table, or countertop space on which to lay out all needed supplies for induction (Fig. 5.3).

This space should include all preop medications, induction agents, IV catheters, tape, syringes of heparinized saline, endotracheal tubes, laryngoscope, endotracheal tube tie, lubrication for the endotracheal tube, ophthalmic lubrication, gauze squares, and fluids with appropriate drip sets.

The premedication and induction agents should be drawn up and labeled. Labeling syringes prevents any confusion if the syringes are accidentally moved. Guessing the drug based on the size and volume of the syringe is not good practice because many drugs look alike. If a patient has a reaction after receiving an injection, it is important to know positively what was given so appropriate treatment can be initiated.

The proper endotracheal tube should be chosen for each patient. It is prudent to choose more than one size, usually a size smaller and one larger than the one that is anticipated, in case the first choice does not fit. If the patient has a potential laryngeal mass, has a congenital anatomic abnormality or is a brachycephalic breed, it is best to have many different sizes of endotracheal tubes available as well as a stylet and/or guide tube. Brachycephalic breeds will generally have a much smaller trachea than other breeds of the same size. Always check that the cuffs of the endotracheal tubes do not leak prior to using them. To check the cuffs, use a 5–10 mL syringe and measure the amount of air it takes to inflate the cuff. After 5–10 minutes, deflate the cuff. There should be the same amount of air taken out of the cuff that was put in. If there is not the same amount of air, the cuff has a leak and should not be used. A leaky cuff prevents a good seal between the tube and the trachea. Failing to adequately protect the airway can potentially increase the risk for aspiration and possibly pneumonia. As with any leak, a leaky cuff will make it difficult to maintain a consistent level of anesthesia and will increase waste gas exposure. A sterile water-soluble lubrication jelly should be used to lubricate the endotracheal tube to minimize trauma when passing the endotracheal tube past the arytenoids and into the trachea. Roll gauze or recycled IV tubing may be used to secure the endotracheal tube to the patient and prevent accidental extubation.

Also on the tray are supplies for IV catheterization. First, decide how many IV catheters the patient will require. Patients likely to require transfusions or multiple infusions will need at least two catheters in case of emergency, and potentially an arterial catheter. Include injection caps or t-sets for the catheters. Catheters should be secured with tape or suture.

Arterial catheters should be clearly identified to avoid accidental intra-arterial injections. Bright-colored labels are commercially available for this purpose. Catheters should be flushed with heparinized saline after placement, and several flush syringes should be available on the tray. Some gauze squares are helpful to clean up any blood and also to hold the tongue during intubation. A laryngoscope is very helpful for intubation (especially with cats) but a pen-light will also work. A small syringe with 0.1 mL of 2% lidocaine is very useful to squirt on the cat's larynx to reduce or eliminate laryngeal spasm.

Anesthetized animals cannot protect their eyes, and certain induction agents can prevent them from closing their eyes, so a mild ophthalmic ointment should be used to lubricate and protect them once the patient is induced.

Prepare the appropriate IV fluids (crystalloid/colloid) and have them ready to connect to the patient. This step will save some time if the patient has a poor response to induction anesthesia and needs immediate resuscitation.

Another important aspect of anesthetic preparation is to prepare for potential emergencies. For example, calculate emergency drug doses for the patient ahead of time. Time is very important during emergency events, and spending even 60 seconds calculating a drug dose can make a difference. Excel worksheets can be designed and stored on the computer so that simply entering the patient's weight results in a complete printable table of all possible emergency drugs needed in an emergency. Drug doses that should be calculated ahead of time include epinephrine, atropine, calcium gluconate, and lidocaine. These calculations should be written down and kept with the patient or anesthetist. Many practices will have a printed list of emergency drugs and their doses posted in operating rooms and any rooms where anesthesia is performed.

Every practice should also have at least one "crash kit" or "crash cart" (Fig. 5.4). A crash cart can be a toolbox or a larger cart with several drawers on wheels, and it should be equipped with everything needed for cardiopulmonary arrest or other emergencies. The crash cart should include many syringes of different sizes, needles of multiple sizes, crystalloids and colloids, IV catheters, heparin flushes, and emergency drugs. These emergency drugs should always include epinephrine, atropine, and lidocaine. Other drugs that could be in a crash cart are calcium, sodium bicarbonate, vasopressors such as dopamine or norepinephrine, dopram, naloxone (narcotic reversal agent), flumazenil, neostigmine, dextrose, heparin, dexemethasone,

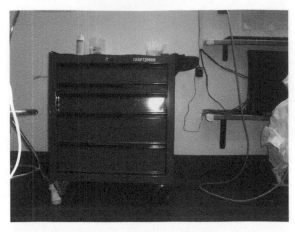

Figure 5.4.   Example of a crash cart model.

and vasopresson. A chart with a list of all the emergency drugs and their doses should also be included. It helps if the crash cart is portable, but there should be at least one crash cart available anywhere there is an anesthesia machine.

For patients in imminent danger of cardiac arrest, or for procedures that seem particularly risky, drug doses should be calculated and readily available. A defibrillator, if available, should also be accessible with a treatment chart attached to it.

If the patient has a status of ASA III, IV, or V, there are some additional steps to take before starting anesthesia. These patients tend to have complicated workups and may need multiple types of fluids, as well as more sophisticated monitoring equipment than a patient with an ASA status of I or II. Administration of different fluid types, such as colloids, (blood products) or constant rate infusions of adjunctive medications is easiest if there are multiple IV catheters. Placing at least two, if not three, of the largest-bore catheters possible in the patient allows for rapid administration of fluids if needed. As an example, consider a patient that is receiving a blood transfusion and also needs a crystalloid fluid, a constant rate infusion (CRI) for pain management, and a CRI of a vasopressor. Patient management is facilitated by having one catheter dedicated to the blood transfusion while the second and/or third catheter is used for other fluids and CRIs. Another option is to use

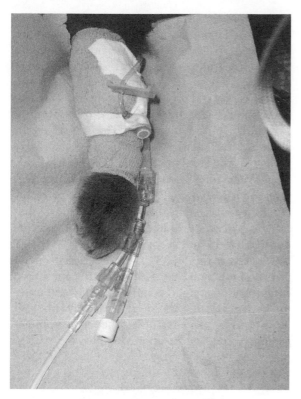

Figure 5.5. Dual port or "Y" adapter for IV catheter.

Y-shaped adaptors (Fig. 5.5), which allow multiple infusions to be given into one catheter.

Many critical patients may benefit from placement of an arterial catheter. With a monometer or pressure transducer and a multiparameter monitor, an arterial line can be used to provide constant and accurate blood pressure readings. In addition, one can quickly and easily obtain an arterial sample for blood gas analysis from the catheter. An arterial catheter will provide the capability to quickly draw blood samples intraoperatively whenever needed.

In critical cases, decreasing the time between induction to surgery is vital. As much patient preparation as possible should be completed before actually anesthetizing the patient. For example, place IV catheters, get fluids set up and ready to start, and place your EKG leads and other monitors if tolerated by the patient. Placing monitors prior to anesthetizing the patient not only decreases anesthesia time but also allows observation of any changes during induction.

CRIs such as dopamine and fentanyl should be prepared in advance. In extremely critical cases, shave and prep as much of the surgery site as possible prior to induction.

It is important to have a good working knowledge of every patient's medical history. This knowledge will help to evaluate potential complications and to determine whether they are caused by surgery, anesthesia, or an underlying disease process. For example, if a patient becomes bradycardic, the cause could be surgical manipulation or too deep a plane of anesthesia, or because the patient is being treated for heart disease and is on medication that slows the heart rate.

The surgery suite should also be prepared prior to induction of anesthesia. The anesthesia machine in the operating room should be pressure checked and set up with the correct size of rebreathing system for the patient. The inhalant anesthesia and CO_2 absorbent should be evaluated as previously discussed.

Monitoring equipment in the surgery room should also be prepared ahead of time to decrease anesthesia time. For example, the EKG leads, pulse oximeter, blood pressure, esophageal stethoscope, end-tidal CO_2, and so forth can be laid out for easy access. The more things that are set up ahead of time, the smoother and quicker the transition from the induction room to the operating room will be. Consider having backup monitors if you are using monitors that can fail due to battery depletion, such as a Doppler instrument. It is always useful to have a roll of tape and a bottle of alcohol near or on the anesthesia machine for easy access when troubleshooting.

Keeping the patient warm is very important; many times this not given the attention it deserves. A severely hypothermic patient is prone to complications. It is important to understand that a patient with a body temperature of just 95 °F has a decrease in anesthetic requirements (Haskins 2007). They are often bradycardic and have decreased perfusion due to vasoconstriction. These patients may show a reduced response to any drug administration, intravenous or intramuscular. For example, extremely hypothermic patients with bradycardia tend not to respond to treatment with an anticholinergic, and the heart rate may stay the same or continue to slow. Finally, patients with a body temperature of 93° or less can not coagulate normally (Robertson 2007).

To prevent hypothermia and its consequences, prepare methods for thermoregulatory support ahead of time. Many clinics will use a recirculating hot water blanket. To be effective, these blankets need to be turned on ahead of time. Another way to warm patients is to use a forced warm-air blower with a disposable blanket. It is important to make sure you have the correctly sized blanket to fit the patient. Forced warm-air blowers should not be turned on until the patient is completely draped because of the possibility of blowing hair and debris onto the surgical site. Warm water bottles are also sometimes used, but they have disadvantages. There have been many patients that have developed severe skin burns after having warm fluid bottles that were too hot next to them. Anesthetized patients are unable to move away from an object that is too hot. Warm water bottles used around patients must be covered with a towel or a couple of layers of drape material or similar paper. A good rule of thumb is objects that are too hot to touch are too hot for use next to even furry patients. Place the bags or bottles against the inside of the anesthetist's arm for 60 seconds. If they can be kept there for the entire 60 seconds without becoming too hot, they should not be hazardous to the patient. Bubble wrap can be placed over any patient area that is not part of the sterile field and can help insulate the patient. Baby socks can be placed on small paws to help prevent heat loss. A fluid warmer also works very well. In place of a fluid warmer warm water bottles or warm fluid bags can be placed around the fluid line. The warm fluid bags will warm the fluid as it runs through the line and into the patient. Placing warm fluid bags above and below the Y-piece can also help warm the cold oxygen being delivered to the patient. Since fresh gas is a major source of patient cooling, this technique can be helpful, provided there is enough space. Be careful not to place tension on the Y-piece that creates tension on the endotracheal tube. Continued tension on the endotracheal tube

could cause tracheal trauma or result in extubation. Heat lamps can also be used but must not be placed so close to the patient as to cause burns. Generally, heat lamps should be kept approximately 6 feet from patients to avoid burns and yet still provide heat benefits. The heat lamp should also be kept away from surgical personnel and equipment. The most recent warming technology available for veterinary patients is the Hot Dog Patient Warmer available from Augustine Biomedical. This product features an energy-efficient controller with heavy duty, cleanable, reusable patient blankets that can be placed over, under, or around patients during surgery and recovery.

Make sure the surgery table is set up properly prior to induction (Fig. 5.6). Once the anesthesia equipment is set up, it is difficult to have to move the patient because the surgery table was not set up properly. For example, the electrocautery ground should be positioned under the patient

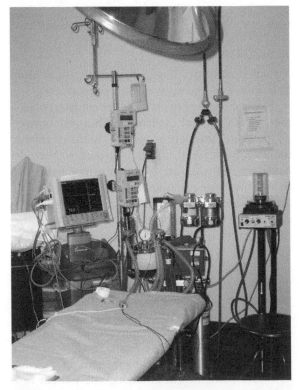

Figure 5.6. The prepared OR table with all anticipated equipment set up and ready for use.

before the surgical prep is complete; otherwise, there is a risk of contaminating the surgical site. This would increase anesthesia time by requiring another surgical scrub with more cold disinfectant on the patient, which can exacerbate and potentiate hypothermia. Any time a patient is moved quickly or dramatically, monitoring equipment can get disconnected, the Y-piece could disconnect, and the endotracheal tube could become kinked or even get pulled out of the patient. If the patient does become extubated, there is a risk of the patient aspirating, becoming hypoxic, and waking up, as well as exposing personnel to anesthetic gas. The patient must be reintubated immediately, a procedure which, depending on the position of the patient, could cause contamination of the surgical site, necessitating yet another surgical scrub of the area. All in all, it could be a potentially stressful situation for the anesthetist, surgeon, and patient. It is wise to keep a laryngoscope and perhaps some additional induction agent nearby in case the patient does become light, extubates, and needs to be reintubated in a hurry.

If available, position anesthesia ventilators for use prior to starting the case. Any patient can potentially require mechanical ventilation. Having the ventilator available is convenient and prevents the need to step away from the patient if the need for the equipment arises suddenly.

Set up any constant rate infusions (CRI) at this time. They should be prepared and hanging with the correct drip rate set. If syringe pumps are available, have them preset and readily available. Extra bags of crystalloids and colloids should be stored in the operating room for easy availability.

Once the patient is in the OR and positioned comfortably on the table, an organized approach is useful. For example, the anesthetist should know where the EKG clips are placed on the patient so that if they stop working well, they can be reached to be reattached or rewetted. All IV access ports should be positioned within reach. Place an extension line on any available IV catheters that will be buried beneath the surgical drape to make them easily accessible, and secure them well to prevent disconnection. Monitoring equipment should be placed so that

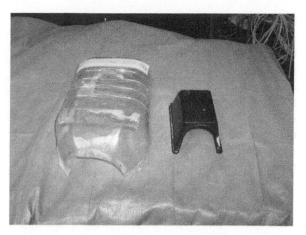

Figure 5.7. Two examples of Doppler guards. Adapted saline bottle on the left and commercially available "mouse house" on the right. These protect the Doppler probe from personnel interference (surgeon's elbows) and interference from the warm air blower.

troubleshooting can be accomplished if needed during surgery. Forced-air heating systems can dry out the alcohol used on the EKG leads, causing interference or failure of the EKG. Placing lubricating jelly on the EKG leads can help prevent this. Placing the Doppler instrument or oscillometric blood pressure cuff on the limb closest to the anesthetist will make it much easier to get to should there be a problem. The Doppler probe can be protected from the surgeon's elbows or interference from a warm air blower by placing a plastic Doppler guard over the probe (Fig. 5.7). Doppler guards can be purchased as "mouse houses" or they can be made by cutting a plastic bottle (500 mL NaCl bottle works well) in half and then cutting an opening in each end to fit over the limb of the patient. Sharp edges should be blunted with tape.

From understanding the procedure being done and the status of the patient, to confirming that the anesthesia machine and monitors are working well, to making sure everything needed is available, preparedness is the name of the game for successful anesthesia. Knowing what possible reactions a patient may have under anesthesia and being prepared to respond to them can make the difference between a positive outcome and a disaster. Good preparation does take time in the beginning of a procedure, but it is important not to get pressured into starting a case before everything is ready. Taking a little extra time in the beginning will be well worth it if there is a crisis—everything needed will be immediately available. Most cases will go smoothly and have few complications, but being ready to handle the one case that goes bad and has multiple complications will boost anesthetist confidence and more than make up for the many that have no complications.

References

Hartsfield, SM. 2007. Anesthetic machines and breathing systems. In Lumb & Jones' Veterinary Anesthesia and Analgesia 4th ed., edited by Tranquilli, WJ, Thurmon, JC, Grimm, KA. Ames, IA: Blackwell Publishing, pp.443–493.

Haskins, SC. 2007. In Lumb & Jones' Veterinary Anesthesia and Analgesia 4th ed., edited by Tranquilli, WJ, Thurmon, JC, Grimm, KA. Ames, IA: Blackwell Publishing, p.552.

Robertson, S. 2007. Hypothermia. The Big Chill, Scientific Proceedings (IVIS) http://www.ivis.org/proceedings/voorjaarsdagen/2007/comp_anim/Robertson6.pdf.

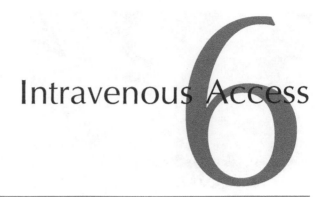

Intravenous Access

Shawn Takada

The intravenous catheter is truly a lifeline for all animals under anesthesia. Used in the safe administration of induction agents to the resuscitation of the critical patient, it is an indispensable tool for the anesthetist. This chapter will cover all aspects of intravenous catheters:

1. Types and sizes
2. Choosing the proper catheter for the patient and procedure
3. Common venous and arterial sites
4. Proper placement and stabilization
5. Care

Types and Sizes of Catheters

There are two basic types of catheters:

1. Over the needle
2. Through the needle

Over the needle catheter

Over the needle catheters are usually placed in peripheral vessels, which include cephalic, lateral saphenous, and medial saphenous veins in the dog, cat, and exotics. Other uses include arterial catheters placed in the medial pedal arteries of the dog and cat and jugular veins in neonates.

An over the needle double lumen catheter for peripheral vessel placement, called the "twin catheter," is now available and is manufactured by Arrow International.

Size: Sizes range from 26 gauge to 16 gauge for most domestic animals. Lengths are available in 3/4 inches to 5-1/2 inches.

Through the needle catheter

Called "central lines," through the needle catheters are used for longer-term fluid therapy and multiple blood sampling. Through the needle catheters are most commonly placed in the jugular vein in the dog and cat, lateral/medial saphenous in the dog, and medial saphenous in the cat.

Size: These catheters are available in 18 and 16 gauge, with lengths in 6 and 12 inches.

Multilumen catheter

Multilumen cathethers are another type of through the needle catheter (Fig. 6.1). They are

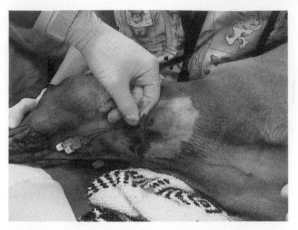

Figure 6.1. Double lumen catheter in the jugular vein of a dog.

used for administration of multiple fluid and drug therapies as well as TPN (total parenteral nutrition). These catheters have two, three, or four separate entrance and exit ports.

Size: A large selection is available in various lengths, gauges, and lumens. Recently manufacturers have impregnated these catheters with silver sulfadiazine and chlorhexidine to lessen the chance of infection.

Catheters also come in many different types of materials; some may be more reactive than others. The anesthetist should take into consideration the possible duration of hospitalization and immune status before choosing the proper catheter. Examples of materials (from least reactive to most) are; silicone, polyurethane, polyvinyl chloride, and Teflon (Battaglia 2001).

Vascular Access Ports (VAP)

These are beneficial for long-term chemotherapy patients. VAPs are surgically placed in the jugular vein with a metal or plastic port that is attached to the extension that runs subcutaneously. The access port is usually located between the scapulas in veterinary patients. Drugs and fluids can be administered by puncturing the port with a noncoring needle recommended by the manufacturer (Battaglia 2001). Single and double access ports are available.

Choosing the Correct Catheter for Patient/Procedure

For the healthy patient undergoing a routine or elective procedure completed within 90 minutes, an over the needle catheter is sufficient. The largest gauge possible should be placed in case of emergencies where rapid fluid administration may be needed. A 22–20 g is recommended in cats and small dogs and up to a 16 g in large dog breeds.

Single Lumen Central Catheters

Single lumen central catheters are manufactured by BD Intracath, Venisystems, and Arrow.

Central venous catheters are useful in cases lasting greater than 90 minutes and/or in patients with one or more metabolic abnormalities. Potassium, sodium, calcium, bicarbonate, glucose, lactate, and pH levels can be assessed easily with central lines. Though possible it is not practical to manually perform venopuncture on a patient draped in for surgery. Although not accurate for oxygen saturation/carbon dioxide levels, central line samples are approximate indicators of SpO_2 and CO_2 concentrations. Long anesthetic procedures on even the healthiest patient can depress the respiratory system, and assisted ventilation (manual or mechanical) may be needed. If more precise levels are warranted (thoracotomies, craniotomies) an arterial sample should be obtained or, ideally, an arterial catheter should be placed.

Double/Triple/Quadruple Lumen Catheters

Arrow, Mila, and Cook are three of the most popular manufacturers of these catheters for veterinary medicine.

A few advantages of multiple lumen catheters are the multiple ports: IV fluids, IV anesthetics, and venous blood gases can all be simultaneously administered and drawn through a dedicated port. Certain drugs may interact adversely with others (i.e., metoclopramide with many antibiotics) when in the same fluid line; a separate port simplifies treatments.

Common Venous and Arterial Sites

The most popular site for peripheral catheterization in the dog, cat, and exotic is the cephalic vein; as stated earlier the largest catheter possible should be placed in case of emergencies. Animals who are declawed, have cherry eyes, have aural hematomas, and so forth (healthy, stable patients with minor upper body surgeries) should have lateral or medial saphenous (short) peripheral catheters. Neonates may only be able to have either an intraosseous or short catheter placed in the jugular.

For central lines the largest vein to choose from is the jugular, though certain issues must be considered before placement. In the case of a splenectomy, liver lobectomy, and hemoabdomen (all patients with possible coagulopathy), jugular venopuncture may not be the best option. The anesthetist should always use good judgment and permission from the veterinarian/surgeon. Possible pancreatic/icteric/diabetic patients may benefit from the placement of a multilumen catheter from the beginning because of the possibility of ongoing treatments and fluid therapy needed. Other venous access sites for sampling/central lines are the lateral saphenous in the dog and lateral/medial saphenous veins in the cat.

Arterial catheter placement is usually done at the medial pedal artery for both canine and feline patients although many other sites are possible (Fig. 6.2). These include the auricular artery in large-eared dogs (bassett hounds, labs), the lingual artery, femoral (not recommended due to the potential for bleeding out should the catheter become dislodged), and even the coccygeal artery in dogs and cats.

As stated previously, arterial catheters are recommended in patients with probable, possible, or known ventilation issues. Critical cases

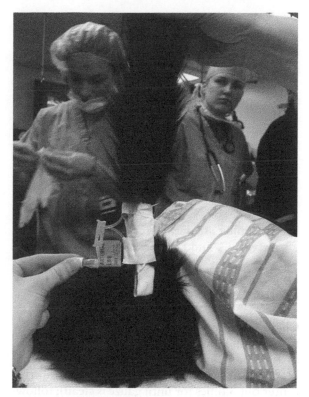

Figure 6.2. Arterial catheter in the coccygeal artery of a cat.

with blood pressure abnormalities will benefit from direct blood pressure monitoring with an arterial line also. BD Angiocath and Arrow Radial Artery catheters are made specifically for arterial placement. A standard peripheral (over the needle, single lumen) catheter can be used just as well. With arterial placement, smaller gauges are preferable due to arterial spasms that may occur. A luer-lock t-port is the better choice with arterial lines; conventional t-ports can give way.

Proper placement and stabilization

Supplies for peripheral catheter placement include the following:

- 1-inch tape; three pieces long enough to encircle the leg 1-1/2 to 2 times; one piece split lengthwise to cross over t-port (approx. 3 inches long)

- Chlorhexadine scrub
- Alcohol-soaked cotton balls
- Catheter
- T-port primed with a 3 mL heparin saline flush
- Clipper with #40 blade
- Gloves (beneficial for immune-compromised patients such as diabetics, cancer/chemotherapy patients, neonates, and so forth)
- Flushes; 2–3 3 mL flushes made of 1 mL of 1000 u heparin per 250 mL sodium chloride
- Wrapping material (cast padding, Kling, Vetwrap®, and tape)

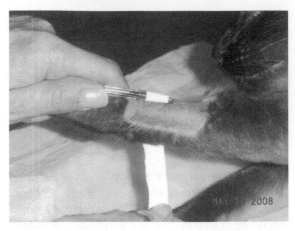

Figure 6.4.   Taping of the cephalic catheter.

Prepping the site

Clip a large-enough area over the vein to ensure no contamination from surrounding fur. Feathers or long hair that may impede the taping should be trimmed. Surgically scrub the area from the center out 3 times (or until gauze is clean); follow with an alcohol wipe.

Proper restraint of the patient is critical for successful catheter placement. The restrainer will usually "hold off" the vein of choice well away from the prepped site (above the elbow for cephalic catheters and above the knee for lateral/medial catheters).

Start in the center of the prepped site above the vein (Fig. 6.3). Using a 30-degree angle, advance the catheter and stylet through the skin and into the vein. Once a flashback is observed the entire unit is advanced a small amount farther to "seat" it into the vein. The catheter is then fed off the stylet into the vessel. Remove the stylet and place the t-port into the catheter hub.

Stabilization

A 1-inch piece of tape is placed over the hub of the catheter and the patient's skin; press down for better contact (Fig. 6.4). Wrap around the leg going over the tape no more than 2 times. Another piece of tape is split vertically 1–2 inches from one edge three-quarters of the way through. This split is placed under the t-port/catheter juncture and partially over the first piece. Wrap around the leg. To stabilize the t-port a piece of tape 1/2 inch wide is placed under (sticky side) and crossed over the t-port and the original tape (Fig. 6.5). A last piece of tape can be used as a tension loop for the t-port; this may help with disconnection problems when moving patients from area to area. Each tape, with the exception of the crossover, should be "courtesy tabbed" for easy removal.

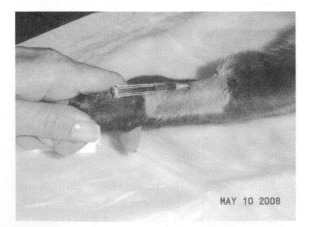

MAY 10 2008

Figure 6.3.   Cephalic over the needle catheter.

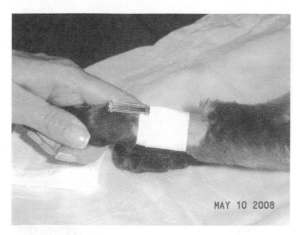

Figure 6.5. Cephalic catheter secured.

Supplies for Central Catheters

Supplies for central catheters include the following:

- 1-inch tape (6–7 pieces long enough to encircle the area 1-1/2 times
- Chlorhexadine scrub
- Alcohol-soaked cotton balls
- Catheter
- T-port primed with a 3 mL heparin saline flush
- Clipper with #40 blade
- Gloves (As mentioned earlier, the immune-compromised patient benefits from aseptic technique; in the case of multilumen catheters that will be used for TPN, sterile placement is mandatory.)
- Heparin flushes. 2–3 3 mL flushes
- Triple antibiotic ointment
- Gauze sponges (3–4)
- Suture (for fractious, obese, active, pendulous skin breeds, and so forth)
- Kling 2–3 rolls

Prepping the site

Clip an area large enough for aseptic placement. A good rule of thumb for jugular placement encompasses the top of the neck to the thoracic inlet for length and the trachea to 1–2 inches above the jugular, depending on the size and species of the patient. Surgically scrub the area from the center out 3 times (or until clean) followed by an alcohol wipe.

The patient is best placed in lateral recumbency for the placement—facing right for the right-handed, and left for the left-handed. The thumb of the opposite hand should be pressed into the thoracic inlet with the other four fingers wrapped around the back of the neck. With the dominant hand, palpate the jugular vein and visualize its location. The skin above the jugular is tented to allow safe puncture of the skin; distend the vein again and advance the needle into it at a 30-degree angle. Depending on the size of the vessel, hydration of the patient, and type of catheter used, there may not be a flash of blood (Fig. 6.6).

If the catheter advances without resistance, the likelihood of success is good. When the catheter is fed almost entirely into the vein the needle should be backed out of the vessel. Use a gauze square over the puncture site for homeostasis if needed. The catheter can then be seated in the needle hub and the stylet removed. Next flush the catheter and secure the needle guard. Flush and return to check the patency of the catheter before wrapping; it may need to be backed out of the vein a small amount if no flash occurs. Loop the excess catheter (be careful of kinks)

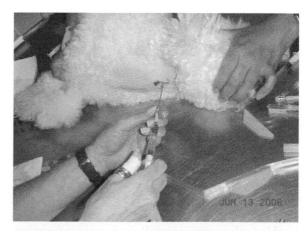

Figure 6.6. Blood flash confirming placement of a single lumen catheter.

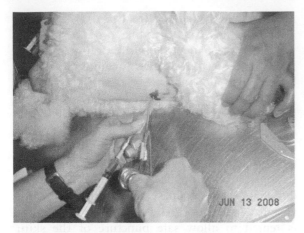

Figure 6.7. Applying the needle guard.

with the needle guard at a 90-degree angle to the neck (Fig. 6.7).

Fold one gauze sponge in half and put it under the guard for patient comfort; the second can be smeared with triple antibiotic ointment and placed over the puncture. Tape, starting at the hub of the catheter (stick both corners to each other), is then brought around the neck securing the needle guard. A second piece is placed around the neck to secure the gauze. Kling is then wrapped around the neck both cranially and caudally to the guard. Place the primed t-port into the catheter and cover the Kling with 1–2 inches of tape (or Vetwrap®, being careful not to wrap tightly) completely. Have tape contact skin on the top and bottom of the bandage to prevent migration of the catheter. Place the last piece of tape over the t-port and needle guard. While bandaging, the technician should check the patency of the catheter between each layer (Fig. 6.8).

Troubleshooting

Dehydrated patients (especially felines) can be challenging when placing central lines. Suggestions to advance a jugular catheter that is giving resistance include the following:

- Feed off the stylet
- Have the restrainer pull the front legs forward while trying to feed.

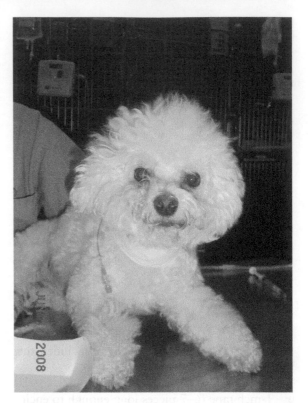

Figure 6.8. Single lumen catheter wrapped with T-set extension.

- Place the patient in dorsal recumbency, first with legs caudal; if still not feeding try pulling the legs cranially.

Care

All catheters are to be watched for reactions on a daily basis. This is easy for peripheral "short" catheters that are not bandage-wrapped. The technician can assess the foot for swelling, flush the catheter to check patency, and check the tape for tightness or slippage. For central lines placed peripherally, the bandage material should be removed and the catheter rewrapped daily for immune-compromised patients; relatively healthy animals can be rewrapped every 2 days. If there is a reaction from the patient when the catheter is flushed, the bandage is soiled, or consistent paw shaking has been observed, the wrap must be broken down to visualize the site. Spiking of a fever may indicate a catheter reaction. If the catheter must be replaced, keep the existing one (if still functional) until the new one has been established; the fluid line and bag should also be changed to reduce cross contamination. T-connectors should be replaced approximately every 3 days.

Conclusion

Veterinary medicine has seen considerable advancement in the uses, type, material, placement, and care of the intravenous catheter within the past few years. We can now tailor the catheter to the patient and its situation. These advances have helped improve the quality of veterinary care that we are able to offer our patients.

Reference

Battaglia, AM. 2001. Small Animal Emergency and Critical Care: A Manual for the Veterinary Technician. Ithaca, NY: WB Saunders Company.

Airway Maintenance

7

Darci Palmer

Airway management is essential for the effective care of the anesthetized veterinary patient. There is always a risk associated with placing an animal under general anesthesia. Protecting and maintaining a patent airway is one way to help minimize the overall anesthetic risk to the patient. This chapter discusses the materials, techniques, and management involved with airway maintenance.

Inhalant anesthetics can be delivered to the patient via a face mask or by endotracheal intubation. A face mask involves placing a cone-shaped mask with a tight-fitting diaphragm over the patient's muzzle. Endotracheal intubation is the process of placing a tube through the oral cavity and into the trachea. This method is considered the most efficient way to manage the airway. Endotracheal intubation offers many advantages over the face mask (Table 7.1).

Types of Endotracheal Tubes

Generally, endotracheal tubes are made from silicone, polyvinyl chloride (PVC) plastic, or rubber. Each type of material has its advantages and disadvantages. Silicone tubes are the most expensive, but they can be cleaned, sterilized, and reused multiple times. A PVC plastic tube is stiffer and contains a curve in the length of the tube to aid in intubation. At body temperature these tubes soften and conform to the shape of the airway (Dorsch and Dorsch 2008a). Most of the PVC tubes are disposable and intended for single use; however, they can be cleaned and reused. Their longevity is less than the silicone tubes. Red rubber tubes are infrequently used in practice. The solid color of the tube lumen makes it impossible to detect occlusions from mucus. They can be reused, but over time the tube becomes hardened, making them more prone to cracking. They are also more likely to cause cross contamination between patients because the rubber is difficult to clean and disinfect.

The three most common types of endotracheal tubes used in veterinary medicine are the Murphy, Magill, and Cole tubes (Fig. 7.1). The Murphy is the most popular style of tube. The Magill tubes are similar to the Murphy tubes except they do not contain the Murphy eye. The red rubber tube shown in Figure 7.1 is an example of the Magill style of tube. The Murphy and Magill tubes can be manufactured with or without a cuff. The Cole tube is uncuffed and has a smaller diameter lumen at the distal end,

Table 7.1. Advantages of endotracheal intubation compared to a face mask for maintenance of general anesthesia with inhalants.

Comparison of Endotracheal Tube and Facemask		
	Endotracheal Tube	Face mask
Patency	Allows anesthetist complete control of airway	Relies on patient to maintain respiratory rate
Efficiency	Oxygen and inhalant are delivered closer to lungs	Uptake of oxygen and inhalant depends on patient's respiratory rate
	Lower oxygen flow rate can be used (decreased cost).	Requires higher oxygen flow rates (increased cost)
Ventilation	Allows for Intermittent Positive Pressure Ventilation (IPPV) during periods of apnea	Cannot assist with ventilation; increased risk of inflating the stomach with anesthetic gases
Dead space	Decreases anatomical dead space	Increases dead space, especially when using a face mask that is too large
Protection	Properly inflated cuffs prevent aspiration of foreign material (blood, saliva, gastric fluid, dental debris) into the lungs (Hughes 2007).	None
Waste anesthetic gas	Little or no exposure to personnel with a properly inflated cuff	High exposure to personnel

compared to the rest of the tube. This tube is designed so that only the narrow distal end fits into the larynx and trachea, thus creating a seal where the larger diameter of the tube meets the laryngotracheal opening (Hartsfield 2007). Cole

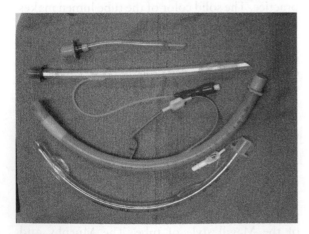

Figure 7.1. Different types of endotracheal tubes. From top to bottom: Cole tube; Murphy silicone tube, HVLP cuff; Magill red rubber, LVHP cuff; Murphy PVC plastic tube, HVLP cuff.

tubes are commonly used in birds, because they have complete tracheal rings that do not expand to accommodate a cuff, and in pediatric patients where tracheal rupture from cuff inflation is a concern.

Special Endotracheal Tubes

Armored or reinforced tubes (Fig. 7.2) contain a wire that spirals around the length of the tube. The wire is embedded in the wall of the tube and helps prevent kinking when the head and neck of the patient are flexed (Hartsfield 2007). These tubes are highly flexible in order to maintain a patent airway. However, the flexibility makes the tube more difficult to handle during intubation, so a stylet is often used to give the tube some stability. Any procedure that involves flexing the head and neck will benefit from the use of these tubes. Such procedures include ophthalmic surgeries, oral surgeries, cervical spinal taps, myelograms, and craniotomies (Hartsfield

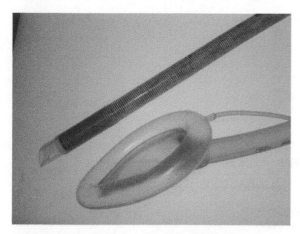

Figure 7.2. Example of a laryngeal mask airway and an armored (reinforced) tube. Note the helical wire located in the armored tube (top). (Courtesy of Susan Bryant, CVT, VTS, Anesthesia.)

2007). There are two major disadvantages with armored tubes. First, the outside wall of the tube is thicker (to accommodate the wire), which makes the internal diameter smaller than a standard tube of the same size. This results in increased resistance to gas flow and subsequent increase in respiratory effort by the patient. For this reason these tubes should be used only when necessary. Secondly, if a patient accidentally bites down on the tube it will become permanently deformed and must be discarded. Bite guards are often present on the proximal end of the tube to prevent this.

Laryngeal mask airways (LMA) (Fig. 7.2) were first developed for use in human medicine as an intermediate between the use of a face mask and endotracheal tube. They are termed *supraglottic devices* because they are positioned proximal to the trachea. They still provide an airtight seal at the larynx and therefore function like an endotracheal tube. They are popular in human medicine because standard intubation with an endotracheal tube can be challenging. Intubation is a much easier technique in animals so the usefulness of an LMA in veterinary medicine is inconclusive (Hughes 2007). There are a few situations, such as surgeries of the trachea, where they might prove to be advantageous. Oncology patients anesthetized consecutive days for radiation therapy will also benefit from the

use of an LMA because the risk of developing tracheitis is decreased. Another benefit is with animals prone to difficult intubations such as brachycephalic breeds of dogs, cats, rabbits, and pigs.

Tube Design

The design of the endotracheal tube is relatively similar for all the different types of tubes. The parts of a cuffed Murphy tube are shown in Figure 7.3. The distal end of the tube, placed in the trachea, is commonly referred to as the "patient end." The end hole is beveled at an angle to help guide the tube past the arytenoids and into the trachea. The Murphy tube contains a unique feature called the "Murphy eye" located opposite the bevel. This extra hole allows for gas flow to continue if the end hole becomes occluded (Dorsch and Dorsch 2008a).

Some endotracheal tubes are equipped with an inflatable cuff system. The purpose of the cuff is to establish an airtight seal against the tracheal wall in order to prevent the mixing of airway gases with room air and to prevent aspiration of foreign material. The cuff system consists of an inflatable cuff, inflating tube, inflating valve, and pilot balloon (Hartsfield 2007). The two most common styles of cuff used in veterinary medicine are the low volume high pressure (LVHP) and the high volume low pressure (HVLP) cuffs. An example of the LVHP cuff is demonstrated on the red rubber tube in Figure 7.1. When not inflated, the LVHP cuff lies flat against the tube. As the name implies, these cuffs require a low volume of air to establish a tight seal with the trachea. The main disadvantage is that the LVHP cuff contacts only a small surface area while exerting a high pressure on the tracheal wall. When this type of cuff is inflated for long periods of time the risk of inducing necrosis to the tracheal wall becomes an issue (Dorsch and Dorsch 2008a). In contrast the HVLP cuff requires a larger amount of air to create a seal with the trachea, but the volume is distributed over a wider surface area, so pressure exerted on the tracheal wall is low. When properly inflated the

Parts of an Endotracheal Tube

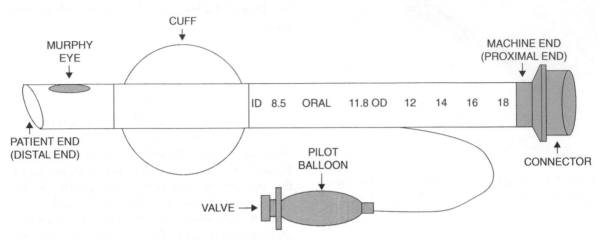

Figure 7.3.   Parts of an endotracheal tube. (Courtesy of Kaitlin Palmer.)

HVLP cuffs are more beneficial for long-term use; however, overinflation of the HVLP cuff can also cause pressure necrosis. Examples of the HVLP cuff are seen on the PVC and silicone tubes listed in Figure 7.1. Note that the HVLP cuff is bulky and contains folds even when deflated.

Most endotracheal tubes have information listed on the tube, such as tube length, diameter, and manufacturer or supplier. The length of the tube starting at the distal end is measured in centimeters. These numbers are located along the tube and help determine the depth of insertion into the trachea. The measurements are universal for all tube sizes and brands. The diameter of the endotracheal tube is measured in millimeters. Some tubes list both the internal (ID) and outside (OD) diameter on the tube. The internal diameter determines the size of the endotracheal tube placed in the patient. The manufacturer or supplier name is usually listed along the length of the tube or on the pilot balloon. Depending on the brand of tube, some contain a radiopaque marker that will show up on radiographs to help confirm placement and length. If the tube is disposable, the caption "Do not reuse" or "Single use only" appears on the tube. In addition the terms "oral," "nasal," or "oral/nasal" may be present and correspond to intended use. The connector is located at the proximal (machine) end of the endotracheal tube. The connector has a standard 15 mm outside diameter that connects the endotracheal tube to the breathing hoses.

Selecting the Appropriate Tube

Since animal sizes and body weights will vary, it is difficult to establish an absolute uniform guideline for selecting an endotracheal tube. However, there are several criteria the anesthetist should take into consideration. The chosen tube should have the widest diameter that will fit comfortably past the larynx and into the trachea without excessive force. The most reliable method to judge the appropriate diameter is by gentle palpation of the trachea. Do not select a tube based solely on body weight. This method can often be misleading for brachycephalic breeds or overweight patients. Brachycephalic breeds usually have a much smaller tracheal diameter for their body weight compared to breeds of similar weight. For example a bulldog that weighs 30 kg may only take a 7.5 mm tube; a 30 kg mixed breed dog could easily take a 10 mm tube (Hartsfield 2007). Another subjective method involves using the width of the nose between the nares as an approximation of tracheal diameter. Regardless of the method used, the only way to get proficient at selecting the appropriate size of tube is with continuous practice. It is helpful to select at least three sizes of tubes for each patient: one that most closely matches the tracheal diameter, one a single size larger, and another one size smaller. This will ensure that there are two additional tubes ready for use should the estimation be incorrect.

It is important to note that a tube that is too small can increase the patient's "work of breathing." According to the Hagen-Poiseuille Law, if the diameter of the airway is reduced, the resistance to gas flow will increase by a factor of four (McDonell and Kerr 2007). For example, if you select a tube that is half the normal diameter of the trachea, resistance to gas flow will increase by a factor of sixteenfold (McDonnell and Kerr 2007). If resistance to gas flow is increased, the patient will have a more difficult time taking in a normal tidal volume, which could result in labored breathing.

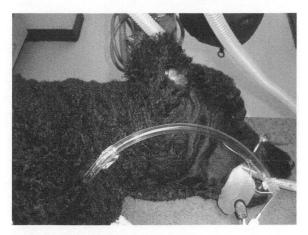

Figure 7.4. Assessing proper length of an endotracheal tube prior to intubation. The distal end should not extend past the point of the shoulder, and the proximal end should not extend past the incisor teeth.

> **Helpful Hint # 1**
>
> As a general guideline:
> - Cats usually take a 3.0–4.5 mm tube.
> - Dogs may take a 3.0–16 mm tube depending on the breed.
> - The veterinary practice should have a large array of tube sizes to accommodate all sizes of animals.
> - Have at least two or more of each size in case one becomes damaged.

Once the diameter of the tube has been selected it is also necessary to ensure that the length of the tube is appropriate for the patient's size. The length of the tube should not extend past the incisors on the proximal end or past the thoracic inlet (point of the shoulder) on the distal end (Fig. 7.4). A tube that extends past the incisors will contribute to excessive mechanical dead space and a decrease in alveolar ventilation. A tube that extends past the thoracic inlet may cause bronchial intubation leading to one-lung

ventilation. This can lead to severe hypoxemia. The tube length should be premeasured to the patient before induction. If the tube is too long it can be cut at the proximal end to accommodate the appropriate length for the patient. Care must be taken not to interfere with the cuff inflating tube when shortening the tube.

Supplies and Equipment for Intubation

Intubation in dogs and cats requires only an endotracheal tube and a good light source to accomplish the task (Hartsfield 2007). However, there are times when it can be challenging (e.g., brachycephalic breeds) and necessitates additional equipment. Figure 7.5 shows the recommended supplies that should be available to intubate a cat. The same supplies can be used for a dog with the adaptation of a larger endotracheal tube, longer laryngoscope blade, and larger stylet.

Laryngoscopes

Laryngoscopes facilitate endotracheal intubation by allowing direct visualization of the larynx and opening to the trachea. They are composed of

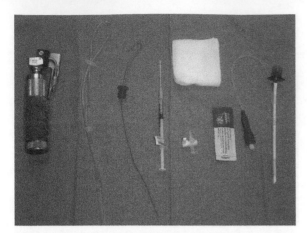

Figure 7.5. Supplies for cat intubation. From left to right: laryngoscope with blade; tube tie made from IV tubing; stylet; lidocaine syringe; 3 × 3 gauze squares; three-way stopcock; KY lube; endotracheal tube.

two basic parts, a handle and a blade that contains a light source. Blades come in many different lengths ranging from 0 (short) to 5 (long) (Hughes 2007; Dorsch and Dorsch 2008b). Longer blades specifically used for sheep, goats, camelids, and swine are also available. The style of blade determines the type of laryngoscope. The two most common types used in veterinary medicine include the Miller (straight blade) and the Macintosh (curved blade) (Fig. 7.6). Both of these blades contain a high ridge along the right side of the blade, the flange. The flange is useful

to divert redundant tissue of the oral cavity away from the field of view, but its location blocks the light source for a person attempting to intubate right-handed. In this regard learning how to intubate with the left hand allows the anesthetist the full advantage of utilizing the light source and visualizing the larynx.

Laryngoscopes are very effective and help expedite intubation in all types of animals; their use is highly recommended. The blade depresses the tongue and manipulates the epiglottis to better expose the glottis and tracheal opening while the light source illuminates the larynx for better visualization. The blade should be placed on the surface of the tongue and only advanced to the base of the tongue immediately rostral to the epiglottis. **Never** place the blade directly on the epiglottis because this can inflict trauma to the tissues leading to edema and inadvertent airway complications. In cats, touching the epiglottis with the laryngoscope blade may induce active closure of the glottis and lead to laryngospasm (Hartsfield 2007).

Stylet and guide tubes

Stylets are usually made of flexible metal and placed inside the lumen of the endotracheal tube to help strengthen and shape the tube for intubation (Fig. 7.7). They are most beneficial with

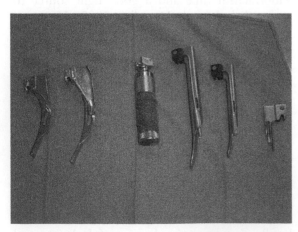

Figure 7.6. Laryngoscope handle and blades. From left to right: Macintosh (curved) blades; laryngoscope handle; Miller (straight) blades.

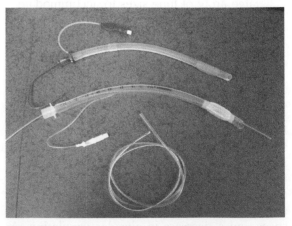

Figure 7.7. Example of stylet and guide tubes. From top to bottom: metal stylet (make sure it **does not** protrude out the distal end); polyethylene urinary catheter used as a guide tube; pediatric stomach tube.

small sizes of tubes because it gives the tube more stability. The entire stylet should remain inside the lumen of the tube and not protrude out the distal end. Improper use of a metal stylet can cause damage to the arytenoids and trachea.

Another method to help facilitate intubation is with the use of a guide tube. Commonly used guide tubes include a canine polyethylene urinary catheter or a pediatric stomach tube (Fig. 7.7). The guide tube is advanced past the arytenoids and into the trachea, and then the endotracheal tube is threaded over the guide tube and follows the path into the trachea. Once the endotracheal tube is properly positioned in the trachea, the guide tube is removed. The smaller diameter of these guide tubes allows for better visualization of the opening to the trachea. They can be especially helpful in brachycephalic breeds where large amounts of redundant tissue often block the full view of the larynx even with the help of a laryngoscope. Guide tubes should be made of soft plastic to avoid injury to the laryngeal tissues and trachea.

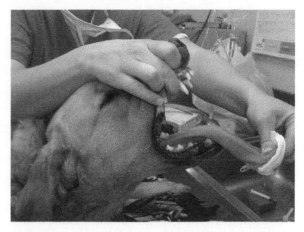

Figure 7.8. Proper way for an assistant to hold the head for intubation.

Intubation

The following steps describe the process of intubation with the patient in sternal recumbency and with the use of an assistant (see also Table 7.2):

1. Preoxygenate the patient with 100% oxygen via face mask 3–5 minutes prior to induction.
2. Once the patient is adequately induced, have the assistant hold the patient's head for intubation (Fig. 7.8).

Table 7.2. Guidelines to help maximize the success and ease of intubation.

Prior to Intubation
Have all supplies ready and within reach **before** inducing the patient.
Have a selection of three different sizes of tubes for each patient.
Inflate the cuff for at least 5–10 minutes prior to use.
• This will test the integrity of the cuff and inflating system.
• The amount of air placed in the cuff as a test should equal the amount of air taken out before the tube is used in the patient.
• If the air taken out is less than what was put in, a slow leak is present and the tube should not be used.
Lubricate the cuff of the tube with a small amount of KY jelly so that a thin layer is present around the cuff. Take care to **not** cover the Murphy eye with lube.
Have an assistant hold the head for intubation.
Place the patient in sternal recumbency with the head and neck extended.
• This position gives the best possible view of the larynx and trachea.
• Intubation can be accomplished in lateral and dorsal recumbency, but these positions are more difficult

Helpful Hint # 2

- The assistant should open the mouth and extend the head and neck by placing the thumb and middle finger of one hand just behind the canine teeth of the maxilla.
- In cats, it is helpful if the assistant places a pinky finger behind the occipital bone to further stabilize and extend the head.
- Keep the lips out of the field of view with the other fingers.
- With the other hand, use a piece of gauze to pull the tongue out of the mouth and gently pull it down so that the mouth opens as much as possible.

Helpful Hint # 4

- Remember: take extreme care **not** to touch the epiglottis with the blade.
- Sometimes, the epiglottis is entrapped within the soft palate. Applying gentle pressure on the soft palate with the blade tip or the endotracheal tube will dislodge the epiglottis.

4. If intubating a cat, consider the use of lidocaine to help prevent laryngospasm (Table 7.3).

Helpful Hint # 3

- If the patient begins to resist this restraint, do not attempt to intubate.
- Administer more anesthetic agent and ensure a good plane of anesthesia before attempting intubation again.
- Inadequate depth will increase the difficulty of intubation, especially in cats.

3. Place the laryngoscope blade on the tongue just in front of the epiglottis. Apply downward pressure to the blade to expose the opening of the trachea (Fig. 7.9).

Table 7.3. Suggestions for how to deal with laryngospasm in cats.

Laryngospasm
Laryngospasm is defined as a reflex closure of the arytenoids in response to stimulus.   It commonly occurs when intubation is attempted before the cat is adequately anesthetized (Quandt 2002). **Prevention:** Apply 1–2 drops of 2% lidocaine on each arytenoid using a 1 mL syringe attached to a 20 g × 1.8 in catheter (stylet removed). Wait 10–20 seconds before attempting intubation. **Treatment:** Do not stimulate the larynx further by attempting to pass the tube. Provide oxygen by mask and administer more induction agent to increase anesthetic depth. As a last resort, a neuromuscular blocking agent such as atracurium may be administered IV to paralyze the laryngeal tissues. NOTE: The diaphragm muscles will also become paralyzed so the cat will be unable to breathe on its own. Intubation MUST be performed immediately to secure the airway and provide manual ventilation until the blocking agent wears off. **Precaution:** Cats are particularly sensitive to the effects of local anesthetics so precise measurement of the lidocaine is very important to prevent toxic doses. Lidocaine sprays are not advocated for use because of inadequate dosage measurements.

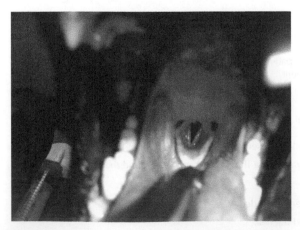

Figure 7.9. Larynx of a dog.

5. Slide the endotracheal tube along the laryngoscope blade, past the arytenoids and into the trachea.

Helpful Hint # 5

- It may help to place the tube with the concave portion facing the hard palate so that the first part of the tube that comes in contact with the arytenoids is the tip of the bevel.
- The bevel can then be used as a wedge right at the base of the larynx to help open the arytenoids.
- Slightly rotating the tube from side to side may help it pass through the larynx more easily.
- The patient may cough as the tube passes through the larynx. Although this is a normal reflex response to intubation, it often indicates that the patient is in a light plane of anesthesia and may need additional induction agent.

---

6. Slide the tube into the trachea to the proper predetermined length.

    The assistant should hold the patient's mouth closed while the anesthetist performs the next three steps.

7. Attach the breathing circuit to the endotracheal tube and then turn on the oxygen flowmeter (to reduce waste gas exposure from residual inhalant in the circuit).
8. Inflate the cuff **before** turning on the inhalant gas to avoid exposure of anesthetic vapors to personnel (Table 7.4).
9. Secure the tube to the patient (Table 7.5).
10. Confirm correct placement of endotracheal tube (Table 7.6).

Table 7.4. Steps for proper cuff inflation and guidelines to prevent overinflation of the cuff.

Proper Cuff Inflation

Steps:

1. Close the pop-off valve and squeeze the reservoir bag until an inspiratory pressure of 20 cm H_2O is reached.
2. Do not hold the breath for longer than 2–3 seconds.
3. While administering the breath, listen for an airway leak (a hissing sound coming from the tracheal tube).
4. Inflate the cuff with air ONLY until the sound stops. Add small increments of air (0.5–2 mL depending on patient size) at a time while listening for the sound to stop.
5. If the reservoir bag deflates before the cuff is sealed, increase the rate of the oxygen flow meter to keep the bag full.
6. Pressure will not hold in the reservoir bag if the cuff is not properly sealed.
7. If you do not hear a leak, then DO NOT put any air into the cuff.
8. Cuff inflation may need to be repeated about 3–5 minutes after the inhalant is turned on because, as the patient's anesthetic depth deepens, the laryngeal and tracheal muscles relax causing a leak to develop.

Additional guidelines:

Always note how much air was placed in the cuff. Double-check that the amount seems appropriate for the size of the endotracheal tube. For example, a 4 mm tube should NOT need more than 3 mL of air to create a seal.

Use an appropriately sized syringe to inflate the cuff depending on patient size. Do not use larger than a 3 mL syringe to inflate the cuff for cats or larger than a 6 mL syringe to inflate the cuff for dogs.

If a leak develops in the cuff during the anesthetic period, it is best to deflate the cuff fully first before adding additional air to reinflate the cuff. This will help prevent overinflation of the cuff.

The fullness of the pilot balloon and the back pressure on the inflation syringe are NOT reliable indicators of proper cuff inflation (Dorsch and Dorsch 2008a; Hardie et al. 1999).

Table 7.5.   An alternative to using gauze for securing the tube to the patient. The IV tubing can be used multiple times and is more economical.

Making a Tube Tie out of IV Tubing
Save the IV tubing from a fluid administration set after it has been used.
Cut into approximately 2-ft portions
Cut the winged portion off a 1 mL syringe (where the plunger inserts). You will need two of these per tube tie.
Fold the IV tubing in half and thread the folded portion through both winged tips.
Separate out the two winged portions so that there are two "circles" in the tubing.
The first circle is used to secure the tie to the tube.
The second circle is used to secure the tube to the patient by placing it around the maxilla, mandible, or behind the ears.

Table 7.6.   Checks that can be performed by the anesthetist to ensure proper placement of the endotracheal tube.

Confirmation of Correct Placement of an Endotracheal Tube
Direct visualization of endotracheal tube passing through the arytenoids is the most reliable indicator of proper tube placement.
Place a tuft of hair or a glass object at the proximal end of the tracheal tube. On expiration the tuft of hair should move or condensation should be present on the glass.
Movement of the reservoir bag and one-way valves should correspond to the inhalation and exhalation of the patient when attached to the breathing circuit.
Palpation of only one tubular structure in the cervical region. The esophagus normally cannot be palpated; if two rigid tubes are felt, there is high likelihood that esophageal intubation has occurred (McKelvey and Hollingshead 2003).
Animals will not be able to vocalize when the tube is placed in the trachea. If patient begins to whine or growl after tube placement, the tube is not in the correct location (McKelvey and Hollingshead 2003).
End tidal carbon dioxide monitor will indicate the presence of carbon dioxide in the expired gases if the tube is correctly placed in the trachea.

Helpful Hint # 6

- Position the tube tie snuggly around the proximal end of the endotracheal tube, taking care not to compress the lumen of the tube.
- Then, secure the endotracheal tube to the patient by placing the tube tie around the maxilla or mandible or behind the ears.
- The tube tie helps prevent movement of the tube (especially important when the cuff is inflated to avoid damage to the tracheal wall).

Extubation

Once the patient is in recovery, the oral cavity should be inspected and cleared of any residual blood or foreign material from surgical or dental procedures. Do not turn off the inhalant until the oral cavity has been examined and cleared. Extubation should occur when the patient has regained the ability to swallow and protect its own airway. The cuff can be deflated manually with a syringe or with a three-way stopcock (Table 7.7). **Do not** deflate the cuff until the patient is showing signs of being able to protect its airway and is ready to extubate (i.e., exhibits multiple swallows, attempts to lift head from table, moves a limb). As soon as the cuff is deflated, the tube should be pulled straight out of the mouth in a steady manner to avoid damage to the tube or cuff as it passes by the teeth. It is advised to place a mouth gag (roll of white tape between the canine teeth) before extubation to help prevent biting of the tube as it is being pulled out of the mouth. If the tube is accidentally bitten in half there is a risk of the distal end being aspirated into the lungs. This will require bronchoscopy or surgery to retrieve the tube. It is also helpful to pull the tongue to the side of

Table 7.7. Usefulness of a three-way stopcock during extubation.

Using a Three-way Stopcock
Place a three-way stopcock on the end of the cuff inflating valve.
The arrow of the stopcock will point toward the closed port allowing the other two ports to communicate.
The arrow should be pointing toward the pilot balloon when placed on a tube that has the cuff inflated.
When deflating the cuff, point the arrow of the stopcock in a direction away from the pilot balloon.
The cuff should deflate immediately if the stopcock is pushed into the valve properly.
The stopcock can be used as an alternative to a syringe to deflate the cuff. This prevents needing an empty syringe at all times to deflate the cuff in recovery.

the patient's mouth. If the patient suddenly wakes up, gently holding the tongue to one side while pulling the tube prevents the patient from biting down on the tube.

Dogs and cats are more easily recovered in lateral recumbency. However, a brachycephalic breed should be recovered in sternal recumbency with its head and neck extended to open up the airway. Extubation is often delayed in a brachycephalic dog breed until it can hold up its head and have better control of its airway. Have all supplies ready for reintubation of a brachycephalic patient in case it begins to show signs of airway obstruction after extubation. It is not recommended that extubation be prolonged in cats. This may result in laryngospasm and subsequent airway obstruction after the tube has been removed.

Gastroesophageal reflux (GER) and regurgitation are additional concerns during recovery. Research studies have shown that some anesthetic drugs (sedatives, opioids, and inhalants) can decrease the lower esophageal sphincter (LES) tone, thus allowing gastric fluid to enter into the esophagus more easily (Wilson et al. 2005; Wilson et al. 2006a; Wilson et al. 2006b). The greater the volume of reflux through the LES, the more likely passive regurgitation into

the pharynx and oral cavity may develop. GER can occur at any time during the anesthetic period and usually goes unnoticed because no clinical signs are apparent. Recognition of regurgitation is usually made by visualization of brown or yellowish fluid coming from the patient's mouth and/or nose. This condition should be treated prior to extubation. Ensure that the cuff is adequately inflated and position the animal so that the head is hanging off the table. Using a red rubber catheter and a 60 mL syringe, lavage the mouth and esophagus with warm water until all the fluid leaving the mouth is clear. Suction the remaining fluid from the mouth and esophagus. Failure to treat regurgitation may lead to esophagitis, esophageal stricture, or pulmonary aspiration (Wilson et al. 2005). Leave the cuff slightly inflated during extubation to help remove any remaining fluid that is left around the laryngeal opening (Kushner 2002). Notify the clinician that regurgitation has occurred because he/she might want to treat systemically with drugs (antibiotics, gastric protectants, and so forth).

Complications

Endotracheal intubation can have grave consequences if performed by an inexperienced person. Table 7.8 lists the complications that the anesthetist should consider.

Cleaning, Sterilization, and Storage

Ideally, the endotracheal tube should be cleaned as soon as possible after extubating the patient. A gentle scrub inside and out using a mild soap detergent followed by a warm water rinse is usually sufficient to remove any mucus, blood, or debris present on or in the tube. A pipe-cleaner brush works well to clean the inside of the tube. Slightly inflate the cuff of the tube while cleaning because the folds in a deflated cuff are a common place for material and debris to hide. If it is not feasible to clean the tube right away, place the tube in a solution of warm soapy water and let it soak until it can be adequately cleaned. Soaking the tube will help prevent any secretions

Table 7.8. Complications that may occur during intubation.

Complications Associated with Intubation

Complication	Cause	Consequence	Prevention
Forceful intubation	Using an endotracheal tube that is too large	Damage to the tissues of the upper airway Edema and airway obstruction Laceration of arytenoids (Hofmeister et al. 2007)	Do not use excessive force when placing tube; tube should glide easily past arytenoids without excessive pressure.
Excessive pressure on tracheal wall	Overinflation of cuff	↓ perfusion of tracheal mucosa May result in necrosis, perforation and/or stricture of tracheal wall	Inflate cuff with the least amount of air to obtain an airtight seal against the tracheal wall.
Tracheal rupture	Changing position of patient without disconnecting breathing circuit (Hardie et al. 1999) Improper use of stylet (Mitchell et al. 2000) Endotracheal tube is too large Removal of tube with cuff inflated	Subcutaneous emphysema (Hardie et al. 1999) Dyspnea (Hardie et al. 1999) Pneumomediastinum (Mitchell et al. 2000) Pneumothorax (Mitchell et al. 2000)	Disconnect patient from circuit before changing position. Use stylet properly. Select tube of proper size. Make sure cuff is fully deflated before extubating the patient (except in the presence of gastroesophageal reflux).
Complete obstruction	Mucus plug inside lumen of tube Accidental kinking when patient is repositioned	Hypoxia Hypercapnia Respiratory arrest	Inspect tube for any occlusions prior to use. Examine tube every time the patient is repositioned.
Esophageal intubation	Not staying ventral enough with tube during intubation (esophagus is located dorsal to the trachea)	Anesthetic gases enter stomach instead of lungs; results in • Hypoxia • Gastric insufflation • Arousal from anesthesia once injectable drugs are metabolized	Use direct visualization of tube entering the trachea. Use a laryngoscope. Have assistant hold and extend the head and neck.

68

or debris from drying on the tube (Shawley and Bednarski 1991).

In human medicine, a new endotracheal tube is used on each patient to eliminate the potential of cross contamination; however, this option is not economically feasible for most veterinary practices. There are no regulations for endotracheal tube sterilization or disinfection in veterinary patients. The following options are available and should be considered to decrease the likelihood of spreading respiratory diseases, such as tracheobronchitis (kennel cough), among veterinary patients (McKelvey and Hollingshead 2003). The two most common disinfectants used are chlorhexidine and glutaraldehyde. Chlorhexidine is an antiseptic and antimicrobial solution and comes in a 2% concentration. According to manufacturer's instructions, it should be diluted by placing 1 ounce (2 tablespoons) of chlorhexidine in 1 gallon of water. Glutaraldehyde is the active ingredient found in products like Cidexplus® and is effective against bacteria, fungi and viruses (Dorsch and Dorsch 2008c). The tubes should be completely submerged in either solution for **no** longer than 30 minutes. After soaking, the tubes must be **thoroughly** rinsed with water and allowed to air dry. Factors such as improper rinsing, soaking for an extended period of time, and using a solution that is too concentrated can all lead to tracheal irritation and should be avoided (McKelvey and Hollingshead 2003).

Sterilization is the most effective way to eliminate all viable sources of organisms that can cause infection and/or disease. The material used to manufacture the tube dictates what type of sterilization can be used. Silicone tubes are the only ones that can be heat sterilized with steam from an autoclave. Red rubber and PVC tubes must be gas sterilized with ethylene oxide (EO) or hydrogen peroxide gas plasma because they break down in the presence of extreme heat. Ethylene oxide is considered the best means of gas sterilization because it penetrates a wide variety of materials, including plastics (Trim and Simpson 1982). However, EO has many disadvantages and due to the health concerns for personnel it is not commonly used in veterinary medicine. Hydrogen peroxide gas plasma sterilization is a good alternative to EO because it is

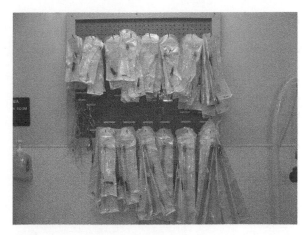

Figure 7.10. Storage of endotracheal tubes in the peel packs and organized on a peg board.

safer for personnel and it does not produce toxic compounds (Yoon et al. 2007).

Optimally, endotracheal tubes should be stored in a place where they are kept clean and readily accessible. One of the most effective ways of ensuring that the tubes remain free of dust and other contaminants is to individually place them inside sterilization pouches used for autoclaving. These pouches can then be labeled with the corresponding size and organized by either hanging them on a peg board on the wall (Fig. 7.10) or placing them into a drawer divided into sections based on size.

Other viable options for storage include using a commercially made rack (Fig. 7.11) or simply

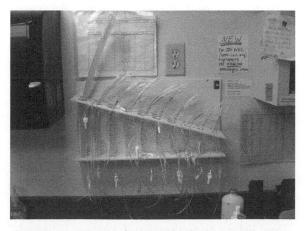

Figure 7.11. Storage of endotracheal tubes using a commercially made rack.

placing the tubes inside a drawer. Both of these methods organize the tubes nicely and allow for easy access; however, the main disadvantage is cleanliness of the tubes. Tubes that are displayed using a wall rack are continuously exposed to dust and other contaminants in the clinic and should not be stored for long periods of time. Likewise, tubes placed inside a drawer are exposed to the atmosphere every time the drawer is opened. Placing a towel underneath the tubes will help keep the drawer and tubes clean, providing the towel is changed frequently.

References

Dorsch, JA, Dorsch, SE. 2008a. Tracheal tubes and associated equipment. In Understanding Anesthesia Equipment, 5th ed., edited by Dorsch, JA, Dorsch, SE. Philadelphia: Lippincott Williams & Wilkins, pp.563–584.

Dorsch, JA, Dorsch, SE. 2008b. Laryngoscopes. In Understanding Anesthesia Equipment, 5th ed., edited by Dorsch, JA, Dorsch, SE. Philadelphia: Lippincott Williams & Wilkins, pp.521–526.

Dorsch, JA, Dorsch, SE. 2008c. Cleaning and sterilization. In Understanding Anesthesia Equipment, 5th ed., edited by Dorsch, JA, Dorsch, SE. Philadelphia: Lippincott Williams & Wilkins, pp.969–981.

Hardie, EM, Spodnick, GJ, Gilson, SD, et al. 1999. Tracheal rupture in cats: 16 cases (1983–1998). J Am Vet Med Assoc 214(4):508–512.

Hartsfield, SM. 2007. Airway management and ventilation. In Lumb and Jones' Veterinary Anesthesia and Analgesia, 4th ed., edited by Tranquilli, WJ, Thurmon, JC, Grimm, KA. Ames, IA: Blackwell Publishing, pp.495–512.

Hofmeister, EH, Trim, CM, Kley, S, Cornell, K. 2007. Traumatic endotracheal intubation in the cat. Vet Anaesth Analges 34:213–216.

Hughes, L. 2007. Breathing systems and ancillary equipment. In BSAVA Manual of Canine and Feline Anaesthesia and Analgesia, 2nd ed., edited by Seymour, C, Duke-Novakovski, T.

Business Park: British Small Animal Veterinary Association, pp.41–45.

Kushner, LI. 2002. Aspiration. In Veterinary Anesthesia and Pain Management Secrets, edited by Greene, SA. Philadelphia: Hanley & Belfus, pp.165–167.

McDonell, WN, Kerr, CL. 2007. Respiratory system. In Lumb and Jones' Veterinary Anesthesia and Analgesia, 4th ed., edited by Tranquilli, WJ, Thurmon, JC, Grimm, KA. Ames: Blackwell Publishing, p.121.

McKelvey, D, Hollingshead, KW. 2003. General anesthesia. In Veterinary Anesthesia and Analgesia, 3rd ed. St. Louis: Mosby, pp.65–74.

Mitchell, SL, McCarthy, R, Rudloff, E, Pernell, RT. 2000. Tracheal rupture associated with intubation in cats: 20 cases (1996–1998). J Am Vet Med Assoc 216(10):1592–1595.

Quandt, JE. 2002. Airway maintenance. In Veterinary Anesthesia and Pain Management Secrets, edited by Greene, SA. Philadelphia: Hanley & Belfus, pp.1–12.

Shawley, RV, Bednarski, RM. 1991. Endotracheal intubation in the horse. In Equine Anesthesia: Monitoring and Emergency Therapy, edited by Muir, WW, Hubbell, JAE. St. Louis: Mosby, p.318.

Trim, CM, Simpson, ST. 1982. Complications following ethylene oxide sterilization: A case report. J Am Anim Hosp Assoc 18:507–510.

Wilson, DV, Boruta, DT, Evans, AT. 2006a. Influence of halothane, isoflurane, and sevoflurane on gastroesophageal reflux during anesthesia in dogs. Am J Vet Res 67(11): 1821–1825.

Wilson, DV, Evans, AT, Mauer, WA. 2006b. Influence of metoclopramide on gastroesophageal reflux in anesthetized dogs. Am J Vet Res 67(1):26–31.

Wilson, DV, Evans, AT, Miller, R. 2005. Effects of preanesthetic administration of morphine on gastroesophageal reflux and regurgitation during anesthesia in dogs. Am J Vet Res 66(3):386–390.

Yoon, SZ, et al. 2007. The safety of reused endotracheal tubes sterilized according to Centers for Disease Control and Prevention guidelines. J Clin Anes 19:360–364.

Anesthesia Equipment 8

Harry Latshaw and Deb Coleman

Functional Components

This chapter discusses the components of the anesthetic machine, their functions, and how to assess the operating condition of the machine. Breathing circuits, bags, and nonrebreathing systems are included in this discussion.

Any anesthetic machine must perform four functions: deliver oxygen, deliver anesthetic, remove carbon dioxide, and remove waste anesthetic gas (WAG).

Delivery of oxygen

The first basic function of an anesthetic machine is to deliver oxygen. Oxygen is most often provided as a compressed gas in cylinders that have a valve in the neck. Cylinders vary in capacity, with the most common two being the small "E" cylinder, which usually attaches to the machine, and a much larger "H" cylinder, which is located remotely from the machine. Oxygen cylinders are considered full when the tank pressure is 2000 pounds per square inch (psi). If a cylinder in use is at 1000 psi, it is 50% full; at 200 psi, it is 10% full. "E" cylinders contain 650 liters and "H" tanks contain 6900 liters at 2000 psi.

A regulator with the proper fittings must be attached to the tank. The regulator should have two gauges—one that reads the remaining pressure in the tank and one that reads the line pressure (Fig. 8.1). The regulator reduces the pressure to a point that is safe for all components of the oxygen system. For most applications this pressure is 40–50 psi.

The valves on O_2 cylinders should be opened very slowly until the pressure on the regulator gauge stops rising. Then the valve can be opened completely. Under no circumstance should a wrench or pliers be used to open the valve.

Oxygen can also be supplied by an oxygen concentrator. This device provides oxygen from room air by introducing compressed air into a molecular sieve that absorbs the nitrogen and allows oxygen to flow to a flowmeter or to a storage tank. The resulting oxygen yield is approximately 96%. If a concentrator is to be used, it is recommended that a compressor and small storage tank be supplied. This provides oxygen at a higher pressure than the concentrator can provide and a reservoir of oxygen for short periods of high demand. Concentrators cannot be used as sources of compressed gas for ventilators.

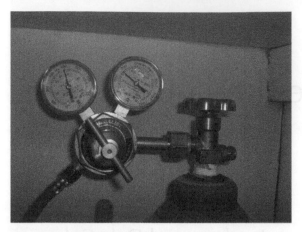

Figure 8.1. Oxygen tank regulator with the gauge on the right indicating tank pressure and the gauge on the left indicating line pressure.

These devices provide oxygen at low cost and eliminate the presence of high-pressure tanks.

Oxygen for the patient breathing system (Fig. 8.2) is delivered either by the flowmeter or the flush valve. The flowmeter delivers oxygen through the vaporizer to the breathing system at a specific rate measured in liters per minute. The flush valve is used to deliver a "burst" of oxygen to the breathing system and should be used only when the patient needs pure oxygen.

Flowmeters are operated with a knob attached to a needle valve. When the needle valve is opened, oxygen flows through a vertical tube that is labeled in milliliters or liters per minute. The flow of oxygen causes an indicator in the tube to rise and the flow rate is read at the appropriate label. The indicators have various shapes, but the most common is a ball. The flow rate is read at the point on the indicator where there is

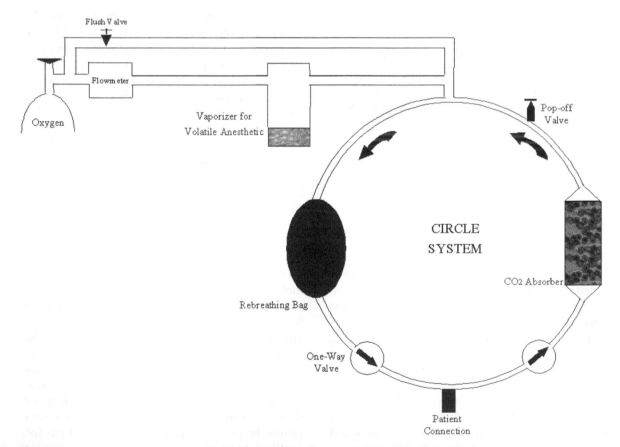

Figure 8.2. Diagram of anesthetic machine with oxygen supply, vaporizer, and breathing system.

the greatest resistance to flow. If a ball is the indicator, this point would be the center of the ball. When operating the flowmeter, the control knob should not be overtightened. Doing so may result in damage or breakage to the needle valve. Always turn the flowmeter off when oxygen is no longer needed. If the flowmeter is on when the oxygen supply is turned on for the next procedure, the sudden pressure in the flow tube may cause the indicator to lodge at the top of the tube and possibly break the tube.

Caution should be exercised when the flush valve is used to deliver oxygen to the breathing system. Always operate the flush valve with the Adjustable Pressure Limiting (APL) valve or pop-off valve open. Stop the oxygen flush before the rebreathing bag is completely filled. Failure to do so may result in high pressure in the system, which in turn could cause damage to the patient's airway and lungs. The same is true when using a nonrebreathing system because the oxygen is delivered directly to the patient connection on the system. It should be noted that some anesthetic machines have flush valves that are either restricted or do not have a high-volume flush. This increases the margin of safety when using these flush valves. To assess the volume of oxygen being flushed, occlude the patient connection on the breathing tube, and then operate the flush valve and observe how quickly the rebreathing bag fills.

At the end of the day, the oxygen supply should be shut off or the machine disconnected if a central oxygen system is in use. This will prevent needless oxygen consumption if a flowmeter is not off or if there are small leaks in any of the connections on the machine.

Delivery of anesthetic

The second basic function is to deliver vaporized anesthetic agent to the breathing system in concentrations that are optimal for the desired effect. Since the liquid agent is in a closed system, a carrier gas must be present to deliver the vaporized agent to the breathing circuit. The gas used to accomplish this is the fresh gas flow of oxygen.

In almost all anesthetic machines used today, the liquid agent is contained in an agent-specific vaporizer that is outside the patient breathing circuit. The fresh gas flows from the flowmeter to the vaporizer. A very precise portion of the oxygen flow is diverted into a vaporization chamber where it is saturated with vaporized anesthetic. It is then mixed with that portion of the flow that bypasses the vaporization chamber and is delivered to the breathing system (Fig. 8.3).

The anesthetic vaporizer also has a thermal compensation device. This is necessary because the liquid anesthetic cools as vaporization occurs and makes vaporization more difficult. This device then diverts more of the flow into the vaporization chamber to compensate for the cooling. Most vaporizers are constructed of brass, which conducts heat from the ambient air to the liquid to minimize the magnitude of the temperature change. This assures that the vaporizer output is constant despite changes in temperature.

Vaporizers have a dial with numbers from 0–5 for isoflurane and 0–8 for sevoflurane. These numbers represent volume percent and indicate the concentration in percent delivered at the output of the vaporizer. If the fresh gas flow is 1 liter per minute and the dial is set at 2%, this means that 0.98 liters per minute of oxygen and 0.02 liters per minute of agent are leaving the vaporizer and are delivered to the breathing system. Doing the math, it is evident that if the fresh gas flow is increased to 2 liters per minute, the amount of agent consumed will be doubled. If the flow rate is 0.5 liters per minute the consumption will be halved. The same relationship is true related to the dial setting on the vaporizer. *It is important to remember that the numbers on the dial do not necessarily indicate depth of anesthesia. That is determined by assessing the patient, not the vaporizer setting.*

Some vaporizers are filled with liquid by using a pin fill device. An agent-specific spout replaces the cap on the agent bottle. A keyed pin fits into the fill manifold on the vaporizer. It is locked into place, and the vaporizer is filled to the desired level on the window. However, most vaporizers have a funnel fill device, and the

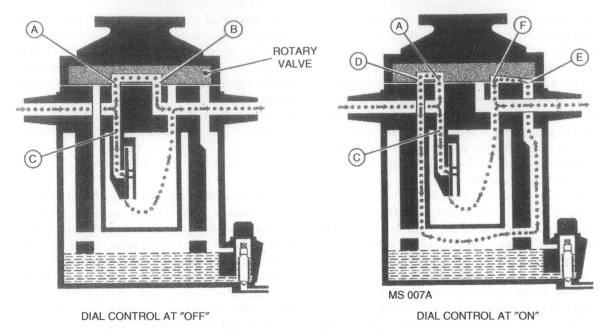

ROTARY VALVE

DIAL CONTROL AT "OFF"   DIAL CONTROL AT "ON"

MS 007A

Schematic-Principle of Operation

Figure 8.3.   The view on the left shows the vaporizer off with all the oxygen bypassing the vapor chamber through thermostat C and rotary valve passage A to rotary valve outlet B. The view on the right shows the vaporizer on with some of the oxygen bypassing through thermostat C and some passing through passage D (B is closed) into the vapor chamber. It passes through calibrated channel E into vaporizer outlet F where it is mixed with bypassed oxygen from C.

liquid agent is simply poured into the vaporizer. Care must be exercised to avoid spillage. Anti-Spil™ adapters are available that replace the cap on the agent bottle and minimize the potential for spillage (Fig. 8.4). The window that indicates

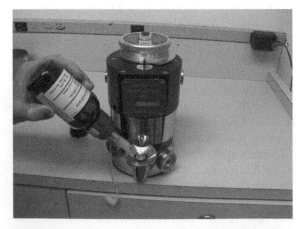

Figure 8.4.   Filling the vaporizer using a device to prevent spillage.

the level of liquid in the vaporizer will help prevent overfilling of the vaporizer and will also indicate when the liquid level is low. Operating the vaporizer with the level too low may result in lower than indicated concentrations.

The fill cap on funnel fill vaporizers has an O-ring that seals against the funnel surface. Each time the cap is removed the O-ring and funnel surface should be wiped with a 4 × 4 gauze pad moistened with alcohol (Fig. 8.5). This prevents the buildup of dirt particles that could cause the O-ring to leak and allow anesthetic vapor into the work environment.

All vaporizers have a drain plug to allow the vaporizer to be drained. This plug is usually in the center of the funnel fill device. Continuous removing of the cap to fill the vaporizer may cause the drain plug to become loose and may result in agent leaking from the drain. The drain plug should be checked periodically to ensure that it is tight.

No vaporizer should be subjected to "blunt force trauma" as a result of moving the anes-

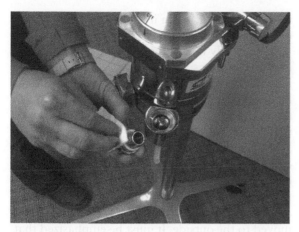

Figure 8.5. Cleaning the O-ring on the fill cap of the vaporizer.

thetic machine or from other portable equipment being moved in the vicinity of the anesthetic machine. Not only can this result in external damage, but internal damage to the thermal compensating device may also occur, resulting in poor performance.

The external surface of the vaporizer should be cleaned periodically using a 4 × 4 gauze pad moistened with alcohol. *No liquid should be poured or sprayed on the vaporizer for the purpose of cleaning.*

The calibration of the vaporizer should be checked periodically, and if necessary, the vaporizer should be serviced. Most vaporizers will provide many years of reliable service with proper care and maintenance.

Removal of carbon dioxide

The third function of the anesthetic machine is to remove carbon dioxide. The following sections discuss the components necessary in a rebreathing system to remove the carbon dioxide.

Canister for carbon dioxide absorber

A container for baralyme or sodalime granules is necessary to chemically remove the carbon dioxide from the circuit. Failure to remove exhaled carbon dioxide from the breathing

circuit results in increased carbon dioxide in the blood. This produces a respiratory acidosis and an increase in respiratory rate. Both conditions are detrimental to a successful anesthetic procedure.

This process utilizes the principle of a base neutralizing an acid. The expired carbon dioxide reacts with water to form carbonic acid, which in turn is neutralized by the alkaline chemicals in the absorbent. The end products of this reaction are water and a carbonate.

The most common absorbent is sodalime. By weight it is 4% sodium hydroxide, 1% potassium hydroxide, 14–19% water and enough calcium hydroxide to make 100% (Dorsch and Dorsch 1999). A small amount of pH sensitive dye is also added. As the absorbent reacts with carbon dioxide, the color changes to purple indicating that the absorbent is exhausted.

The water in the absorbent is necessary for the chemical reaction that takes place between the carbon dioxide and the absorbent. The high-moisture absorbents (14–19%) have a slower rate of absorption and do not exhaust as rapidly as low-moisture absorbents. The humidity of the breathed gases does not affect the capacity of the sodalime to absorb carbon dioxide (Dorsch and Dorsch 1999).

This chemical reaction is exothermic, meaning that heat is released as the reaction takes place. This heat can be detected on the outside of the canister. If heat is not present, it may mean that absorption is not taking place. The amount of carbon dioxide absorption is about 26 liters/100 grams of absorbent. Efficiency may vary depending on the design of the canister and the method of packing (Hartsfield 1996). If the absorbent is working properly there should be a negligible amount of carbon dioxide being rebreathed by the patient.

One-way valves

One-way valves serve as another functional component necessary to remove carbon dioxide. These are check valves that allow the gas in the circuit to move in only one direction. Therefore, fresh gas is always being moved toward the patient and expired gas away from the patient.

Most valves are horizontal discs that rest on top of open tubes. They open and close individually based on patient inspiration and expiration. On most machines, the discs are enclosed in a clear chamber that allows visual verification of proper function. The one-way valves, in effect, minimize the amount of mechanical dead space that is created by the machine. In a properly functioning rebreathing circuit, this space is where the inspiratory and expiratory tubes join to where the endotracheal tube attaches.

APL valve

The final component on the machine that removes carbon dioxide is the adjustable pressure limiting (APL) valve or pop-off valve. Since the flow of fresh gas into the system is greater than what the patient removes, there must be a way for the excess gas to be removed. With a high fresh gas flow, more carbon dioxide will be removed through the APL valve and vice versa. This valve is usually located near the expiratory valve or the rebreathing bag. It is very important to keep the valve open unless positive pressure is being used to inflate the lungs. If the valve remains closed, pressures that will be fatal to the patient will be created in the system.

Removing Waste Anesthetic Gas

Since anesthetic gas is removed through the APL valve, it also performs the final function of the anesthetic machine—to remove waste anesthetic gas (WAG) from the work environment. All APL valves are designed to receive a 19 mm diameter evacuation tube that carries the WAG to the evacuation device.

Passive system

The evacuation tube can be connected to a canister containing activated charcoal, which absorbs the anesthetic gas. This passive method is effective only if the canister is replaced according to the directions. Most often the canister

must be replaced when it has absorbed 50 grams of agent.

If relatively high flow rates are used, the canister will expire sooner than if a lower flow rate is used. As more of the canister becomes expired, higher flow rates might move some of the WAG through the canister without being captured by the charcoal.

This tube can also be directed into a nonrecirculating ventilation exhaust duct. The exhausted air will move the WAG from the tube to the outside. This method is preferred over the charcoal canister because the WAG is being moved to the outside. It must be emphasized that the WAG is vented into an exhaust duct and that the air in the duct is not being recirculated to other areas in the hospital but is going directly to the outside.

Active system

In this system, the WAG is moved passively from the APL valve to a duct system that removes the gas through a vacuum or other device that draws the WAG to the outside. This system requires the use of an atmospheric interface that allows the system to draw room air and prevent the system from actively removing gas from the APL, which results in the collapse of the rebreathing bag (Fig. 8.6).

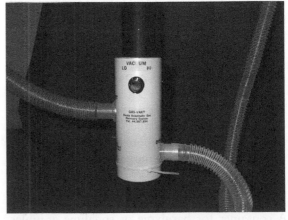

Figure 8.6. An atmospheric equalizer device with the WAG hose on the left from the machine and on the right to the evacuation device. Room air enters at the top of the canister.

These interfaces are different depending upon the evacuation system in use. The interface has a connection to receive the 19 mm tube from the APL and another connection to receive a tube that removes the gas to the evacuation device, which may be a vacuum pump or an enclosed fan that is vented to the outside. If a vacuum pump is used, there must be a way to adjust the vacuum so the atmospheric interface will function properly.

Troubleshooting before a Procedure

The assessment of the machine includes the oxygen supply system, the flowmeter, the flush valve, the breathing system, the WAG removal system, and all hose and tubing connections on the machine.

Oxygen supply

The O_2 regulator on the tank should be set at 40–60 pounds per square inch (psi), and all connections should be free of leaks. A large leak can usually be heard and should be corrected to prevent loss of oxygen. Small leaks can be detected by applying a solution containing surfactant and watching for bubbles. Many older machines have solid plumbing from the O_2 supply connection to the flowmeter. It is difficult to assess the presence of leaks in that situation, but if a leak is discovered it may require the attention of a service representative. The connections to the flush valve should be secure and free from leaks.

The breathing system

This portion of the machine needs to be assessed very carefully because any leaks present will likely include anesthetic vapor. This part of the machine is most susceptible to problems, but they are usually easy to correct. The process of discovering these problems utilizes visual and auditory inspection and a pressure test. The assessment should focus on the one-way valves, sodalime canister, breathing bag and circuit, and WAG connections and tubing.

One-way valves

Valves that can be dissembled will have either a rubber O-ring or gasket that forms a seal between the dome and the valve body. If this O-ring or gasket is torn, deformed or missing, it should be replaced. The plastic dome should be examined for chips or cracks and if any are found, the dome should be replaced. The threaded rings that hold the dome against the O-ring or gasket can be easily cross-threaded when assembling the one-way valve. When the ring becomes difficult to turn, the operator thinks it is tight and stops tightening the ring. This results in failure to seal the dome and can be a major leak in the system. If enough force is applied, the threads can be permanently damaged and new parts are required.

On some machines, it is possible to impinge the one-way disc between the dome and the valve body in such a way that it remains open all the time or it fails to open when the patient breathes. The one-way valves can be tested by using a surgeon's mask or by curling one's hand around the Y-piece, breathing into the circuit, and observing that the one-way valves move in the proper sequence.

Sodalime canister

There are many different styles of canisters, but functionally there are only two types. If the gases go only one way through the canister, the canister will be open on top and will have a perforated bottom with a gasket or O-ring that seals both the top and bottom surfaces of the canister. If the canister contains a baffle or a return tube in the center of the canister so that gas comes in the top and then flows to the bottom, around the baffle, and back to the top, there will be a seal only on the top surface. These two types of canisters can be described either as one-way or two-way canisters.

Since the one-way canister has a seal on both the top and bottom surfaces there is a greater potential for leaks. Soda sorb granules and dust can accumulate on the lower gasket or sealing surface and prevent the canister from forming a tight seal. This is one of the most common causes of leaks in an anesthetic circuit, and care must be taken to assure that all surfaces are clean and free of soda sorb dust and granules.

The two-way canister has less potential for leaks because it seals only at the top of the canister. However, since there is usually a tube down the center of the canister, the tube should be covered or plugged when being filled to prevent spilling of granules into the tube. Failure to remove the plug before attaching the canister to the machine will result in very high resistance to breathing. Some two-way canisters that have a baffle in the center have a threaded insert that fastens the canister to the machine. This insert must be covered when filling the canister to prevent soda sorb from getting into the threads. It is not necessary to fill soda sorb canisters to the very top. This can result in granules falling off or rubbing against the surface of the absorber gasket as the canister is placed into position on the absorber assembly. A 1/2–3/4 inch space should be left at the top of the canister.

Breathing bags and circuit

The major area of concern is where the tubes and bag connect to the machine. The stress created by repeatedly connecting and disconnecting the parts will cause breaks or cracks that will eventually cause leaks. These are usually visible by careful inspection prior to using the machine. To discover a hole in the bag, it will be necessary to do a pressure test so that the bag becomes distended and the hole is visible or audible. A hole in the breathing tubes can also be discovered during the pressure test, but it sometimes requires the use of a leak test solution to disclose the hole.

WAG tubing and connections

The most common problem is a poor connection to the APL valve on the machine. All connections should be made with the correct tubing size and with the proper adapters. The evacuation tubing should also be inspected for holes or tears and replaced if necessary. If the tubing lies on the floor and the anesthetic machine is moved frequently, the wheels may run over the tubing causing damage. One of the most common problems with the WAG tubing is the presence of very small holes, probably caused by cats that play with the tubing. In this case the tubing should be replaced at least once a year.

Many of these problems can be discovered by visual examination. Components that are broken, installed improperly, or disconnected can be discovered if the technician is familiar with the machine and understands the flow of fresh and breathed gases, as well as the correct placement and orientation of all components.

Performing a Pressure Test

A pressure test is performed by attaching the breathing circuit and bag, closing the pop-off valve, and occluding the patient end of the breathing circuit. Pressurize the circuit to 30 cm H_2O, setting the flowmeter to 200 cc/minute, and observe the manometer for decreasing pressure. If the pressure holds or rises very slowly there is no leak, but if the pressure drops there is a leak greater than 200 cc/minute and it should be isolated.

To isolate the leak by auditory inspection, pressurize the circuit to 60 cm H_2O and set the flowmeter to maintain the pressure. Put one ear close to any point on the circuit where there is a joint or connection and listen for the leak. It is possible that the leak cannot be discovered in this manner because either the leak does not create any sound or it is in a place that is difficult to get close enough to hear.

The leak can also be isolated by using a solution-containing surfactant. It is sprayed on the machine at any point where a leak is possible. In the presence of a leak the solution will bubble. Sometimes there is a delay of several seconds between the time the solution makes contact and the appearance of bubbles. Once the leak is discovered the problem can be corrected.

At this point the vaporizer can be tested for external leaks. Once the pressure is holding and stabilized, turn the vaporizer dial to 0.5%. This will pressurize the vaporization chamber and will create a slight drop in pressure on the manometer. The pressure should stabilize again. If the pressure, however, continues to drop, this is an indication of a leak in the vaporizer. This leak most likely will be in the fill spout and is easily corrected by cleaning or replacing the O-ring on the fill spout cap.

Following the pressure test of the breathing circuit, the evacuation tubing should also be tested for leaks. To check 22 mm tubing simply connect each end of the tubing to the inspiratory and expiratory valve connections and then pressurize the circuit to 30 cm H_2O as before. If the tubing is 19 mm, appropriate adapters can be used to connect the tubing in the same way as the 22 mm tubing; then perform the test. Before testing the evacuation tubing, verify that the breathing circuit does not have leaks.

Troubleshooting during a Procedure

Sometimes problems may not be discovered before a procedure and are discovered during the procedure by observing the patient. Therefore it is necessary to ask several relevant questions related to the patient and potential problems with the machine, and not problems related to technique—i.e., improper intubation.

Frequently it is difficult to keep patients anesthetized. There are several possible explanations for this. The most obvious is that there is a leak somewhere in the breathing circuit that is allowing room air to enter and dilute the concentration of anesthesia.

There may also be a one-way valve that is not functioning properly and is allowing the patient to rebreathe expired gases, resulting in lower anesthetic concentration and higher carbon dioxide levels. This is a persistent problem in some machines that have one-way valves that are

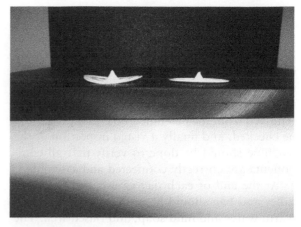

Figure 8.7. Warped one-way valve disc on the left and normal disc on the right.

vertically oriented and become warped due to the effect of gravity. The valve, therefore, doesn't close properly. Occasionally, horizontal one-way valves will become warped or curled and will not seat properly (Fig 8.7). This problem must be discovered visually unless inspired CO_2 levels are monitored.

Finally, there could be a problem with the vaporizer calibration. If outputs are extremely low, the result will be anesthetic concentrations that will not keep the patient anesthetized. This problem will need to be verified by having the calibration of the vaporizer checked.

Another problem is that patients get too deep. This problem (remember it's not related to technique) can only be a vaporizer that is out of calibration. The only answer for increasing depth of anesthesia, if the vaporizer setting is appropriate, is that the output is significantly higher than it should be. The calibration should also be verified in this situation.

A frequent problem during the procedure is the presence of anesthetic agent odor. This is simply a leak somewhere in the system (as long as ET tube cuff leaks have been ruled out). If there is an odor present, this means that the level present is above tolerable limits; if this problem persists, the machine should be removed from service until the problem is isolated.

Troubleshooting after a Procedure

Assessment of the machine following anesthesia is as important as doing it before. This is the time to observe the CO_2 absorbent and change it if necessary. Excess moisture should also be removed from the machine, the O_2 supply should be checked, and finally a visual inspection of the machine should be done to verify that all components are correctly connected and assembled.

At the end of each day of use, the breathing tubes and bag should be removed, washed with warm water and mild soap, and rinsed well. The breathing tubes should be hung so that they will drain and the bag should be hung upside down to allow it to drain. Do not use any soap used for surgical scrub to wash these parts because any residue left in the tubes or bag may result in patient airway irritation.

If the one-way valve domes have condensation on the inside they should be removed, dried, and replaced on the machine.

Once a week, the soda sorb canister should be removed for 12–24 hours to allow any condensation on the interior parts of the machine to dry. The presence of water and soda sorb dust is a caustic combination and results in deterioration of parts of the machine in contact with this combination. Allowing this time to dry once a week will prolong the components of the machine.

Correcting Problems

Correcting the problem is the final step in the process of troubleshooting. Three questions need to be answered to successfully accomplish the correction.

Can the problem be corrected without tools or parts? If the fresh gas tubing has a crack at one end, it is very easy to remove the tubing, cut it behind the hole, and reattach it to the circuit. However, if a one-way valve dome is cracked, it requires parts and the correction will be delayed.

Is it safe to use the machine or should it be removed from service? If the machine can be operated without risk to the patient or the operator, it may not be necessary to remove it from service. However, risk to either patient or user requires that the machine not be used.

Can the problem be corrected by staff or does it require a service representative? The answer to this question will be determined by the skills and desires of the hospital staff.

Breathing Systems

The general purpose of the anesthetic breathing system is to deliver oxygen and anesthetic gases to the patient and remove expired carbon dioxide. An additional function is to provide a means of manual intermittent positive pressure ventilation (IPPV) to the patient.

Many classifications of breathing systems have been used since the first clinical anesthetics were administered (Hartsfield 2007). In the U.K., a basic classification divided the breathing systems into open, semiopen, semiclosed, or closed (Hall et al. 2001). In North America the same classification is used for different systems, making the terminology confusing and impractical.

The most commonly used classification of breathing systems are *rebreathing* and *nonrebreathing*.

Rebreathing systems remove carbon dioxide from the exhaled gases by passing through an absorber filled with sodalime or Baralyme. Once the extraction of carbon dioxide occurs, all or part of the exhaled gases flow back to the patient allowing *rebreathing* of the gases.

Nonrebreathing systems remove carbon dioxide by the use of high fresh gas flow rates to flush the carbon dioxide into the scavenger system. The exhaled gases are removed from the system and do *not* allow the patient to rebreathe the exhaled gases.

Rebreathing systems

The circle rebreathing systems commonly used today include the pediatric circle, standard adult circle, and large animal circle. Each of these systems differ in its internal diameter (ID) and volume. Rebreathing systems conserve anesthetic, oxygen, heat, and moisture, but they impart more resistance to ventilation (Watney 1998–2003).

The rebreathing circles consist of two breathing tubes and a Y-piece. The tubes are made of plastic or rubber and channel the gases between the one-way valves and the Y-piece. The breathing tubes are flexible and corrugated to reduce the possibility of obstruction if bent. The tubes should have an ID larger than the ID of the patient's endotracheal tube (Hartsfield 2007).

Pediatric circles have been recommended for veterinary patients <7 kg (15.4 lb) or used by some for patients 7–12 kg (15.4–26.4 lb). The ID of the pediatric breathing tubes is smaller (15 mm) than the standard adult circle (22 mm). Because the tubes are smaller, the total volume of the circle is decreased. This allows a more rapid change in anesthetic concentration when adjusting the vaporizer setting. The Y-piece also has an ID of 15 mm to connect to the endotracheal tube or to a mask.

Standard adult circles have been recommended for veterinary patients that weigh 7–135 kg (15.4–297 lb).

The *Universal-F* circuit is a coaxial system with the inspiratory tube running inside the corrugated expiratory tube. The purpose of the coaxial system is to aid in the warming and humidification of inspired gases. The Universal-F is also less cumbersome than the standard circle systems in that only one tube connects to the endotracheal tube.

The Universal-F is available in pediatric and adult circuit sizes. This system is identical in appearance and function to other coaxial systems, but it is not considered an economical alternative to the Bain system (see next section).

One of the major problems with all coaxial circuits is the possibility of the inner tube breaking, kinking (Quandt 2005) or becoming disconnected from the absorber end. Once this disconnection occurs the entire volume of the tube becomes apparatus dead space (Hartsfield 2007). Daily vigilant inspections of the breathing circuit, rebreathing bag, and anesthetic

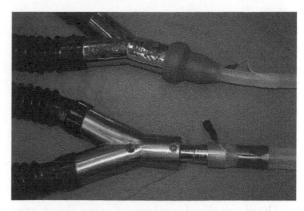

Figure 8.8.   Large-animal Y-piece with blue funnel endotracheal tube connector (top). Large-animal Y-piece with insert and endotracheal tube with stainless steel adapter (bottom).

machine will prevent potential life-threatening complications.

The large animal circles are recommended for patients >135 kg (300 lb). The Y-piece can be connected to the endotracheal tube by using the outside of the Y or the inside depending on the type of endotracheal tube connector. Endotracheal tubes with a blue funnel on the end can be connected to the outside of the Y-piece. Endotracheal tubes with a stainless steel adapter can be connected to the inside of the Y-piece if it contains an insert (see Fig 8.8).

Mechanical dead space is not a factor with the breathing tubes if the one-way valves are working properly (Hartsfield 2007).

Nonrebreathing systems

Breathing systems that eliminate carbon dioxide by high fresh gas flow rates and not a chemical absorbent are classified as Mapleson systems. In 1954, Dr. Mapleson further classified the systems into five groups (A through E). The five groups are functionally similar and differ by the fresh gas flow required to prevent rebreathing and the ease to perform manual ventilation. A diagram and list of characteristics for the Mapleson systems can be found in Hartsfield (2007, p. 482).

The Mapleson systems are called *nonrebreathing systems*. A nonrebreathing circuit relies on high fresh gas flow rates to eliminate carbon dioxide from the system, therefore eliminating the need for a chemical absorbent. The systems are easy to use and lightweight, which can reduce the anesthetic equipment drag on the endotracheal tube. Patients weighing <7 kg (15.4 lb) are recommended for the nonrebreathing system.

Nonrebreathing systems add minimal mechanical dead space and impart little resistance to respiration. One of the major advantages with this system is the ability to rapidly change the inspired anesthetic concentration.

There are disadvantages of using the nonrebreathing systems. Due to the high fresh gas flow rates required in the system there is an increase in cost. The high flow rates also exacerbate hypothermia and drying of the respiratory tract. The nonrebreathing systems require scavenging systems to protect the personnel from the large amounts of waste anesthetic and carrier gases.

Two of the commonly used nonrebreathing systems are the *Bain Coaxial* system and the *Modified Jackson Rees.*

The *Bain Coaxial* system is a tube within a tube. The Bain circuit consists of a tube that carries the fresh gas directly from the vaporizer outlet or from the fresh gas outlet from the anesthetic machine to near the reservoir bag. The fresh gas then enters the Bain system via the small inner tube and is delivered near the patient end. When the patient exhales, the expired gases move down the external corrugated tube and to the reservoir bag. In order to scavenge the excess gases, the reservoir bag needs a means to attach to the scavenger system. A *bag-tail valve* can be used on the tail end of the reservoir bag and then be connected to the scavenger tubing. The bag-tail valve also acts as a pop-off valve, which allows the anesthetist to assist ventilation (Fig. 8.9).

A *Bain block* can be purchased and added to an anesthetic machine. The block ports provide a means to attach the Bain circuit and the reservoir bag. It is also equipped with a manometer, a pop-off valve, and a connection for a scavenging system (Fig. 8.10).

The *Modified Jackson Rees* is another type of nonrebreathing system that is constructed in a different way. The modified Jackson Rees has a tube to deliver the fresh gases much like the Bain

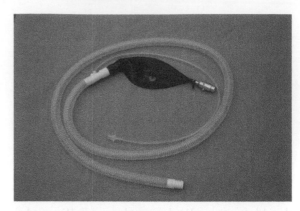

Figure 8.9.   Bain coaxial system with a bag-tail valve on the end of the reservoir bag.

circuit, but it is *not* a coaxial system. Instead, the fresh gas tube is independent of the system and connects to the patient elbow adapter. The exhaled gases travel through a short corrugated tube, pop-off valve, and reservoir bag. Waste gases are evacuated by a hose from the pop-off valve. The pop-off valve is built into this system and allows the patient to be manually ventilated.

When a patient is connected to any nonrebreathing system the anesthetic machine's flush valve should not be used. The high flow (35–

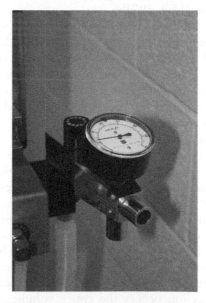

Figure 8.10.   Moduflex Bain circuit adapter (Moduflex Anesthesia Equipment, San Diego, CA) with a manometer, pop-off valve, and ports for the Bain circuit and reservoir bag. The scavenger tubing is connected at the bottom of the circuit/block.

75 L/min) from a flush valve into a nonre-breathing system can cause volutrauma (rapid overpressure of the lungs) (Hartsfield 2007).

Inadvertently leaving the pop-off valve closed can cause volutrauma and possibly a pneumothorax. The use of a *high pressure alarm* is a means to prevent such a trauma. Most alarms are preset to alarm when the pressure in the breathing circuit exceeds 20 cm H2O. The alarms can be added to the rebreathing or non-rebreathing circuits on all types of anesthesia machines.

Reservoir bag

The reservoir or rebreathing bag can be used during spontaneous ventilation to determine respiratory rate and estimate tidal volume. The bag can act as a reservoir if the pop-off valve is inadvertently left closed therefore preventing the immediate buildup of pressure within the circuit.

The appropriate size of rebreathing bag for each patient can be calculated by multiplying the patient's tidal volume (10–15 mL/kg) times 6. Rebreathing bags are available in sizes of 0.5, 1, 2, 3, and 5 L for small animals and sizes of 15, 20, and 30 L for large animals.

The following is a guideline to determine the appropriate size rebreathing bag for veterinary patients:

0.5–1 L   Patients ≤7 kg (15.4 lb)
2 L   Patients >7–20 kg (15.4–44 lb)
3 L   Patients >20–34 kg (44–74.8 kg)
5 L   Patients >34–90 kg (74.8–198 lb)
15 L   Patients >90–250 kg (198–550 lb)
30 L   Patients >250 kg (>550 lb)

Fresh gas flow rates

Closed, *low-flow*, and *semiclosed* are the terms used to describe circle breathing systems. The terms reflect the fresh gas inflow rate compared to the patient's metabolic needs. These three terms do *not* relate to the position of the pop-off valve.

When determining the fresh gas flow rate for circle systems, the patient's metabolic rate and oxygen consumption are just two of the factors considered.

The oxygen consumption for small animal patients is considered 4–7 mL/kg/min. This number is used as a guideline to determine the fresh gas flow rate for circle systems.

Closed circle system

The fresh gas flow rate for a closed circle system is equal to the uptake and metabolism of oxygen by the patient. A range of 4–11 mL/kg/min has been suggested for this system.

The advantages of a closed system include the following: it retains heat and humidity, it is economical, and it is safe for the environment.

The major disadvantage is the inability to change the anesthetic concentrations rapidly. This can be accomplished only by increasing the fresh gas flow rate and the vaporizer setting simultaneously.

Another consideration when using a closed circle system is the flow requirement for the vaporizer accuracy. Variable-bypass vaporizers (VOCs) require a minimum flow to assure proper performance; otherwise, erratic output of anesthetic can occur.

The quality of carbon dioxide absorbent should be checked before using a closed system. The removal of carbon dioxide from the closed system is completely dependent on the chemical absorption.

Due to the possibility of developing a hypoxic gas mixture, nitrous oxide is *not* used in a closed circle system.

Low-flow circle system

Low-flow anesthesia has an oxygen flow greater than the patient's oxygen consumption (4–7 mL/kg/min) but <22 mL/kg/min (22 mL/kg/min is the traditional lower limit for a semiclosed circle) (Hartsfield 2007). The suggested flow rate for small animal patients on a low-flow circle system is 10–15 mL/kg/min.

Low-flow and closed systems have the same advantages. They are economical, save heat and humidity, and reduce waste gases.

The major disadvantage of low-flow anesthesia is the transition from induction (short-acting injectable anesthetics or mask induction) to maintenance of an inhalant. To help with this transition higher fresh gas flow rates may need to be used for the first 15–30 minutes of anesthesia. Once the patient reaches a light surgical plane of anesthesia, the low-flow technique can be used to maintain anesthesia.

Semiclosed circle systems

The flow rate for a semiclosed circle system is traditionally 22–44 mL/kg/min. This flow rate exceeds the patient's uptake of oxygen and anesthetic for this system.

With the higher flow rates for the semiclosed system a significant amount of excess gas is exhausted through the pop-off. The increase of waste gases and the less retention of heat and humidity make this system less economical when compared to the closed and low-flow system.

The advantage of using higher flow rates is the ability to rapidly change the anesthetic concentration within the circle system. Nitrous oxide can safely be used with the semiclosed circle system. The high flow rate assures adequate flow for the proper performance of the variable-bypass vaporizer.

Nonrebreathing system flow rates

The exact flow rate for a nonrebreathing system differs with each individual patient and type of system. Ranges have been reported from 100 to >600 mL/kg/min for patients <7 kg (15.4 lb). An approximate range of 100–300 mL/kg/min with a minimum of 500 mL/min and a maximum of 3 L/min has been recommended for patients <6.8 kg (15 lb) (Hartsfield 2007).

Continuous monitoring of expired carbon dioxide values (with a capnograph) is the ideal mode to determine the flow rate for an individual patient. The purpose of the high fresh gas flow rate is to eliminate the rebreathing of carbon dioxide during spontaneous ventilation.

Selecting a breathing system

Determining a breathing circuit for a patient involves more than the weight of the animal. An overweight 8.2 kg (18 lb) cat technically falls into the range for a pediatric circle and a 1 L rebreathing bag. The cat's tidal volume is likely diminished due to the adipose tissue within the lungs, possibly making the effort to open the valves on the circle system difficult and ineffective. This cat could benefit from the nonrebreathing system's reduced resistance and lower mechanical dead space.

However, healthy patients <7 kg (15.4 lb) have been safely anesthetized with a pediatric circle.

Knowing the advantages and disadvantages of the breathing circuits, the patient's physical status, length of the procedure, and the comfort level with the anesthetic equipment are some of the factors to consider when selecting an appropriate breathing system.

References

Dorsch, JA, Dorsch, SE. 1999. Understanding Anesthesia Equipment, 4th ed. Baltimore: Williams and Wilkins, p.234.

Hall, LW, Clarke, KW, Trim, CM. 2001. Apparatus for the administration of anaesthetic. In Veterinary Anaesthesia, 10th ed. London: WB Saunders, pp.208–218.

Hartsfield, SM. 1996. Anesthetic equipment and monitoring. In Lumb and Jones' Veterinary Anesthesia, 3rd ed., edited by Thurmon, JC, Tranquilli, WJ, Benson, GJ. Baltimore: Williams and Wilkins, pp.393–394.

Hartsfield, SM. 2007. Anesthetic machines and breathing systems. In Lumb and Jones' Veterinary Anesthesia and Analgesia, 4th ed., edited by Tranquilli, WJ, Thurmon, JC, Grimm, KA. Ames, IA: Blackwell Publishing, pp.453–493.

Quandt, JE. 2005. Anesthesia case of the month. J Am Vet Med Assoc 227(12):1902–1904.

Watney, G. 1998–2003. www.asevet.com/resources/index.htm. Breathing circuits, nonrebreathing circuits, Ayre's T-piece, Bain circuit, Rebreathing circuits.

Introduction to Monitoring: Monitoring the ECG and Blood Gases

Jennifer Keefe

Monitoring anesthetized patients is imperative for all procedures. All anesthetic drugs act as cardiovascular and respiratory depressants on varying levels, and they can compromise a patient's homeostasis at unpredictable times in unpredictable ways. Crises are rapid in onset and devastating in nature. The term "young and healthy" never implies that the animal is exempt from a crisis while under anesthesia. There is always the potential of underlying disease that routine and even thorough screening can miss. Therefore, the goal of the anesthetist is to maximize the beneficial aspects of anesthesia while minimizing the effects on the organs. This vastly increases the potential for a full and uneventful recovery.

There are guidelines approved by the Diplomates of the American College of Veterinary Anesthesiologists (DACVA) as to what needs to be monitored on every anesthetized patient. These guidelines were approved by the Diplomates of the ACVA in December of 1994 and published in the *Journal of American Veterinary Medical Association* on April 1, 1995 (JAVMA, Vol. 206, No. 7, 936–937). Guidelines include monitoring *circulation, oxygenation, and ventilation*. The monitoring chapters cover methods that the anesthetist can use to monitor and also stresses the importance of keeping accurate anesthetic records.

The Anesthesiologist Society of America (ASA) has set a physical status scale that is used to rate patients for potential anesthetic risk:

- ASA status I is a healthy patient.
- ASA status II is a patient with mild systemic disease with no functional limitations.
- ASA status III is a patient with severe systemic disease with functional limitations.
- ASA status IV is a patient with severe systemic disease that is a constant threat to life.
- ASA status V is a moribund patient that is not expected to survive 24 hours with or without surgery.
- E denotes an emergency.

The ACVA added *personnel* to the guidelines in anesthetic monitoring for patients rated as ASA status III, IV, V, and E. This means there is one person aware of and responsible for the patient at all times.

Information can be quantitative, meaning there is a specific value to assign, or nonquantitative, meaning there is no specific value. Nonquantitative information is not reliable in anesthetic monitoring, although it can complement or contradict the quantitative information the instrument gives, perhaps warranting further investigation. The collection of information allows the anesthetist to properly assess the anesthetic patient.

ECG

Applications for monitoring

The electrocardiogram (ECG) is a graphic representation of electrical impulses as they move through the heart. This type of monitor is used to watch the heart rate and rhythm, which is imperative in anesthesia because many anesthetic agents predispose the patient to cardiac arrhythmias. Stress before induction and lack of oxygenation can also cause arrhythmias. It should be noted that ECGs indicate nothing about cardiac function; therefore, the anesthetist still needs to monitor blood pressure. Auscultating the patient throughout the anesthetic procedure is also indicated. An esophageal stethoscope is an economical and effective instrument for auscultation during anesthesia (Devey and Crowe 2002).

Physiology

The following traces the path the electrical impulse travels in normal conductivity:

1. The impulse starts in the sinoatrial (SA) node, which is located in the right atrium.
2. The impulse then travels through the atrium to the atrioventricular (AV) node, which is located in an area between the atria and ventricles.
3. The impulse then passes through the purkinje fibers that are located in the inner ventricular walls of the heart.
4. The impulse then travels throughout the ventricles.

Monitoring information

The readout of the ECG consists of the following:

- *P wave.* The P wave represents atrial depolarization (contraction), which occurs when blood is being pumped from the atria into the ventricles. The P wave should be positive (above the baseline) in small animal patients, and the size and configuration correlate to atrial activity.
- *QRS complex.* The QRS complex represents ventricular depolarization, which occurs when blood leaves the heart to travel to the lungs (from the right ventricle) or to the rest of the body (from the left ventricle). It also occurs when the pulse is generated. The R should be positive, and the size and configuration of the QRS complex correlates to ventricular activity.
- *T wave.* The T wave represents ventricular repolarization (relaxation), which occurs when the passive filling of the ventricles occurs. This wave can be either positive or negative.

The monitoring process

The most common lead used in anesthetic monitoring of veterinary patients is Lead II. An esophageal probe is a convenient way to obtain an ECG on an anesthetized patient. If a probe is unavailable, alligator clips can be attached to the skin where the limbs connect to the thorax and abdomen, or this skin can be pierced with a 22-gauge needle, secured with injection caps, and the clips can be attached to the needles. Standard ECG cables for veterinary monitoring contain three lead wires. One lead wire each is placed on the front limbs and one is attached to the left rear limb. Electrical activity is measured across the body from the right front to the left rear leg, which most closely represents the axis of the heart. The third lead wire is a ground lead.

Isopropyl alcohol can be used for conduction, but it evaporates quickly and may need to be reapplied. This can be difficult after the patient is draped for surgery, especially for a long anesthetic procedure. Ultrasonic gel will prolong conduction and will not likely need reapplication. Be sure to wipe excess gel off of the clips after

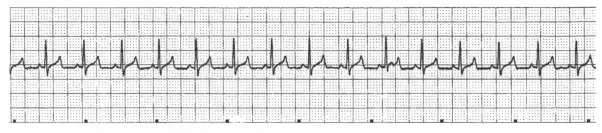

Figure 9.1. Increased amplitude of T waves.

each use because the buildup of gel can affect conduction.

Interpreting data: clinical significance

When assessing a rhythm strip, one should first see whether the rhythm is a normal sinus rhythm (regular) or some type of arrhythmia (irregular). It should also be noted whether the heart rate is normal, fast (tachycardic), or slow (bradycardic). The next step is to assess the P, QRS, and T waves by determining whether the intervals are the same distance (Tilley 2004):

■ Determine the P-P and R-R intervals, which are the distance between each P wave and each R wave, respectively. That distance should be equal with each heartbeat. There is an exception with a normal condition called a *sinus arrhythmia*. That occurs when the P-R interval remains the same, but the heart rate changes with breathing. The rhythm is considered "regularly irregular."
■ Determine whether each wave is uniform in size and shape. Then observe the relationship between waves:
  ■ Determine whether every P wave is followed by a QRS complex.
  ■ Determine whether every QRS complex is preceded by a P wave.
  ■ Determine whether the P-Q interval, which is the distance between each P wave and subsequent QRS complex, is the same distance for each beat (Tilley 2004). Variances can indicate AV block. (See arrhythmia section that follows.)

■ T waves should be the same distance from the QRS and uniform in size.
  ■ A progressive increase in T wave size can indicate myocardial hypoxia. It is important to remember that T waves can be either positive or negative (Fig. 9.1). When this is seen, anesthesia should be lowered or stopped, and the patient needs to be ventilated. Anesthesia should be discontinued if the wave configuration does not improve (Devey and Crowe 2002).

Progressive changes in the S-T segment and T wave configuration can also indicate electrolyte imbalances. The most common imbalances associated with these ECG changes are hyperkalemia and hypocalcemia. Determine what the imbalance is and treat accordingly (Kittleson and Kienle 1998).

What makes monitoring inaccurate?

The anesthetist should also be aware of the following:

■ *Electrical equipment*, such as cautery, interferes with conduction (Battaglia 2001).
■ *Electromechanical dissociation* can occur. This is a situation in which an animal can have no cardiac contraction for up to 5 minutes and still show a normal ECG. This is another reason the anesthetist should auscultate the patient (McKelvey and Hollingshead 2003).

Arrhythmia

An ECG will detect an arrhythmia, which is any electrical activity that differs from normal. Since the literal translation is "no rhythm," some prefer to use the term "dysrhythmia" (Kittleson and Kienle 1998). The arrhythmia's significance varies with age and preexisting condition. The anesthetist should be able to recognize arrhythmias, alert the veterinarian, and be knowledgeable about treatments (McKelvey/Hollingshead 2003).

Sinus tachycardia

Sinus tachycardia on an ECG will show a fast, regular rhythm with normal morphology (shape) (Fig. 9.2). It is defined as the following:

- A heart rate greater than 200 beats per minute (bpm) in a cat
- A heart rate greater than 180 bpm in a small dog
- A heart rate greater than 160 bpm in a large dog (McKelvey/Hollingshead 2003)

   Potential causes include the administration of drugs such as ketamine or anticholinergenics, heart disease, hyperthyroidism, surgical stimulation, hypotension, shock, sepsis, anemia, and hypoxia (McKelvey/Hollingshead 2003). Tachycardia can decrease cardiac output because there is less time for filling of the ventricles. The workload on the heart is increased, as is the myocardial oxygen consumption. This can progress to harmful arrhythmias if untreated (Hartsfield 2006).

After determining the cause, appropriate treatments are as follows:

- Drug-induced tachycardia usually does not necessitate treatment unless there are negative effects (blood pressure is affected).
- Metabolic causes can indicate the administration of drugs to slow the heart.
- Surgical stimulation/pain indicates the administration of analgesia and/or increasing anesthesia (Battaglia 2001).
- Hypotension or shock indicates a need for an increase in fluid administration. If that is ineffective, consider sympathomimetics, although these can worsen tachycardia if the patient is hypovolemic.
- Anemia can indicate that a blood transfusion is needed (Battaglia 2001).
- Hypoxia needs to be treated with increased ventilation. The heart is trying to optimize oxygen delivery by working harder. Check mucous membrane color because cyanosis (blue/gray) indicates severe hypoxia. Ensure that there is not an airway obstruction, and discontinue anesthesia if ventilation is ineffective (Battaglia 2001).

Sinus bradycardia

Sinus bradycardia on an ECG will show a slow regular rhythm that has a normal morphology. It is defined as the following:

- A heart rate lower than 100 bpm in a cat
- A heart rate lower than 70 bpm in a small dog

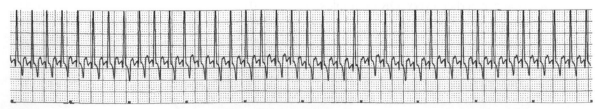

Figure 9.2.   Tachycardia.

- A heart rate lower than 60 bpm in a large dog (McKelvey and Hollingshead 2003)

Potential causes include excessive anesthetic depth, hypoxia, hypothermia, increased vagal tone, and the administration of alpha-2 agonists (such as medetomidine) (McKelvey and Hollingshead 2003). Bradycardia can also be a sign of severe hypotension (Battaglia 2001), and the decrease in heart rate can lessen cardiac output (Hartsfield 2006).

The anesthetist can lower inhalant anesthesia, ventilate the patient, and apply/increase external heat. Jaw tone can show excessive anesthetic depth as a loose, flaccid jaw. The surgeon can stop stimulation of the vagus nerve if that appears to be the cause (McKelvey and Hollingshead 2003). Bradycardia can usually be treated successfully with the administration of an anticholinergic although these drugs will not work in hypothermic patients. The doses for anticholinergics are as follows:

- Atropine 0.02–0.04 mg/kg IV (Plumb 2005)
- Glycopyrrolate 0.011 mg/kg IV (Plumb 2005)

If the patient was administered an alpha 2 agonist (such as medetomidine), anticholinergic administration is contraindicated. The heart rate is slowed to compensate for the vasoconstriction (and subsequent increased blood pressure) that occurs with alpha-2 agonists. Therefore, increasing the heart rate will put undue pressure on the heart.

If these efforts fail to improve heart rate, reversal of opioid-induced bradycardia can be facilitated by administering naloxone at a dose of 0.002–0.02 IV titrated to effect. Be aware that analgesic effects will also be reduced or eliminated so the administration of other analgesics will be indicated.

Atrioventricular block (AV block)

Atrioventricular (AV) block occurs when there is a disruption in the conduction between the sinus node and ventricles (Kittleson and Kienle 1998).

Causes include the administration of alpha-2 agonists, high vagal tone, hyperkalemia, and cardiac disease in which AV block is the primary problem (McKelvey and Hollingshead 2003). There are three degrees to be concerned with in anesthesia: 1st degree AV block, 2nd degree AV block, 3rd degree AV block.

1st degree AV block

A 1st degree AV block is present when there is a prolonged P-R interval (Kittleson and Kienle 1998). The ECG shows a slow, regular rhythm with normal morphology. Treatment is usually not necessary, but the patient should be monitored closely for 2nd or 3rd degree block.

2nd degree AV block

A 2nd degree AV block is present when there are P waves that lack QRS complexes (Fig. 9.3). Treatment with an anticholinergic is indicated if the animal becomes bradycardic and blood pressure lowers. Sometimes the problem can worsen before it gets better after the dose of anticholinergic is given. Again, these drugs will not be effective in hypothermic patients.

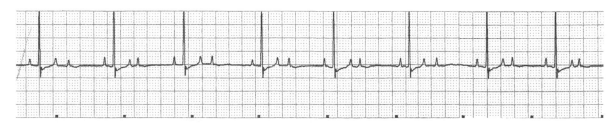

Figure 9.3. Second-degree AV block indicated by P waves without a QRS complex to follow.

3rd degree AV block

A 3rd degree AV block is identified when the P-wave and QRS complex occur completely independent of each other. The ECG shows a slow, regular rhythm with a QRS complex that is wide and bizarre. The ventricles are not receiving the signal to contract from the AV node, and a signal to depolarize is generated in the ventricles themselves. The ventricles can usually contract at a rate of 50–60 beats per minute. Because the signal does not follow the normal pathway through the purkinje fibers, the QRS complex looks wide and bizarre. The appearance is similar to a VPC, which is described in the next section, but treatment for VPCs (such as lidocaine) is contraindicated and may cause the heart to stop.

A 3rd degree AV block occurs only when there is a defect in the heart and is not related to anesthesia. The animal needs either a temporary or permanent pacemaker. Therefore, anticholinergics may be ineffective.

Ventricular premature contraction (VPC) or premature ventricular contraction (PVC)

A ventricular premature contraction is defined as a contraction originating in the ventricle that happens before a contraction is expected (prematurely). This can result in an ineffective and uncoordinated contraction with pulse deficits because there is a lack of ventricular filling. A pulse deficit occurs when the heart beats, but no pulse is generated. The ECG shows a normal rhythm interrupted by one or more wide and bizarre QRS complexes. Though VPCs are not uncommon, the patient should still be monitored closely when they are seen because there is an association between VPCs and cardiac muscle dysfunction. VPCs can progress to life-threatening arrhythmias (Battaglia 2001).

Causes for VPCs include the administration of barbiturates or halothane, hypoxia, gastric dilation and volvulus (GDV), possibly secondary to ischemia/reperfusion (I/R) injury, pain (also often seen in splenectomy patients), hypercarbia (increased CO_2) and trauma to the heart. Excitement, fear, or pain on induction can cause a catecholamine release that sensitizes the myocardium to arrhythmias (McKelvey and Hollingshead 2003).

Treatment with medication is indicated when there are more than 15 VPCs per minute with a subsequent drop in blood pressure. The most common medications used are lidocaine and procainamide (McKelvey and Hollingshead 2003).

The canine dose for lidocaine is a slow bolus of 2 mg/kg IV with a maximum of 8 mg/kg, followed by a constant rate infusion (CRI) at 25–80 mcg/kg/min if necessary.

Use lidocaine with extreme caution in cats because they are very sensitive to its effects on the central nervous system. The feline dose is one-tenth to one-quarter of the canine dose.

If hypoxia may be the cause of the arrhythmia, the patient should be ventilated. Ensure that there is not an airway obstruction, and discontinue anesthesia if the arrhythmia persists (Battaglia 2001).

Ventricular tachycardia (V-tach)

Ventricular tachycardia is defined as more than three VPCs in a row (Fig. 9.4). It is a fast, irregular rhythm with wide and bizarre QRS complexes. Often, the P wave is lost in the QRS complexes.

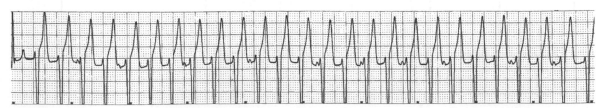

Figure 9.4.   Ventricular tachycardia.

The causes are the same as for VPCs. Treatment is indicated when the heart rate is greater than 160–180 bpm, if the patient's blood pressure is affected, or if there is "Q on T." Q on T occurs when the arrhythmia is so rapid the T wave is lost in the QRS complex. There is almost a complete lack of passive ventricular filling and this can be a precursor to ventricular fibrillation. Use the doses listed above for lidocaine. Refractory ventricular arrythmias may require treatment with procainamide.

Ventricular fibrillation (V-fib)

Ventricular fibrillation is defined by chaotic electrical activity and no mechanical activity (meaning there is no heartbeat) (Battaglia 2001). The ECG shows no definable pattern (Battaglia 2001). It is a terminal rhythm that is considered a form of cardiac arrest (Kittleson and Kienle 1998).

The patient needs immediate defibrillation. The energy level for external defibrillation starts at 3 joules (J)/kg, and internal defibrillation starts at 0.2 J/kg. If a defibrillator is not available, a chemical defibrillation of 1 mEq/kg potassium chloride (KCl) followed by 0.6 mL/kg of calcium gluconate (or 0.2 mL/kg of calcium chloride) can be administered IV. A precordial thump, which is a sharp blow over the precordium, can also be attempted (Battaglia 2001).

Performing a precordial thump

The patient should be placed on its right side. Locate the left apex; Strike this region with a fist while recording the ECG. The strength of the blow required depends on the size of the patient. A forceful blow is required in large dogs; smaller dogs and cats require a softer blow. A firmer thump should be applied if the initial thump is unsuccessful (Kittleson and Kienle 1998).

Atrial fibrillation (A-fib)

Atrial fibrillation occurs when there is contraction of small muscle bundles within the atria

(McKelvey and Hollingshead 2003). There is a "shoes in dryer" sound on auscultation. The ECG shows a fast, irregular rhythm with no discernible P waves, and the baseline is trembling or undulating. The QRS complex is normal. A-fib results in decreased cardiac output because there is no coordinated atrial contraction to fill the ventricles.

A-fib is always associated with atrial enlargement. In cats it is usually associated with severe enlargement of at least one atrium, and that has a very poor prognosis (Kittleson and Kienle 1998). Causes of atrial enlargement include severe mitral regurgitation (MR) or dilated cardiomyopathy (DCM). DCM occurs when the myocardium is weakened, thereby inhibiting the heart's ability to pump.

Treatment is usually with digoxin and a beta blocker to slow the ventricular rate and improve cardiac function (Battaglia 2001).

Atrial premature complex (APC)

Atrial premature complexes do not usually cause instability, so therapy is not often necessary. Though they can precipitate supraventricular tachyarrhythmias such as atrial tachycardia or atrial flutter (an atrial rate exceeding 300 beats per minute), these arrhythmias can be of concern if there is a lack of atrial filling.

Causes of APCs include atrial enlargement, myocardial disease, sepsis, neoplasia (particularly hemangiosarcoma), hyperthyroidism, and drug toxicities such as digitalis (Fox et al. 1988).

Blood Gas Analysis

The purpose of blood gas analysis in anesthesia is to give an accurate representation of a patient's respiratory function and acid-base status. The acid-base status refers to the mechanisms the body uses to maintain a normal pH (i.e. neither acidotic nor alkalotic).

Physiology

Thorough analysis of blood gases is intricate and complicated. The systems that regulate acid-base balance are the renal and respiratory systems. If a patient has a metabolic alkalosis, the respiratory system will slow respirations to retain carbon dioxide (CO_2), therefore, increasing the acid level in the body. On the same note, if a patient has a respiratory acidosis, the renal system will retain bicarbonate (HCO_3^-) to buffer excess acid, therefore lowering the acid level in the body. The acidotic patient may also pant to "blow off" CO_2. The respiratory response adjusts very quickly to changes in the acid-base status because it takes only minutes in normal circumstances. This is in opposition to the renal response, which takes hours (Battaglia 2001). Therefore, the ability to monitor blood gases gives the anesthetist a tool in helping the compromised patient undergoing anesthesia. Small changes in ventilation can make a big difference in acid-base regulation.

There are two types of blood gas sampling: arterial and venous. This section concentrates on arterial sampling; arterial blood is much more informative regarding respiratory status because it is oxygenated. If an artery is inaccessible, the lingual vein can be used because lingual values are closer to arterial readings due to the extensive anastomoses with the arteries in the tongue (McKelvey and Hollingshead 2003).

Blood gas analysis components

The following sections define the components in blood gas analysis as they apply to respiratory assessment.

pH

pH is a mathematical representation of hydrogen ion concentration. The normal range is 7.35–7.45. A low value indicates acidosis, and a high value indicates alkalosis. The pH is inversely proportional to CO_2, meaning that if the CO_2 is elevated, the pH is decreased and vice versa (Battaglia 2001).

Partial pressure of carbon dioxide ($PaCO_2$)

The partial pressure of carbon dioxide is the major ventilation parameter. The normal range is 35–45 mm Hg. A value of less than 35 mm Hg indicates hyperventilation, hypocapnia, and/or metabolic alkalosis, and values greater than 45 mm Hg generally lead to respiratory acidosis as they indicate a ventilation deficit, hypoventilation, and/or hypercapnia (an excess of carbon dioxide)(Battaglia 2001).

End-tidal carbon dioxide ($ETCO_2$)

End-tidal carbon dioxide is the amount of carbon dioxide an anesthetized patient exhales. It is measured with a capnograph and a device attached to the end of the endotracheal tube. This value is estimated to read 5–10 mm Hg less than the $PaCO_2$. $ETCO_2$ is covered in more detail in chapter 11.

Partial pressure of oxygen (PaO_2)

The partial pressure of oxygen determines the physiologic response to ventilation and oxygen (Battaglia 2001). It should be approximately five times the inspired oxygen concentration (FiO_2). The FiO_2 in room air is 21%; mask delivery, nasal oxygen cannula, or an oxygen chamber is usually about 35–40%. The FiO_2 is 100% in a patient that is intubated with the cuff inflated and on 100% oxygen (with or without inhalant anesthetic) (Willard 2002). In patients breathing room air, the normal PaO_2 values in a healthy awake patient are 90–115 mm Hg, and a value of less than 80 mm Hg indicates hypoxemia (McKelvey and Hollingshead 2003). A patient that is intubated with the cuff inflated should have a PaO_2 of nearly 500 mm Hg (five times inspired oxygen percentage) when being administered 100% oxygen if it is ventilating adequately.

Oxygen saturation (SaO_2)

Oxygen saturation measures the percentage of hemoglobin binding sites in the bloodstream that are occupied by oxygen. The value should be greater than 95%, and that is equivalent to a PaO_2 of 85–100 mm Hg. When the patient is hypoxemic with a SaO_2 of between 75–90%, the PaO_2 is that percentage minus 30 (McKelvey and Hollingshead 2003).

Bicarbonate level (HCO₃⁻)

The bicarbonate level represents the metabolic (or nonrespiratory) component of acid-base regulation. This regulation is achieved by the renal tubules balancing bicarbonate ions with hydrogen ions (Willard 2002). The normal range is 18–26 mEq/L. Metabolic acidosis occurs when the bicarbonate is less than 18 mEq/L, and alkalosis occurs when it is greater than 26 mEq/L (Battaglia 2001).

Base excess (BE)/base deficit

Base excess (BE)/base deficit refers to the total of bases (alkalis) in the blood and is usually affected by metabolic processes (Willard 2002). A negative number is a base deficit and is considered acidotic, while a positive reading is base excess and is considered alkalotic. The normal range is −2 to +2 (Battaglia 2001).

Analysis and Errors in Sampling

The two most common analyzers used in veterinary medicine are point-of-care and countertop units. Point-of-care units are handheld and use a disposable cartridge for each test. Calibration usually involves using a pH buffered aqueous solution of the analytes at known concentrations. This is contained in a cartridge within a foil pouch. Countertop units usually use a touch screen to initiate testing. Maintenance and calibration are done internally when the operator prompts it.

Errors in blood gas sampling tend to be due to improper sampling, but there are other causes, such as inadequate machine maintenance and microclots and/or air bubbles in the sample.

Sample Collection

Proper sample collection is imperative because accuracy is paramount in blood gas analysis (Willard 2002):

1. Take the patient's temperature if the analyzer adjusts for it. Temperature can affect PaO_2, $PaCO_2$, and pH.
2. Heparinize a 3 mL syringe with a 25-gauge needle attached by filling the syringe with heparin and expelling it back into the bottle so there is just the remainder in the hub. There are also syringes made specifically for blood gas collection.
3. If the animal does *NOT* have an arterial line:
   a. Common sites for sample acquisition are the femoral or dorsal pedal arteries.
   b. Locate the site, clip, and prepare with surgical scrub.
   c. Palpate and isolate the pulse with the nondrawing hand's index and middle fingers.
   d. Direct the needle at a 45 degree angle between fingers, and insert the needle into the site. A flash should be seen upon entering the artery.
   e. Hold the needle steady and slowly draw at least one mL into the syringe. One mL is needed to prevent dilutional effects from the heparin.
4. If the animal does have an arterial line:
   a. Wipe hub of catheter with isopropyl alcohol.
   b. Insert needle and draw at least one mL into the syringe.
   c. Flush catheter with saline.
5. Immediately expel air bubbles from the syringe and cap the needle with a rubber stopper. Redraw if the blood has a frothy appearance or many air bubbles, because room air will alter values.
6. Have the restrainer apply direct digital pressure to the draw site for at least 2 minutes.
7. Run the sample right away, or place on ice and run within 2 hours.

Acknowledgment

Special acknowledgment to Marrit Meesters, DVM, for her help in writing the ECG section and to Lois Ann Wetmore, DVM, DACVA, for her help in writing this chapter.

References

Battaglia, AM. 2001. Small Animal Emergency and Critical Care: A Manual for the Veterinary Technician. Philadelphia: WB Saunders Company.

Devey, J, Crowe, DT. 2002. Western Veterinary Conference 2002. Practical Monitoring Techniques and Equipment.

Fox, PR, Sisson, D, Moise, NS. 1988. Textbook of Canine and Feline Cardiology: Principles and Clinical Practice. Philadelphia: WB Saunders Company.

Hartsfield, SM. 2006. Western Veterinary Conference 2006. Cardiovascular Support during Anesthesia.

Kittleson, MD, Kienle, RD. 1998. Small Animal Cardiovascular Medicine. St. Louis: Mosby.

McKelvey, D, Hollingshead, KW. 2003. Veterinary Anesthesia and Analgesia, 3rd ed. St. Louis: Mosby.

Plumb, D. 2005. Veterinary Drug Handbook, 5th edition. Ames, IA: Wiley-Blackwell.

Tilley, LP. 2004. Western Veterinary Conference 2004. The Electrocardiogram.

Willard, S. 2002. American College Veterinary Internal Medicine (ACVIM) Forum 2002. Tips in Obtaining Blood Gases & Interpreting Results.

Monitoring: Pulse Oximetry, Temperature, and Hands-On

Amy Levensaler

Pulse Oximetry

A pulse oximeter is one of the most common monitors used in veterinary anesthesia and critical care medicine. It is generally easy to use, does not require special training, requires minimal site preparation, and is reasonably priced. It is a noninvasive monitor that uses infrared and visible light absorption in tissues to calculate the oxygen saturation of arterial hemoglobin. Pulse oximeters also measure the pulse rate of the patient and may provide visual pulse waveforms or bar graphs that provide information about the strength of the signal that the pulse oximeter is receiving (Grubb 2002). Pulse oximeters are commonly attached in small animals to unpigmented tissues such as the tongue, ear, lip, vulva, tail, prepuce, and digits. The tongue, nasal septum, and nostrils are the most effective locations used in equines. Haired areas can be used if the animals have minimal hair growth or if the hair is first clipped. Pulse oximeters work well on all species of veterinary patients (Wright and Hellyer 1996).

Physiology and how the monitor works

Pulse oximetry is based on the fact that oxyhemoglobin (hemoglobin bound to oxygen) and deoxyhemoglobin (hemoglobin not attached to oxygen) absorb infrared and red light at different wavelengths. The probe of the oximeter emits infrared light (920–940 nm) and red light (660 nm) several hundred times per second by two light-emitting diodes (LEDs). Sensitive photodetectors placed across an arterial bed measure the amount of light absorbed at each wavelength. The data is calculated and is expressed as a percentage of oxygenated hemoglobin to total hemoglobin (SpO_2). Arterial blood is pulsatile (venous blood and tissue beds are not) and oximeters are designed to restrict readings to areas that pulsate due to arterial blood flow, hence the name pulse oximetry. Although the pulse oximeter appears to be directly measuring arterial hemoglobin saturation, it is measuring light absorption in tissues with pulsatile flow during systole and subtracting that measured during diastole (Grubb 2002). Therefore, in a still patient, because arteries are pulsating, arterial saturation only is calculated (Wright and Hellyer 1996; Grubb 2002).

Pulse oximeters require no calibration by the user since the units are empirically calibrated by the manufacturer. There is a wide variety of brands of pulse oximeters currently available, some of which are specific to the veterinary market. Each manufacturer uses its own unique calibration method, and as a result, different brands may display slightly different saturation values when being used on the same patient (Grubb 2002).

Types of pulse oximeter probes

There are two different types of pulse oximeter probes. *Transmittance probes* are the most common and are designed with the LEDs and photodetectors placed on opposite sides of the tissue beds. The probes are available as C-clamps (which can be used on the nasal septum of large animals) and as clips designed for the human earlobe. Finger probes are also available but do not make good tissue contact due to their concave surface (Grubb 2002). Finger probes have some success at obtaining values using a cat's entire paw if the paw is not completely pigmented and may also be used successfully on equine tongues. There are also *reflectance probes* in which the photodetector and LEDs are positioned side by side on the emitting surface of the probe, which is placed in contact with the mucosa or skin (Grubb 2002) (Fig. 10.1).

In order to obtain measurements, pulse oximeters require that patients have reasonable cardiovascular function and hemoglobin concentrations. Normal physiologic SpO_2 values range between 90 and 100% (Grubb 2002). Values in this range indicate that the patient's ventilation and circulation are adequate (the

hemoglobin is adequately oxygenated and blood is being delivered to the tissue being monitored that meets the tissue's oxygen demands). It is common that we extrapolate a normal SpO_2 value to indicate that the entire patient is being adequately perfused. This assumption holds true most of the time but in unique situations where there is regional impedance of blood flow, this assumption cannot be made.

Factors that influence accuracy

Like many monitoring techniques used today pulse oximetry is also susceptible to inaccuracies. There are intrinsic and extrinsic factors that can provide inaccurate saturation data. Intrinsic factors include intravascular dyes (methylene blue) and dysfunctional hemoglobin (hemoglobin that does not carry oxygen, such as that bound to carbon monoxide, called *carboxyhemoglobin*). Extrinsic factors include ambient lights or heat lamps, use of electrocautery units, and more commonly patient movement or motion. Sources of ambient light can cause failure of the pulse oximeter to produce data or display erroneous SpO_2 readings. If possible, shielding the pulse oximeter probe (with dark material) from light sources may help eliminate inaccuracies. During measurement patients need to remain still because most of the currently used pulse oximeter probes are sensitive to pulsating motion. Movement may affect the unit's ability to detect a pulse as well as differentiate between movement and normal arterial pulsations. If the pulse oximeter does not detect a pulse at all or senses motion artifacts, it may audibly alarm and display an erratic heart rate. When the unit detects a pulse and displays a heart rate that matches the patient's actual heart rate you can be assured the pulse oximeter is accurately detecting a pulse. Proper fitting and size-appropriate probes may help to decrease motion artifacts. Improving cardiac output during low perfusion states may also help decrease inaccuracies due to patient motion (Wright and Hellyer 1996; Grubb 2002), as will using pulse oximeters that are motion insensitive (such as many of those made by Massimo Corporation).

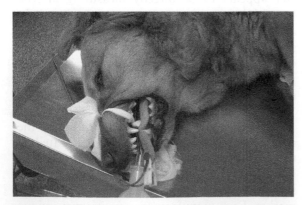

Figure 10.1.   Pulse oximeter transmittance probe placed on the tongue of a dog.

Interpretation of data

Pulse oximeters are known to be accurate in the 80–100% saturation range within 2–6%. At an oxygen hemoglobin saturation of greater than 90%, pulse oximetry saturation (SpO_2) tends to be slightly lower than actual arterial oxygen hemoglobin saturation (SaO_2). With saturations of less than 70%, SpO_2 tends to be higher than SaO_2. As SaO_2 continues to decrease, the accuracy of SpO_2 may decrease. The pulse oximeter probe must be in place for a minimum of 30 seconds before it will read and display an SpO_2 value. The displayed pulse rate must match the palpable pulse rate (except in horses in which the pulse rate may double on the unit as a result of the large dicrotic notch), and the waveform should be consistent and smooth for the reading to be considered acceptable (Wright and Hellyer 1996; Grubb 2002).

Pulse oximetry data should be interpreted in conjunction with the status of the entire animal as well as other monitored patient parameters. For example, anemia may cause a low SpO_2 reading despite a normal PaO_2, and shocky animals may have poor perfusion, which may cause a falsely low SpO_2. If the animal is breathing 100% oxygen, saturation should be maintained between 95–100%. Rapid response by the anesthetist is required when the saturation is less than 90% in the presence of a pulsating and strong signal. This can indicate severe shock, anemia, or significant desaturation and hypoxemia. The first response to a low saturation is to ensure that ventilation is adequate. Evaluate respiratory rate (RR) and tidal volume, and ensure a patent airway. Check that there are no interruptions of the flow of oxygen and that the nitrous oxide flow, if being used, is not in excess of 2/3 of the total fresh gas flow. To improve or treat a low SpO_2 the anesthetist can institute mechanical or intermittent positive pressure ventilation, provide oxygen supplementation, correct ventilation-perfusion mismatches (by changing patient position), and administer diuretics if indicated. When high inspired oxygen concentrations are being used it is important to note that normal oxygen saturation is often achieved in a hypoventilating patient. SpO_2 may not warn the anesthetist that the patient has extreme and non-physiologic elevations in $PaCO_2$. A pulse oximeter is not a reliable indicator for hypercapnia or hypoventilation. Therefore, the adequacy of ventilation and the adequacy of saturation should be assessed separately (Wright and Hellyer 1996; Grubb 2002).

Patient assessment/treatment of decreased SpO_2

If ventilation and arterial oxygenation are adequate but the SpO_2 is decreasing, assess the patient's cardiac output using some of the following indicators: capillary refill time (CRT) and mucous membrane color, pulse quality, and arterial blood pressure. An attentive anesthetist must rapidly respond to treat the problem if any of these indicators appear abnormal. Hypothermic, hypovolemic, vasoconstricted, and poorly perfused patients have decreased pulsatile flow, and this may result in a poor signal. Warming the patient, improving cardiac output first by reducing anesthetic concentrations and second by administering fluids and repositioning the sensor may help to improve the signal (Wright and Hellyer 1996; Grubb 2002). When the probe is being used on the tongue, periodic repositioning of the probe, massaging the tongue, and keeping it moist with water appear to help increase the signal (although the latter probably acts to increase perfusion at the site as well).

Conclusion

A veterinary practice is likely to purchase and use a pulse oximeter if the staff is familiar with it and comfortable recognizing and responding to abnormal values. A pulse oximeter has many advantages, and using it provides a higher level of care for veterinary patients.

Body Temperature

Heat loss is an almost inevitable consequence of anesthesia. The volatile anesthetics used in general anesthesia change the set point for thermoregulation (Harvey 2002). This change results in the patient's inability to respond to changes in body temperature. If a response is initiated it may be ineffective at restoring normal body temperature.

Temperature normals

The normal rectal temperature in the cat is 100.5 °F to 102.5 °F. The normal rectal temperature in the dog is 101.0 °F to 102.5 °F (Eddlestone 2006).

Hypothermia

Hypothermia, decreased body temperature, is known to cause postanesthetic shivering (resulting in increased oxygen consumption), prolonged recoveries, decreased anesthetic requirements, electrocardiographic changes, coagulation deficiencies, impaired platelet function, increases in fibrinolysis, decreased activity of the pathways of coagulation, and death (Harvey 2002). Animals frequently become hypothermic during anesthesia due to the reduced heat production by skeletal muscles, open body cavities, cold intravenous fluids, cold environment (prep tables, cool air) and prolonged anesthetic periods where the shivering response is inhibited. Most healthy patients can tolerate the physiologic challenges brought on by mild to moderate hypothermia. Unlike healthy patients, a decrease in body core temperature of 2 °F (1 °C) can adversely affect the critical or significantly compromised patient. This patient population is of increased risk of morbidity and mortality as a result of anesthetic-induced hypothermia (Haskins 1999; Harvey 2002).

Monitoring body temperature

As mentioned earlier, hypothermia decreases the requirements for general anesthesia. For each 2 °F decrease in body temperature there is a 5% decrease in the minimal alveolar concentration (MAC) of the volatile anesthetics. Hypothermia

also causes a decrease in the clearance of anesthetic drugs as well as an increase in the solubility of volatile anesthetics in the body. Diligence by the anesthetist is warranted because the combined result of the processes can be a significant potential for anesthetic overdoses. Therefore, perioperative monitoring of body temperature is strongly encouraged. It is easy to do and is relatively inexpensive. The attentive anesthetist who monitors body temperature is then able to adjust vaporizer settings and anesthetic doses in order to minimize the anesthetic complications of hypothermia. A thermometer probe in the esophagus or rectum allows constant temperature measurement. Accidental placement in the stomach or oral cavity reduces accuracy of core body temperature estimate. These probes can be cleaned between patients with a diluted chlorhexidine diacetate solution and allowed to dry. Thermometers (mercury or digital) placed in the rectum for intermittent measurement can also be used. Thermometers can be cleaned with isopropyl alcohol and allowed to dry between patients. Mercury thermometers are easily broken and cleanup of the mercury is expensive and potentially dangerous, and disposal is hazardous to the environment. As a result, digital thermometers are strongly preferred (Haskins 1999; Harvey 2002).

Prevention of hypothermia

Prevention of hypothermia includes minimizing patient heat loss. The easiest thing to do to control radiant heat loss is to shield the patient from its cool environment with towels or blankets. When permitted, place a warm blanket or towel on the cold surgical or prep table to shield the patient from its surface and/or place warm blankets or towels directly on the patient on the nonsurgical areas to help minimize convective losses. Wrapping limbs in commercial bubble wrap or placing baby booties on the paws of the smaller patients seems to help in the prevention of heat loss. When possible the use of low flow gas techniques is also helpful. Keep prep time to a minimum and warm the antiseptic preparations used if at all possible. Minimizing surgical time will also help in preventing hypothermia but may not always be feasible (Haskins 1999; Harvey 2002).

Active patient warming

There are several active warming strategies that can be used during the patient's perioperative period to maintain or restore body temperature. Turning up the heat in the operating suites as well as the recovery areas is recommended. Employing the use of circulating warm water blankets, not electric heating pads, as well as use of convective warm air devices are suggested. Electric heating pads are not recommended due to the very high temperatures reached, which increases the risk of iatrogenic thermal injuries. Tissue burns may been seen on patients warmed with electric heating pads due to the uneven distribution of heat and their inability to recognize excessive heat and remove themselves from the source. These pads are designed to be used on human patients who are conscious and able to remove the pad when they feel overheated. In addition, use of hot water bottles and gloves filled with warm or hot water is also dangerous for the anesthetized, comatose, or sedated patient. Thermal burns may be caused, and as these devices continue to cool, they contribute to the loss of body heat. In contrast, the circulating warm water blankets are less likely to cause thermal burns and can be used to prevent or minimize hypothermia when used correctly. Covering the patient's cage floor with half of the warm water blanket allows the patient to move away from the heat source, when able, to prevent injury (Haskins 1999; Harvey 2002).

Convective warm air devices are very effective in preventing and treating hypothermia. Units such as the Bair Hugger® by Gaymar Industries, blow warm air through porous blankets to surround the patient in warm air (Harvey 2002). There are many sizes and configurations of blankets on today's market. Use the best one to fit your patient to maximize the heat available to them. The Hot Dog Warming System® by Augustine Biomedical + Design features reusable, easy to clean, heavyweight nylon outer shell blankets that are flexible so they can be used around, under, or over the patient. Any of these blankets can also be covered with commercial bubble wrap or blankets and towels to help prevent the loss of heat. Body temperature must be monitored while using these units as it may increase rapidly. Use the blower units in the operating suites with caution as they work by "blowing" warm air and may blow debris and hair onto sterile fields, thereby contaminating various surfaces. If convective warm air devices are allowed in the operating suite, the anesthetist can decrease contamination risk by waiting until the patient is completely draped in before turning the unit on.

Warmed intravenous fluids or irrigation fluids must be used with caution. Overzealous warming of these fluids can be damaging to tissues. Fluid line warmers are available and act by heating the IV fluids as they run through the drip set. These may work better to control overheating of fluids but testing the temperature of the fluid first on one's wrist is recommended. Depending on the fluid drip rate and where the warmer is positioned on the drip set, fluids can again cool off before reaching the patient. Radiant heat via a heat lamp above the patient and the surgical field can also damage tissues when used carelessly in operating suites and recovery areas. Radiant heat sources can overheat tissues and burn through oxygen hoses and breathing circuits when not used properly. Temperature monitoring is again mandatory to decrease the risk of thermal injury when using active heating systems. Whatever active heating methods are employed, they should be started early to prevent hypothermia and their use should be controlled. Monitoring of patient body temperature should be mandatory (Haskins 1999; Harvey 2002).

Hyperthermia

Hyperthermia, increased body temperature, may be an iatrogenically induced response to specific drug combinations in certain species (cats) or with overzealous use of heating devices (e.g., circulating hot water blanket) in an effort to prevent the animal from cooling. Disruption of the normal processes for heat loss may also cause abnormal increases in body temperature due to anesthesia. Particularly in the small animal patient, increased body temperature is a less common sequela of general anesthesia and surgery but nonetheless is important to watch for (Haskins 1999; Harvey 2002).

Causes of hyperthermia

Patients' body temperatures may rise to above normal levels during anesthetic events. Decreased loss of body heat due to increased insulation (e.g., blankets, insulating hair coats), excessive or poorly monitored active heating devices, and increased metabolic production of heat (e.g., increased muscle tone) are mechanisms that may contribute to hyperthermia. Adverse effects of hyperthermia include increased metabolic rate, consumption of energy, and an increase in oxygen utilization, which may result in cellular hypoxia. Potential brain, kidney, liver, and blood damage may occur. Mild to moderate hyperthermia requires immediate intervention by the anesthetist. Active cooling of the patient and organ function monitoring are required to identify any complications from the hyperthermic event (Haskins 1999; Harvey 2002).

Treatment of hyperthermia

The underlying cause or causes should be identified and corrected during moderate hyperthermic events. Usually external active warming devices are to blame, but not always. Remove all external warming devices and begin to cool the patient immediately. Increasing oxygen flow can help cool the patient and prevent rebreathing of carbon dioxide and its retention. The application of cool water or alcohol to the footpads and skin may help to increase evaporative cooling. Judicious use of cold packs while avoiding tissue damage may help increase conductive heat loss. Cool intravenous fluids help to increase peripheral perfusion and heat loss. Cool enemas, cool abdominal lavage, and cool water submersion are some more aggressive methods of cooling. Whatever methods for cooling are employed, body temperature must be monitored continuously in order to remove the cooling methods before the return of normal body temperature. It may be difficult to anticipate the continued drop of body temperature once cooling methods are removed. Therefore, continued monitoring of temperature and evaluation of organ function for signs of compromise or failure is mandatory. Any adverse sequelae should be identified and treated appropriately (Haskins 1999; Harvey 2002).

Malignant hyperthermia

True malignant hyperthermia (MH) syndromes are rare but have been reported in humans, pigs, and dogs. MH is based on an abnormal release of calcium from the sarcoplasmic reticulum as well as abnormal calcium function. This excess concentration of calcium in the myoplasm causes extraordinary catabolic anaerobic and anaerobic metabolic reactions and is thought to be the functional defect in MH. In MH, patients may develop a syndrome of progressive and possibly fatal increased body temperature that is "triggered" by general anesthetics, particularly the volatile agents and succinocholine. Signs of MH include rapid increases in body temperature, increased end-tidal carbon dioxide levels in canines, and acidosis and muscle rigidity in porcines and humans. Fatalities may result from cardiac arrest, brain damage, failure of other body systems, and internal hemorrhage (Haskins 1999; Harvey 2002).

Rapid and aggressive response by the anesthetist is required in suspect cases of MH. Removal of the triggering agent, active cooling, intravenous fluid therapy, treatment for hypoxia, management of acidosis, and administration of dantrolene sodium, if possible, are imperative. Dantrolene is expensive and the results are variable in animal patients. Dantrolene is seen as a lifesaving component in human medicine and works by preventing the ongoing release of calcium from the sarcoplasmic reticulum storage sites in muscle tissue. Whatever therapies are initiated, intensive patient monitoring is required (Haskins 1999; Harvey 2002).

Conclusion

Monitoring body temperature during anesthesia and the postoperative period is recommended.

Despite the fact that hypothermia is almost inevitable during anesthesia, there are many methods the anesthetist may employ to limit the loss of heat and/or to safely and actively warm the patient. Monitoring body temperature may also alert the anesthetist to an increase in body temperature, hyperthermia from overzealous active heating methods, or hyperthermia from the rare, but life-threatening, malignant hyperthermia syndrome.

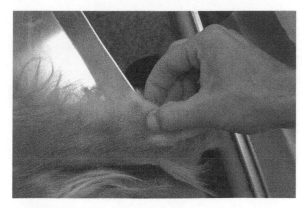

Figure 10.3. Toe pinch used to assess the withdrawal reflex in a dog.

Hands-on Monitoring

Anesthetic depth

The depth of anesthesia can be indirectly assessed by the *position of the eye* and the degree of depression of the eye's protective reflexes. During a surgical plane of anesthesia, the eyes roll ventrally in most species (Fig. 10.2). The eye is centered in the globe during light and deep planes of anesthesia. Dissociative anesthetics (e.g., ketamine) keep the eye centered in the globe during all planes of anesthesia (Haskins 1999).

The *palpebral reflex* is absent in most species during a deeper level of surgical anesthesia (Haskins 1999). In small animals it is elicited by tapping the eyelids or medial/lateral canthus.

The *corneal reflex* should always be present during anesthesia. Since this reflex is lost rela-

tively late and there is risk in causing trauma to the cornea, this reflex should never be used in an animal unless confirming complete cardiovascular arrest.

The *swallowing reflex* is occasionally maintained under surgical planes of anesthesia and may be elicited by passing a tube (e.g., esophageal stethoscope) into the esophagus.

The *withdrawal reflex* is elicited by a hard toe pinch, which results in withdrawal of the limb (Fig. 10.3). This reflex is useful when performing mask inductions to indicate whether an animal is deep enough to attempt endotracheal intubation.

The degree of muscle relaxation may be used to assess depth of anesthesia. However, it may not be a reliable indicator in animals given ketamine because this drug can increase muscle tone (Haskins 1999). *Jaw tone* is an indicator of muscle relaxation, which varies with the depth of anesthesia and is very subjective (Fig. 10.4).

Mucous membrane color (MM) and *capillary refill time (CRT)* are indicators of respiratory as well as cardiovascular status. MM and CRT provide subjective information regarding hemoglobin oxygenation, peripheral vascular tone, and tissue perfusion. Normal CRT is less than 1 to 2 seconds (Muir 2000). The gingiva, vulva, and eyelids are sites where MM and CRT can be evaluated (Fig. 10.5). Assessment may be difficult in animals with pigmented mucus membranes. CRT and MM are variably affected by

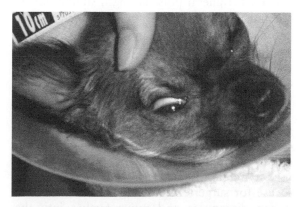

Figure 10.2. The canine eye rotates ventrally and medially during light planes of anesthesia.

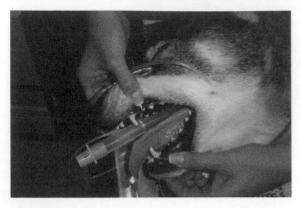

Figure 10.4.   Technique used to assess jaw tone in a dog.

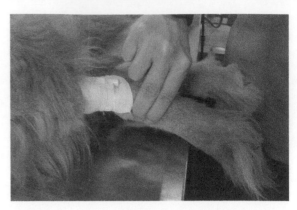

Figure 10.6.   Dorsal pedal palpation in the dog.

anesthetic drugs. Drugs that cause vasodilation may decrease CRT by improving peripheral perfusion. Anesthetic agents also affect MM. Drugs that cause vasodilation may result in pink MM and normal CRT, although cardiac output and blood pressure are decreased. Drugs that cause vasoconstriction may result in pale MM, but the hemodynamic status may be OK. Under anesthesia a normal CRT may not be a reliable indicator that perfusion is adequate, although a prolonged CRT is significant. Prolonged CRT (>3 seconds) is indicative of low cardiac output and poor tissue perfusion (Hackett 2009). Pale MM may indicate vasoconstriction due to pain, decreased cardiac output, blood loss, hypoxia, and decreasing circulating red blood cells. Dark pink MM may indicate vasodilation due to anesthetic

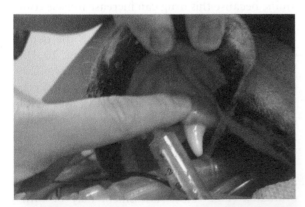

Figure 10.5.   Technique used to assess capillary refill time (CRT).

agents, sludging of blood in the capillaries (endotoxemia), and increased CO_2. Cyanotic MM indicates severe hypoxemia. Brown MM can be seen with methemoglobinemia, and a yellowish hue to the MM indicates increased serum bilirubin from hemolysis or hepatic disease (Hackett 2009).

Direct palpation of arteries provides an opportunity to assess pulse rate and rhythm as well as qualitative assessment of pulse pressure. In lean, narrow-chested or small animals (cats), the heartbeat can also be palpated through the chest wall. Pulse rate changes vary with anesthetic depth in small animals. Pulse pressure is the difference between systolic and diastolic arterial blood pressure (Hackett 2009). Pulse pressure does not indicate perfusion pressure, which is usually measured by the mean arterial pressure (MAP). Peripheral pulse strength should not be overinterpreted because anesthetic drugs alter peripheral vascular tone and therefore alter pulse pressure. Palpable arteries in the dog and cat include the femoral, lingual, dorsal pedal, digital, and buccal artery or lingual artery (Muir 2000) (Fig. 10.6).

Used primarily in small animals, an *esophageal stethoscope*, with the tip placed at the level of the heart, is coupled to earpieces or to an electronic amplifier (Fig. 10.7). It can also be used to monitor breath sounds. It can be difficult to use for surgeries involving the neck because it can disconnect and move farther into the gastrointestinal tract. In large-breed dogs,

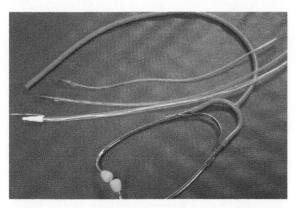

Figure 10.7. An esophageal stethoscope is a relatively simple device that allows auscultation of heart sounds during anesthesia.

securely taping the probe to the stethoscope ears is recommended to help prevent this.

Conclusion

The patient's cardiovascular and respiratory systems, anesthetic depth, and body temperature should be monitored during anesthesia. This can be done using monitoring equipment; but equipment alone, although able to alert when a problem has occurred or is occurring, is less likely to warn about trends in physiologic parameters that precede an anesthetic crisis. Regular subjective evaluations by a trained and attentive anesthetist and the use of electronic monitors that can be observed by the anesthetist are the most effective tools for preventing complications in anesthetized patients.

Acknowledgment

Special thanks to Lois Wetmore, DVM, DACVA, for her help and guidance in the writing of this chapter.

References

Eddlestone, S. 2006. Small animal medical nursing. In Clinical Textbook for Veterinary Technicians, edited by McCurnin, B, 6th ed. St. Louis: Elsevier Inc., p.787.

Grubb, T. 2002. Pulse oximetry. In Veterinary Anesthesia and Pain Management Secrets, edited by Greene, SA. Philadelphia: Hanley & Belfus, Inc., pp.121–126.

Hackett, T. 2009. Physical examination. In Small Animal Critical Care Medicine, edited by Hopper, S. St. Louis: WB Saunders Company, pp.2–4.

Harvey, R. 2002. Hypothermia; Hyperthermia. In Veterinary Anesthesia and Pain Management Secrets, edited by Greene, SA. Philadelphia: Hanley & Belfus, Inc., pp.149–152, 153–156.

Haskins, S. 1999. Perioperative monitoring. In Manual of Small Animal Anesthesia, 2nd ed. edited by Paddleford, R. Philadelphia: WB Saunders, pp.123–146.

Muir, WW, Hubbell, JAE, Skarda, RT, Bednarski, RM. 2000. Patient monitoring during anesthesia. In Handbook of Veterinary Anesthesia, 3rd ed. St. Louis: Mosby. pp.250–283.

Wright, M, Hellyer, PR. 1996. Respiratory monitoring during anesthesia: Pulse oximetry and capnography. Compendium 18(10):1083–1096.

Monitoring Blood Pressure and End-Tidal CO_2 in the Anesthetized Patient

Heidi L. Reuss-Lamky

Intraoperative monitoring is imperative for optimizing all anesthetic procedures. In addition to allowing informed, flexible, and well-timed responses to changes in the patient's status it also serves as a database for comparison prior to subsequent anesthetic episodes and facilitates legal documentation of the anesthetic care provided (McCurnin 1994; Muir et al. 2000; Seahorn 2004; Baetge 2007). Monitoring can be divided into two categories: *physical* and *technical*. While physical methods involve the perceptible skills of the anesthetist (e.g., observing chest excursions, assessing eye position), technological methods employ the use of sophisticated equipment (McCurnin 1994).

It is well known that inhalant anesthetics cause respiratory depression, especially when used in combination with opiate analgesics or induction agents such as barbiturates or propofol (McCurnin 1994, Taylor and McGehee 1995; Greene 2002; Seahorn 2004; Weil 2005). Moreover, hypotension is a frequently observed complication in anesthetized patients due to the fact that many injectable anesthetic drugs (e.g., acepromazine, thiobarbiturates, propofol) and inhalant anesthetics decrease cardiac output, systemic vascular resistance, or both, in a dose-dependent manner (Greene 2002; Weil 2005;

Love and Harvey 2006; Wagner and Ryan 2006; Baetge 2007). Anesthesia-induced hypotension can be exacerbated in hypovolemic, critically ill, or compromised patients and can lead to acute renal failure, especially in geriatric patients (Mosley 2006; Stokes and Bartages 2006, Baetge 2007; Tefend 2007). Other direct effects of inhalant anesthetics include central nervous depression, muscle relaxation, and impaired thermoregulation. Consequently, technological monitoring of the cardiovascular and pulmonary systems can provide the anesthetist invaluable information regarding the status of the anesthetized patient (McCurnin 1994).

Blood Pressure

Blood pressure assessment can be a crucial component of patient care during anesthesia and surgery since *all* patients will experience some degree of hypotension during general anesthesia. In fact, the American College of Veterinary Anesthesiologists recommends blood pressure monitoring as a minimum standard for managing the anesthesia care of moderate to severely ill patients (Love and Harvey 2006).

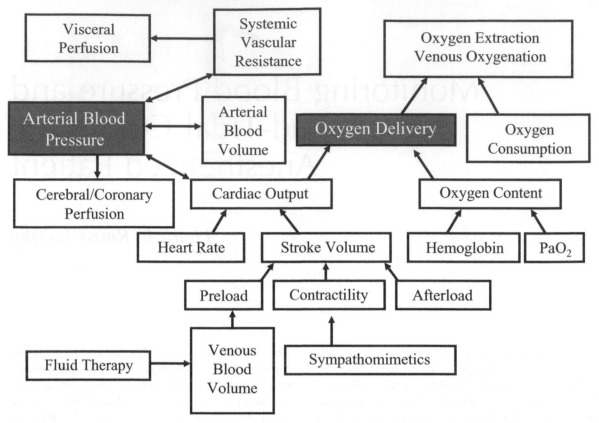

Figure 11.1. This diagram demonstrates all of the factors that determine blood pressure. Reprinted with permission from Thurmon J, et al. 1996. Lumb and Jones' Veterinary Anesthesia, 3rd ed. Baltimore: Lippincott Williams & Wilkens.

In summary there are two factors that affect blood pressure and two factors that affect cardiac output (Fig. 11.1). Blood pressure is determined by *total peripheral resistance* and *cardiac output*. Total peripheral resistance is defined as the resistance to blood flow created by the peripheral arterial system as well as capillary beds. Cardiac output is determined by a combination of the *heart rate* and *stroke volume*. The heart rate is the speed at which the heart is pumping, or the number of contractions per minute. The stroke volume is the amount of blood ejected with one contraction of the heart. Cardiac contractility, preload, and afterload are all factors that can influence the stroke volume. Blood pressure itself may be defined as "the lateral force on the arterial wall" (Love and Harvey 2006). Additionally, blood volume is a major determinant of blood pressure (Durham 2005). Baroreceptors located

in the carotid sinus and aortic arch help regulate blood pressure through the sympathetic nervous system control centers. Furthermore, many other factors can impact blood pressure homeostasis, including chemoreceptors, hormonal influences, and the renal sensing systems (Durham 2005; Tefend 2007).

Normal arterial blood pressure values for dogs and cats are indicated in Table 11.1.

Systole represents cardiac contraction, and diastole occurs during cardiac filling. Pulse pressure is a result of the difference between the systolic and diastolic pressures. The mean arterial pressure (MAP) is determined by the following equation:

$$\text{Diastolic} + 1/3 \text{ Pulse Pressure}$$
$$(\text{Systolic} - \text{Diastolic}) = \text{MAP}$$

Table 11.1.   Normal arterial pressure values.

Canine	Feline
Systolic: 110–190 mm Hg	Systolic: 120–170 mm Hg
Diastolic: 55–110 mm Hg	Diastolic: 70–120 mm Hg

Blood pressure monitoring for the critically ill. Proceedings Western Veterinary Conference (Waddell L. 2004).

Blood Pressure Monitoring

There are two techniques available for measuring blood pressure—*directly* utilizing invasive methods or *indirectly* via noninvasive methods such as Doppler ultrasonography and DINAMAP (Device for Indirect, Noninvasive, Automatic Mean Arterial Pressure) oscillometric devices (Waddell 2004, Durham 2005). It has been demonstrated that although the heart rate can be reliably and repeatedly predicted there is great variability regarding the indirectly obtained measurements of the diastolic, systolic, and mean arterial pressures as compared to the telemetrically acquired direct blood pressure (Data Sciences International, DSI) readings obtained within a given (3–4 minutes) time frame in a conscious dog. All brands compared in one head-to-head study (using Cardell® 9401 and Dinamap® 1846 SX oscillometric devices) ranged consistently 10% (or as much as 20–30%) lower than the direct, telemetric recordings (Durham 2005; Cowgill 2006; Love and Harvey 2006). Experienced personnel using Doppler (Parks Model 811-BTS) methods to record systolic pressures ranged from 18% to nearly 28% lower than the referenced measurements, demonstrating the lowest level of accuracy. The results of this study found that 1) in normal dogs, "spot" blood pressure measurements may not accurately reflect the patient's physiologic or pathologic state as accurately as time-averaged blood pressure readings over larger segments of the day; 2) although blood pressure trends were accurately predicted among the indirect oscillometric methods tested, each one provided unique values that were not consistently comparable to the validated standard; and 3) as compared to the referenced measurements, there were wide deviations in recorded blood pressure values when trained and experienced personnel in a clinical setting used oscillometric or Doppler techniques. The apparent inability to accurately gauge blood pressure in veterinary patients using currently available indirect methods led the American College of Veterinary Internal Medicine Consensus Panel to proclaim the following (Cowgill 2006):

> ⋯ for the diagnosis of systemic hypertension, the indirect device used should be one that is commonly employed or designed for veterinary use, and has been previously validated in conscious animals of the species of interest. However, no indirect device has met these criteria for use in conscious dogs or cats.

These are just a few examples as to why direct arterial blood pressure (DABP) monitoring, proven to be the most accurate method of measuring blood pressure in both human and veterinary patients, is considered the gold standard.

Direct (invasive) blood pressure monitoring

Although a thorough understanding of the regional anatomy and an advanced skill level are necessary to place arterial catheters, their use for DABP monitoring has many advantages when used in critically ill or high-risk anesthetic patients. Preserving blood pressure during anesthesia is imperative to ensure adequate perfusion of tissues and vital organs such as the heart, lungs, kidneys, and brain (McCurnin 1994; Glerum 2005; Love and Harvey 2006). Untreated hypotension can lead to organ failure, shock, and death (Durham 2005; Baetge 2007).

The administration of intravenous crystalloids, colloids, or positive inotropes can be an integral part of maintaining blood pressure in anesthetized patients (Love and Harvey 2006). As such, direct blood pressure monitoring is extremely helpful in assessing the progress of fluid resuscitation, or inotropic or pressor therapy in patients with hypovolemic or septic shock (Waddell 2004). Arterial catheters can also be used for arterial blood gas analysis, considered the gold standard for assessing a patient's ventilatory function or acid/base status (Marshall 2004; Beal 2006; Tegtmeyer 2006; Terry 2006; Wagner and Ryan 2006).

There are numerous arteries that may be selected as the placement site for an arterial catheter. The dorsal pedal/metatarsal artery is most commonly used and is one of the easiest to maintain on a long-term basis (Beal 2006). Other arteries that are suitable for short-term use in veterinary patients include the radial, brachial, palmar, femoral, auricular, carotid, coccygeal, and sublingual (ventral tongue) arteries. The femoral artery may be used in smaller patients such as cats and small dogs, and the auricular artery (located on midline of the dorsal surface of the pinna) can be utilized in larger dogs with big, pendulous pinnae (e.g., basset hound, beagle) (Waddell 2004; Beal 2006; Love and Harvey 2006; Terry 2006).

Other considerations when selecting the site for an arterial catheter include avoiding compromise of the circulation distal to the placement site (e.g., end arteries or other areas with known deficiencies in collateral circulation) and avoid infected areas or areas that have sustained trauma proximal to the proposed insertion site (Tegtmeyer et al. 2006).

Arterial catheters used for DABP measurements must be connected to a continuous flush system via the shortest possible length of noncompliant extension tubing and to either an aneroid manometer or to an oscilloscope with a strain gauge pressure transducer (Love and Harvey 2006; Wagner et al. 2006; Baetge 2007). Both DABP methods will provide the anesthetist with continuous readings even during extreme physiologic adversities that may be associated with hypotension, vasoconstriction, tachycardia, and arrhythmias (Baetge 2007). Although the less expensive aneroid manometer is capable of recording only the mean arterial pressure value, an oscilloscope monitor displays values for the systolic, diastolic, and mean arterial pressure as well as a series of real-time waveforms (McCurnin

1994; Love and Harvey 2006; Baetge 2007). There is a reported 2–4% level of inaccuracy associated with DABP measurements; 1–2% of the inaccuracy arises from the transducers, and another 1–2% occurs from the amplifier (Waddell 2004).

Not all brands of anesthetic monitors are capable of obtaining DABP measurements. Consult the manufacturer's instruction manual to find out whether a particular model of anesthetic monitor is capable of performing invasive blood pressure monitoring as well as which type of transducer kit or other equipment may be necessary, and how to correctly assemble and operate it.

DABP waveform interpretation

Understanding the DABP waveform is essential for assessing cardiac function, particularly as it relates to left ventricular ejection. Used in conjunction with an ECG, evaluation of the DABP waveform permits the anesthetist to determine when cardiac arrhythmias may be causing poor pressures or when pulse deficits become detrimental to the patient, thereby allowing timely institution of interventional drugs. For example, a state of poor perfusion exists when cardiac arrhythmias (e.g., premature ventricular contractions) are associated with a dampened waveform appearance in conjunction with an abnormal MAP (Tefend 2003a).

Peak ejection occurs during the highest point on the waveform and is associated with systole (Fig. 11.2). The downstroke of the waveform is associated with a drop in pressure. Midway through the downstroke the dicrotic notch may be visible and indicates closure of the aortic valve. The dicrotic notch also represents the beginning of diastole. The remainder of the waveform downstroke represents the flow of blood into the arterial tree, with the lowest point of the waveform representing diastole. What's more, it is possible to identify physiologic abnormalities such as vasoconstriction or vasodilation based on the appearance of the DABP waveform (Fig. 11.3) (Muir et al. 2000; Tefend 2003a; Love and Harvey 2006).

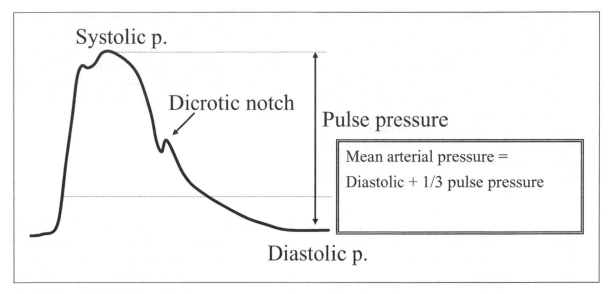

Figure 11.2. DABP waveform—normal.

Troubleshooting DABP

A thorough knowledge of the potential complications and limitations associated with arterial catheters can simplify the troubleshooting process and ensure their continued use for DABP

monitoring. Some of the most common problems encountered include:

■ *Waveform dampening or loss:* This may indicate actual hypotension or loss of pulse. Assess the patient. It may be associated with

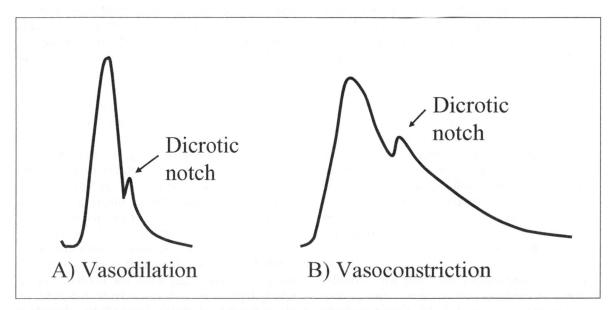

Figure 11.3. Affects of vasoconstriction and vasodilation on the DABP waveform.

air bubbles or blood clots, or excessive blood or kinks present in the catheter or tubing line (Mazzaferro 2004). Additionally, the artery may be in spasm. During arterial spasms the MAP is generally correct even without a good tracing. In all cases, flush the line and catheter after ensuring that the line has not been clamped off. If the catheter has migrated up against the vessel wall, a change of the patient's position may resolve the problem (Tefend 2003a; Waddell 2004; Love and Harvey 2006).

- *The line flows and can be aspirated, but the waveform is not visible:* Ensure that the cable is still attached to the monitor and that the stopcock is not in the OFF position toward the patient.
- *Sudden change in pressure:* Ensure the transducer has not moved and is still at the level of the heart, and that the surgeon is not leaning on the patient line or a major blood vessel. More importantly, a sudden change in pressure can indicate that cardiac arrest has occurred or is imminent: Assess the patient's pulse and monitor end-tidal carbon dioxide production.
- *Inaccurate readings:* Lower systolic and higher diastolic values may be present whenever the waveform becomes dampened. Artificially increased pressure readings may occur if the catheter itself obstructs blood flow in smaller arteries (Love and Harvey 2006). Furthermore, inaccurately low readings may be evident in patients with severe peripheral vasoconstriction (e.g., severe hypovolemia or due to higher doses of pressor agents) (Waddell 2004).
- *Waveform amplification:* Reflections of the waveform from a peripheral catheter may amplify the systolic pressure, resulting in falsely elevated systolic values. Although less common in veterinary medicine, this phenomenon occurs routinely in geriatric human patients when arteries are noncompliant (Waddell 2004).

Do not waste unnecessary time with troubleshooting techniques when there are doubts regarding the accuracy of DABP. Always perform a thorough exam and assessment of the patient first and combine those findings with an indirect blood pressure reading. Although differences will be evident between indirect and DABP measurements, the patient's clinical management may be affected by large disparities (Tefend 2003a).

Indirect (Noninvasive) Blood Pressure Monitoring

There are three commonly recognized methods used to measure blood pressure indirectly: *Doppler ultrasonography*, *photoplethysmography*, and *oscillometrically* with a DINAMAP device (e.g., Dinamap®, Cardell®, petMAP®) (Acierno and Labato 2004; Durham 2005; Love and Harvey 2006). All indirect methods tend to underestimate the actual blood pressure, and all work best when the MAP is 60–100 mm Hg (Seahorn 2004; Durham 2005; Cowgill 2006; Love and Harvey 2006). However, because they are consistent over a wide range of pressures, they are considered reliable (Durham 2005; Cowgill 2006).

Regardless of the method used, cuff selection is *imperative* for obtaining the most accurate results. Inappropriate cuff size and placement are the most common sources of errors. The width of the cuff should extend 40% around the circumference of the limb. When the cuff is determined to be too small, the next wider size should be selected. In cats it is acceptable to use a cuff that is only 30% of the circumference of the limb (Fig. 11.4) (Acierno and Labato 2004; Durham 2005; Love and Harvey 2006).

The cuff should be snug but not too tight (Durham 2005). It is acceptable to secure the cuff using a piece of tape to prevent it from becoming dislodged during inflation (Seahorn 2004). Due to the effects of gravity on arterial blood pressure the cuff should ideally be positioned at the level of the heart (Love and Harvey 2006; Duffy 2007). If the cuff is too narrow, too loose, or below heart level, the reading will be falsely high. If the cuff is too wide, too tight, or above heart level, the reading will be falsely low

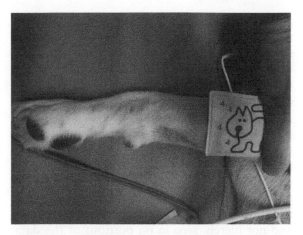

Figure 11.4. Measuring correct cuff size.

(Durham 2005; Love and Harvey 2006). Additionally, a cuff placed over a joint is less likely to compress the artery, and a hole in the cuff may result in rapid cuff deflation that thwarts machine interpretation (Durham 2005; Duffy 2007). Acceptable cuff locations include the forelimb, tail, and hindlimbs. The areas proximal to the carpus and tarsus work best. The ventral tail is a good choice in cats as well as short-legged dog breeds, such as the bassett hound and dachshund (Durham 2005). In cats the author has had satisfactory results with oscillometric devices by using the distal humeral area, proximal to the elbow.

Doppler ultrasonography

Doppler ultrasonography uses a Ravi-Ricci return-to-flow principle to detect the systolic blood pressure and is most accurate when the systolic pressure is within normal limits and the patient has good peripheral perfusion (Valverde 2003; Seahorn 2004; Durham 2005; Love and Harvey 2006). Doppler ultrasonography is also more useful in small patients and short-legged dog breeds (Durham 2005).

Using the Doppler method to measure blood pressure is very easy, and all technicians should be able to proficiently perform this simple task. Arterial sites commonly used for Doppler measurements include the caudal metacarpal and metatarsal areas, and ventral tail (Love and

Harvey 2006). Preferably the area directly over the selected artery should be shaved, but wetting the haircoat with alcohol may be adequate (Love and Harvey 2006). A dollop of ultrasonic coupling gel is placed over the artery. The Doppler piezoelectric crystal (a 10 MHz ultrasound probe) is held or secured directly over the artery until an audible pulse "swoosh" sound is detected. An appropriately sized cuff is then placed proximally to the Doppler crystal. The cuff is inflated with an aneroid manometer until blood flow can no longer be heard, and then pressure is slowly released until the "swoosh" sound returns. During the first audible pulse sound, the manometer reading corresponds to the systolic blood pressure measurement (Tefend 2003b; Love and Harvey 2006). For best results, inflate the cuff 20–30 mm Hg past the highest point where blood flow was last detected (Acierno and Labato 2004).

Doppler methods tend to underestimate systolic blood pressure (Cowgill 2006; Love and Harvey 2006). In cats weighing <4–5 kg, it is hypothesized that the resultant reading probably represents the MAP (Taylor and McGehee 1995; Greene 2002; Love and Harvey 2006). As a result, a correction factor of 14 mm Hg is added to the reading to more accurately reflect the actual systolic blood pressure of cats (Taylor and McGehee 1995).

Doppler devices are becoming commonplace in veterinary facilities because they are easy to use, noninvasive, portable, and less expensive than oscillometric machines (Love and Harvey 2006). Therefore use of a Doppler device is an excellent alternative for obtaining periodic blood pressure readings in anesthetized patients if an oscillometric unit is unavailable (Love and Harvey 2006).

Care should be taken when using Doppler ultrasonography. Ensure good probe contact and adequate coupling gel. Be warned that Doppler methods can mistake heavy respirations for blood flow. Additionally, operator inexperience, profound arrhythmias, hypothermia, patient motion, low batteries, and electrical interference can also impede obtaining valid readings (Tefend 2003b; Welsh 2003; Durham 2005; Glerum 2005; Love and Harvey 2006).

Photoplethysmographic methods

Also relying on the Ravi-Ricci principle of detecting flow, photoplethysmographic methods estimate the MAP by measuring the penetration of an infrared beam through tissues. Arterial volume is controlled with an aneroid manometer attached to a pressure cuff placed around the metatarsal region (just distal to the hock) (Durham 2005; Love and Harvey 2006). Although used predominantly in humans, the advantages of this method include its ability to provide continuous blood pressure measurements with a waveform, a low incidence of motion artifacts, and relative accuracy in cats and small patients (<4–10 kg) (Acierno and Labato 2004; Durham 2005; Love and Harvey 2006). Drawbacks to photoplethysmography include limited patient candidacy (≤10 kg), poor cuff fit due to human designed finger cuffs, poor readings on cats with darkly pigmented skin, and up to a 60-second delay in signal interpretation (Acierno and Labato 2004; Durham 2005; Love and Harvey 2006).

Oscillometric methods

These methods detect intracuff changes caused by arterial pulsations. They calculate the systolic, diastolic, and MAP as well as the heart rate. Oscillometric devices often can be programmed to obtain readings at various time intervals (once per minute, once per hour, etc.) Most of these monitors are reasonably accurate in animals weighing more than 5 kg and when the blood pressure is within normal range (Acierno and Labato 2004; Seahorn 2004; Love and Harvey 2006).

It is important to understand and properly interpret the data provided by *all* blood pressure monitors. If the systolic blood pressure is >90–100 mm Hg and the MAP is >60–70 mm Hg, it is assumed that a state for adequate tissue perfusion exists (Seahorn 2004). Let's consider two patients: One patient has a blood pressure reading of 85/79 mm Hg, and the second patient has a blood pressure reading of 105/69 mm Hg. Both patients have a MAP of 81 mm Hg. Is one patient "better off" than the other? The first patient is suffering from a condition called *narrow margins*, meaning the systolic and diastolic values are very close together; this indicates that the heart is neither contracting nor relaxing with much vigor. This patient will have cold extremities, pale mucous membranes, and a poor pulse quality as compared to the second patient. This phenomenon is the result of decreased cardiac output with a compensatory peripheral vasoconstriction and occurs as a response by the body to maintain adequate blood pressure (Tefend 2003a,b). This explains why it is critical to carefully evaluate the *whole patient* and not merely zero in on portions of the data provided by the anesthetic monitor.

There are many caveats associated with indirect blood pressure measurement methods. Results may vary greatly based on the selection of the cuff size, fit, and location, patient size (<5 kg) or movement, presence of excessive skin, limb edema, or significant arrhythmias, and the experience of the operator (Tefend 2003b; Seahorn 2004; Waddell 2004; Cowgill 2006). Furthermore, all external methods of obtaining blood pressure measurements are the least accurate when results would be most revered, such as in small patients or those with vasoconstriction, hypotension, hypothermia, tachycardia, bradycardia, or ventricular arrhythmias (Welsh 2003; Seahorn 2004; Macintire et al. 2005). Most concerning, some oscillometric devices will provide readings even when the cuff becomes inadvertently disconnected from the patient (Baetge 2007).

Capnography

Capnography provides a noninvasive method for assessing systemic metabolism, cardiac output, pulmonary perfusion, and the adequacy of patient ventilation in a variety of clinical situations, such as during anesthesia when effects of drugs and inhalants can cause respiratory depression or during long-term ventilatory assistance, as with the use of a mechanical ventilator (Marshall 2004; Weil 2005). Furthermore, capnography is superior over pulse oximetry for the prompt identification of apnea and airway mishaps since changes in the percentage of hemoglobin saturated with oxygen (SpO_2) will be delayed as compared to the instantaneous changes that are visible with end-tidal carbon dioxide ($ETCO_2$) monitoring (Marshall 2004). When alveoli are not perfused, carbon dioxide is unable to diffuse out of the bloodstream. But as blood flow improves and alveoli are perfused, carbon dioxide can then be excreted (Haldane and Marks 2004). Therefore, an abrupt decrease in $ETCO_2$ can be an early and reliable indication of an impending cardiovascular collapse or cardiac arrest (Greene 2002; Tefend 2003b; Marshall 2004). Conversely, since delivery of carbon dioxide from the lungs requires blood flow, cellular metabolism, and alveolar ventilation, the presence of $ETCO_2$ can be used to assess the effectiveness of cardiopulmonary and cerebral resuscitation (CPCR) efforts (Lerche 2000; Haldane and Marks 2004; Marshall 2004; Seahorn 2004).

Carbon dioxide is transported in the body in three forms: after conversion in the red blood cells, 60–70% is transported as bicarbonate ion, another 20–30% is transported while bound to proteins, and the remaining 5–10% is dissolved in plasma. The latter is what is actually measured during blood gas analysis and is known as the arterial partial pressure of carbon dioxide ($PaCO_2$) (Marshall 2004).

Normal $ETCO_2$ values are 35–45 mm Hg (Dodam 1996; Marshall 2004). Under normal circumstances, $ETCO_2$ typically underestimates the $PaCO_2$ by a clinically insignificant 2–5 mm Hg. This difference occurs when there is a slight variance (usually a value of 0.8 in the normal lung) in the ventilation:perfusion ratio (V_A/Q) due to alveolar dead space ventilation where alveoli are ventilated but not perfused (Martin 1999; Marshall 2004). End-tidal carbon dioxide values above 45 mm Hg indicate inadequate ventilation requiring ventilatory assistance via manual or mechanical means. On the contrary by temporarily allowing modest increases in $ETCO_2$ (>45 mm Hg) the anesthetist can bolster arterial blood pressure via endogenous catecholamine release. However be warned that prolonged increases in $ETCO_2$ may cause respiratory acidosis that can eventually lead to narcosis, arrhythmias, subsequent myocardial depression, and heart failure (Taylor and McGehee 1995; Welsh 2003; Seahorn 2004; Weil 2005; Perkowski 2007). Therefore, the highest $ETCO_2$ permissible should be 60 mm Hg (Greene 2002).

End-Tidal Carbon Dioxide Monitoring

The two primary methods for measuring end-tidal carbon dioxide in respiratory gases consist of either *mass spectroscopy* or *infrared light absorption* (Martin 1999; Greene 2002; Marshall 2004). Mass spectrometers function by separating gases and vapors of various molecular weights and determining their elemental composition, but they are deemed impractical due to their expense and bulkiness (Marshall 2004). Therefore, infrared light analyzers are most commonly utilized in veterinary medicine for measuring carbon dioxide in respiratory gases (Marshall 2004).

There are two types of monitors available for assessing end-tidal carbon dioxide: the *capnometer* and the *capnograph*. Both monitors obtain samples of the patient's respiratory gases from the anesthetic circuit via sensing devices placed on the proximal end of the endotracheal tube (Dodam 1996; Seahorn 2004). The sensing device must be placed precisely at the end of the patient's nose to eliminate excessive dead space and prevent rebreathing of carbon dioxide (McCurnin 1994; Greene 2002). Dead space gas is air that is not available for gas exchange and tends to remain relatively constant (Weil 2005). *Anatomic dead space* may consist of air in the nasal passages, mouth, and trachea, while *mechanical dead space* can be the result of an excessively long endotracheal tube or the respiratory monitor itself (Weil 2005). Therefore, it is prudent to eliminate excessive mechanical dead space by trimming the proximal endotracheal tube to a shorter length, thereby allowing it to sit level with the incisors while the distal (cuff) end is located beyond the larynx but no further than the thoracic inlet (Fig. 11.5) (Thurmon et al. 1996; Lukasik 2006).

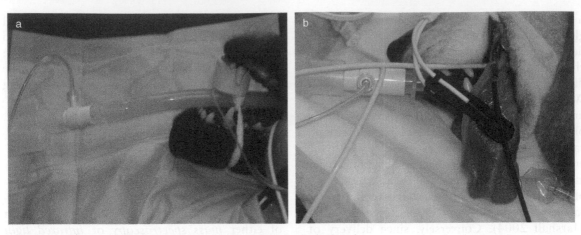

Figure 11.5.   Photos of improper (a) and proper (b) endotracheal tube lengths.

Capnometers provide only numeric ETCO$_2$ values, while capnographs can provide a graphic representation of exhaled carbon dioxide in respiratory gases over time (Fig. 11.6). A normal capnogram is represented by four phases: three expiratory phases and one inspiratory phase. Phase 0 occurs as the inspiratory downstroke and contains CO$_2$ free gas, phase I is the expiratory baseline (which should be zero) and represents the beginning of exhalation, phase II occurs during the expiratory upstroke and includes a rapidly increasing level of CO$_2$, and phase III represents the expiratory plateau when alveolar air is expelled. The highest point of phase III correlates with the actual ETCO$_2$ value (Marshall 2004).

Recognizing abnormalities in ventilation or anesthetic circuit function (e.g., breathing system leaks, apnea, and bronchospasm) is easier using the graphical data provided by a capnogram (Figs. 11.7–12) (Dodam 1996; Thurmon et al. 1996; Greene 2002; Marshall 2004).

Capnometers and capnographs may be categorized as *mainstream* or *sidestream*, based on the location of the sensing device (Greene 2002; Marshall 2004).

Mainstream (nondiverting) monitors

Mainstream (nondiverting) monitors analyze the respiratory gases locally at the endotracheal tube breathing system interface using infrared light rays that distinguish respiratory gases in a photodetector, located within a heated cuvette that prevents water condensation (Marshall 2004). Mainstream monitors provide rapid (<100 milliseconds) results and encounter few problems secondary to secretions or moisture buildup as compared to sidestream technologies. Furthermore, mainstream monitors utilize few disposable supplies and do not require scavenging of sampled gases.

Nonetheless, there are drawbacks associated with mainstream monitors. Due to the weight and location of the monitor, they are prone to accidental disconnection, leaks, and damage, and can cause kinking of the endotracheal tube. Mainstream monitors also require a longer warm-up period (Greene 2002; Marshall 2004). Furthermore, the heated cuvette may cause patient burns (Marshall 2004).

Sidestream (diverting) monitors

Sidestream (diverting) monitors employ small, lightweight, sensing tees placed at the endotracheal tube breathing system interface and pump respiratory gases for analysis up into the measurement chamber via a length of tubing. Sidestream monitors warm up quickly thereby, allowing immediate ETCO$_2$ results and are amendable to remote use (e.g., MRI).

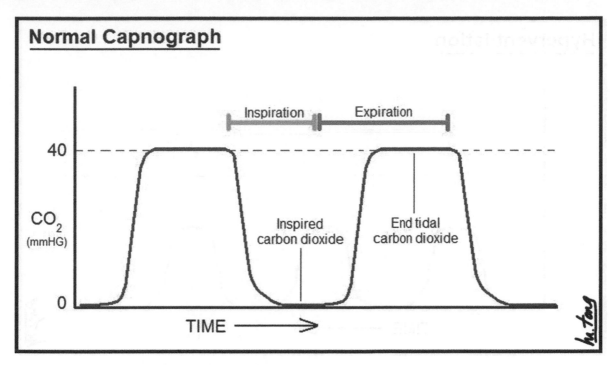

Figure 11.6. Normal capnograph. (Drawing by Mele Tong.)

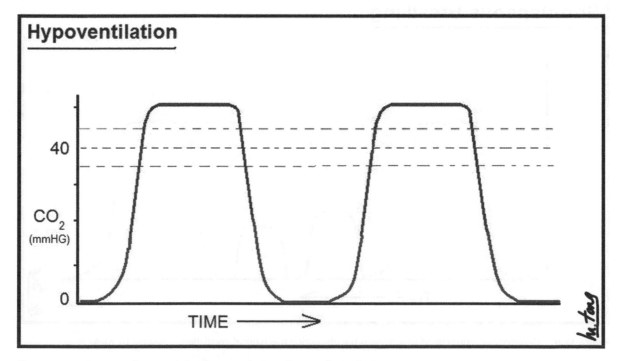

Figure 11.7. Capnograph representing hypoventilation. (Drawing by Mele Tong.)

115

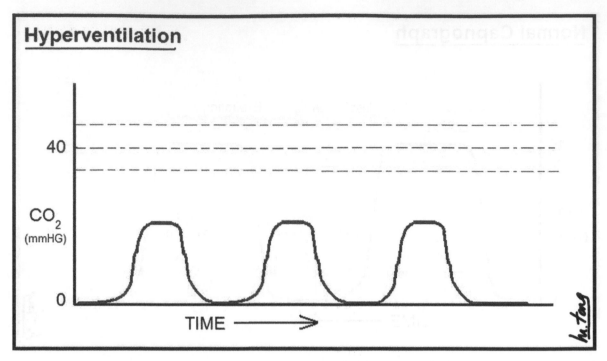

Figure 11.8. Capnograph representing hyperventilation. (Drawing by Mele Tong.)

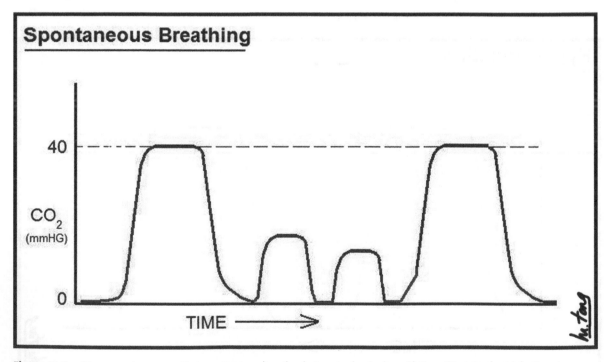

Figure 11.9. Capnograph representing spontaneous breaths during mechanical ventilation. (Drawing by Mele Tong.)

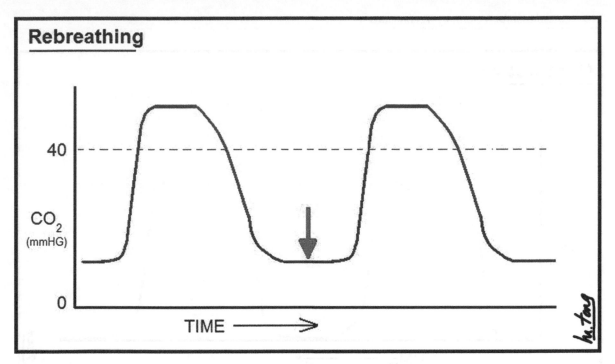

Figure 11.10   Capnograph representing rebreathing of CO_2. (Drawing by Mele Tong.)

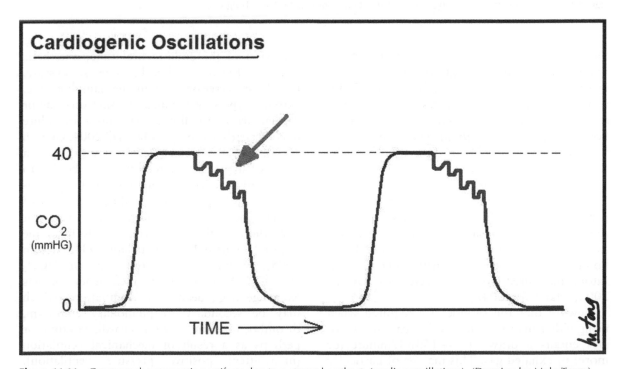

Figure 11.11   Capnograph representing artifacts due to a strong heartbeat. (cardiac oscillations). (Drawing by Mele Tong.)

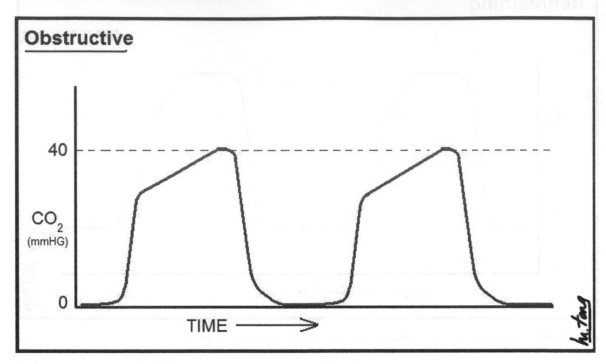

Figure 11.12.   Capnograph showing airway obstruction. (Drawing by Mele Tong.)

Furthermore, they can be used on intubated and nonintubated patients. High fresh gas flow rates in small patients may yield falsely low $ETCO_2$ values and waveform changes due to sample dilution. A moderate reduction in the fresh gas flow rate (10–30 mL/kg/min) can help increase the accuracy of $ETCO_2$ in these small patients (Marshall 2004).

The disadvantages of sidestream monitors include a 2–3 second delay in response time, periodic calibration requirements, frequent replacement of disposable supplies (e.g., sample tubing and sensing tees), and an increased likelihood of sample tubing obstruction due to respiratory moisture, blood, or secretions (Greene 2002; Marshall 2004).

Beware that the sample size required when using either mainstream or sidestream technologies entails a draw of 50–150 mL/minute (or more) of exhaled gas. This may be of particular importance when utilizing low-flow anesthetic techniques (Welsh 2003; Marshall 2004).

There are caveats to $ETCO_2$ monitoring. Esophageal intubation, an inadequate seal or occlusion of the endotracheal tube, anesthetic circuit dysfunction and/or disconnects, moisture, blood, or secretions within the sampling line, extreme hyperventilation, and respiratory and/or cardiac arrest are all potential causes for failure to detect carbon dioxide (Marshall 2004; Glerum 2005). Elevated $ETCO_2$ levels may occur as a result of hypoventilation, which may be due to airway obstruction, pneumothorax, body positioning, or lung disease, or during periods of acutely increased metabolism (e.g., malignant hyperthermia, thyroid storm, or catecholamine release) (Dodam 1996; Marshall 2004; Glerum 2005). Significant disparities between $PaCO_2$ and $ETCO_2$ indicate an inefficiency of gas exchange (e.g., dead space ventilation), which may be secondary to pulmonary embolism, thromboembolism, decreased cardiac output, or perhaps as a result of mechanical ventilation (intermittent positive pressure ventilation). Explanations for elevated $ETCO_2$ along with *inspiratory* carbon dioxide may include faulty anesthetic equipment (e.g., malfunctioning valves within the breathing circuit), unsuitable fresh gas

Table 11.2. Potential causes of changes in the capnogram.

End-Tidal CO$_2$ Change	Potential Causes
Sudden decrease to zero	Airway obstruction Airway disconnection Ventilator failure Capnograph malfunction Obstructed aspirating tube
Sudden decrease to low plateau values	Airway leaks
Exponential decrease in plateau values	Severe cardiovascular disturbance Inadvertent sudden hyperventilation
Slow decrease in plateau values	Hyperventilation Hypothermia Vasoconstriction
Low measurement without good plateau—slow rate of rise	Low aspirating flow rate Fresh gas contamination Incomplete exhalation prior to next inhalation (partial obstruction; bronchospasm, rapid breathing rates)
Low measurement with a good plateau	Uncalibrated capnograph Large physiologic dead space
Increased plateau	Hypoventilation Increased rate of metabolism
Increased baseline	Contaminated sample cell
Increased baseline and plateau	Rebreathing
Increased P(a-A)CO$_2$	Dead space ventilation

Reprinted with permission from Thurmon J, et al. 1996. Lumb and Jones' Veterinary Anesthesia, 3rd ed. Baltimore: Lippincott Williams & Wilkins, pp.413.

flow rates (e.g., nonrebreathing circuits), or exhausted sodalime absorber (Table 11.2).

Furthermore, ETCO$_2$ measurements can at times be simply unreliable; such as when the PaCO$_2$ is greater than 55 mm Hg or during thoracotomy procedures when altered gradients occur due to altered V$_A$/Q (Greene 2002; Marshall 2004; Wagner and Ryan 2006).

Therefore ETCO$_2$ is best used as a trend study tool and ideally should be analyzed in conjunction with an arterial blood gas sample to yield the most complete status of respiratory function (Dodam 1996; Glerum 2005; Wagner and Ryan 2006).

General Care and Maintenance of Blood Pressure and ETCO$_2$ Monitoring Equipment

Proper care and maintenance of all monitoring devices is paramount to ensure their reliable, long-term function. However, there are inherently equipment pieces or parts that will become worn or damaged with time and frequent use. All equipment should be regularly inspected, and worn or damaged parts should be repaired or replaced to ensure many years of dependable service. Blood pressure cuffs may develop holes and should be inspected often and replaced as necessary.

The moisture trap on capnometers or capnographs may overfill, causing monitor malfunction, so they should be checked frequently and emptied or replaced as needed. Additionally, it is important to ensure that sampling lines do not become damaged, clogged, or kinked. Many capnometers and capnographs require periodic calibration for optimal performance and accuracy (Greene 2002). Consult the manufacturer's instruction manual for specific instructions on calibration.

Keep all monitoring equipment clean and free of blood, saline, dust, and dirt. The use of alcohol is to be avoided due to surface damage that may occur, especially with repeated use. A clean, soft cloth slightly moistened with a mild soap and water is all that is usually necessary for the exterior spot cleaning of most monitoring devices.

Always consult the manufacturer's instruction manual for proper care and maintenance guidelines. For older or discontinued monitoring units it may be worthwhile to contact the manufacturer regarding instruction manuals; they may still be available (even if supplied as copies or in an Internet downloadable format).

Although it is advisable to take advantage of manufacturer warranties, it may be prudent to learn whether the manufacturer offers a service contract with equipment purchases. These contracts may include regularly scheduled maintenance, service calls, and minor repairs when necessary.

Acknowledgments

The author would like to thank Mele Tong, CVT, for supplying all of the capnogram diagrams, and the National Association of Veterinary Technicians in America (NAVTA) Journal (Spring 2008) for allowing portions of this article to be reprinted for this publication.

References

Acierno, M, Labato, MA. 2004. Hypertension in dogs and cats. Compendium 26, No. 5.

Baetge, C. 2007. Back to basics: Monitoring the anesthetized patient. Vet Tech 28, No. 1.

Beal, MW. 2006. Vascular Access in the Trauma Patient. Proceedings Michigan Veterinary Conference.

Cowgill, LD. 2006. Accuracy of Methods for Blood Pressure Measurement. Proceedings American College of Veterinary Internal Medicine, pp.658–659.

Dodam, JR. 1996. Monitoring the Anesthetized Patient. Proceedings American College of Veterinary Surgeons, pp.535–537.

Duffy, T. 2007. Hemodynamic Monitoring. Proceedings American College of Veterinary Surgeons, pp.621–626.

Durham, HE. 2005. Arterial blood pressure measurement. Vet Tech May:324–339.

Glerum, LE. 2005. Anesthetic Monitoring: Interpreting the Data. Proceedings American College of Veterinary Surgeons, pp.652–655.

Greene, S. 2002. Veterinary Anesthesia and Pain Management Secrets. Philadelphia: Hanley & Belfus, Inc., pp.1, 17–18, 113–119, 135–136.

Haldane, S, Marks, SL. 2004. Cardiopulmonary cerebral resuscitation: Techniques. Compendium 26, No. 10.

Lerche, P. 2000. Monitoring Small Animal Patients. Proceedings American College of Veterinary Surgeons, pp.162–166.

Love, L, Harvey, R. 2006. Arterial blood pressure measurement; Physiology, tools and techniques. Compendium 28, No. 6.

Lukasik, VM. 2006. Anesthesia of the Pediatric Patient. NAVTA J Fall:52–57.

Macintire, DK, et al. 2005. Monitoring Critical Patients, Manual of Small Animal Emergency and Critical Care Medicine. Baltimore: Lippincott Williams & Wilkins, pp.73–74.

Marshall, M. 2004. Capnography in dogs. Compendium 26, No. 10.

Martin, L. 1999. All You Really Need to Know to Interpret Arterial Blood Gases. Baltimore: Lippincott Williams & Wilkins, pp.15, 35, 37.

Mazzaferro, EM. 2004. Arterial Catheterization. Proceedings International Veterinary Emergency & Critical Care Symposium.

McCurnin, D. 1994. Clinical Textbook for Veterinary Technicians, 3rd ed. Philadelphia: WB Saunders, pp.234–240.

Mosley, C. 2006. Anesthetic Management of the Geriatric Patient, NAVTA J Summer:52–58.

Muir, W, et al. 2000. Handbook of Veterinary Anesthesia, 3rd ed. St. Louis: Mosby, pp.251, 276–278, 455.

Perkowski, S. 2007. Anesthetic Crises. Proceedings American College of Veterinary Surgeons, pp.595.

Seahorn, J. 2004. Monitoring the Anesthetized Small Animal Patient. NAVTA J Winter: 53–58.

Stokes, JE, Bartages, JW. 2006. Causes of acute renal failure. Compendium 28, No. 5.

Taylor, R, McGehee, R. 1995. Manual of Small Animal Postoperative Care. Media, PA: Williams & Wilkins, pp.12, 93–97.

Tefend, M. 2003a. Blood pressure monitoring: What you may not know. Proceedings American College of Veterinary Internal Medicine.

Tefend, M. 2003b. Hemodynamic Monitoring in the Postoperative Patient. Proceedings American College of Veterinary Surgeons.

Tefend, M. 2007. Acute renal failure—Causes and treatment. Vet Tech 28, No. 2.

Tegtmeyer, K, et al. 2006. Placement of an arterial line. N Eng J Med 354:15.

Terry, B. 2006. Step by step: Arterial catheter placement. Vet Tech 27, No. 7.

Thurmon, J, et al. 1996. Lumb and Jones' Veterinary Anesthesia and Analgesia, 3rd ed. Baltimore: Lippincott Williams & Wilkins, pp.411, 413, 414, 417, 859.

Valverde, A. 2003. Monitoring the Anesthetized Patient: What Do the Numbers Mean? Proceedings American College of Veterinary Surgeons.

Waddell, LS. 2004. Blood Pressure Monitoring for the Critically Ill. Proceedings Western Veterinary Conference.

Wagner, AE, Ryan, SD. 2006. An in-depth look: Cesarean section in dogs: Anesthetic management. Compendium 28, No 1.

Weil, A. 2005. Anesthetic emergencies. NAVTA J Spring:42–48.

Welsh, E. 2003. Anaesthesia for Veterinary Nurses. London: Blackwell Science Ltd., pp. 230–231, 236.

12

Fluid Therapy and Blood Products

Courtney Beiter

Before selecting the appropriate fluid therapy for each patient, it is important to understand the body compartments that retain the fluid being administered. Roughly 60% of the patient's body weight is water. Of that 60%, 66.6% is intracellular and 33.3% is extracellular. The extracellular compartment is composed of 25% intravascular water and 75% interstitial water (Kirby and Rudloff 2000).

Transcellular fluid is another type and includes cerebrospinal fluid, gastrointestinal fluid, lymph, bile, glandular and respiratory secretions, and synovial fluid. Transcellular fluid is produced through specific cell actions. It is not a transudate from plasma, meaning it should have a higher protein and cell count. Transcellular fluids are not taken into account when assessing extracellular fluid volume.

The intracellular compartment is the space within a cell membrane, which is permeable to water. The intravascular fluid is contained within the arteries, veins, and capillaries. The capillaries are the sites of fluid exchange between the intravascular and interstitial spaces, with the interstitial space being the extravascular space between vasculature and cells. The size of the solute will determine whether it can move freely across capillary membranes. Lipid soluble molecules such as oxygen and carbon dioxide can move easily. Nonlipid soluble particles must diffuse through "endothelial intercellular clefts" (Kirby and Rudloff 2000).

The interstitium, which comprises less than 1% of free fluid in normal tissues uses kinetic motion to diffuse solutes. The diffusion of electrolytes, nutrients, cellular waste material, oxygen, carbon dioxide, and proteins occurs rapidly. The lymphatic system removes excess fluid, protein molecules, and debris from the interstitial fluid compartments to systemic circulation. The movement of surrounding tissues propels this. Cellular metabolism depends upon the filtering and exchange of interstitial fluid. This filtration of water and solutes from the capillaries to the interstitium allows delivery of water, nutrients, oxygen, and electrolytes to cells for metabolism. The waste-containing fluid diffuses from the interstitium to venous capillaries where it is then transported to the liver, lung, and kidneys for degradation and excretion.

Interstitial edema occurs when the lymphatic system is overwhelmed. It is a result of a decrease in oncotic pressure and an increase in hydrostatic pressure. This can occur due to shock, illness, or trauma. The capillary endothelial junctions can become separated when previously hypoxic tissues become reperfused. This then results in the leaking of albumin and fluids out of the intravascular space. Shock states can also lead to edema formation. This is caused when the intracellular water content is increased. The resultant hypovolemia and edema then lead to a decrease in oxygen transport and therefore a decrease in oxygen diffusion to cells (Kirby and Rudloff 2000).

The number, charge, and size of the particles determine the movement of fluid across the mentioned compartments. Capillary dynamics also play a role in this. Osmosis is the movement of water from a solution of lesser solute concentration to a solution of greater solute concentration across a semipermeable membrane (Blood and Studdert 1999). Osmotic pressure is the amount of pressure needed on the opposite side of the membrane to oppose the movement of solutes. An equal number of cations and anions needs to be on either side to ensure electrochemical neutrality between the intravascular and interstitial compartments.

Classifications of Fluids

There are two main classifications of fluids: crystalloids and colloids. Within each of these classifications there are many different types of fluids. The type of fluid therapy chosen for administration should be based upon the current needs of the patient.

Crystalloids

Any solutions that contain electrolyte and non-electrolyte solutes can be classified as crystalloids. They can enter all body fluid compartments but have their main effect on the interstitial and intracellular spaces.

Crystalloids can be further broken down into isotonic, hypertonic, and hypotonic preparations. Isotonic fluids, Normosol-R and Plasma-Lyte 148, have a similar sodium and chloride concentration to that of the extracellular fluid, as well as a similar osmolarity. Normal saline is also said to be isotonic (although not balanced),

due to the sodium and chloride content. Hypotonic solutions, 0.45% NaCl, 5% dextrose, Normosol-M, and Plasma-Lyte 56, have a lower sodium and chloride content and a higher potassium content. Hypertonic crystalloids, such as 3% NaCl, 7.2% NaCl, or 23.7% NaCl, have much higher sodium and chloride content than that of the extracellular fluid.

Crystalloids can be further classified as balanced or unbalanced solutions. Balanced solutions have a fluid composition that closely resembles the patient's extracellular fluid. Some examples of this would be lactated Ringer's solution, Normosol-R, and Plasma-Lyte 148. Unbalanced solutions do not have a fluid composition that resembles the patient's extracellular fluid. Normal/physiologic saline (0.9%) would be an example of an unbalanced solution.

Crystalloids are used to expand the plasma compartment. However, 2.5–3 times as much crystalloid, compared to colloid, must be given because they are rapidly redistributed to the intracellular and interstitial spaces (DiBartola and Bateman 2006).

Colloids

Colloid preparations contain large molecular weight substances that, in a patient with an uncompromised endothelium, will stay within the plasma compartment. They are predominantly used as expanders of the intravascular space. There are natural and synthetic colloids. Plasma, whole blood, and concentrated albumin are examples of natural colloids. Dextrans, hydroxyethyl starch (hetastarch and pentastarch), and hemoglobin-based oxygen-carrying (HBOC) fluids are all examples of synthetic colloids. Colloids may be preferred for use in fluid resuscitation due to the smaller volumes that are required when compared to fluid resuscitation with crystalloids alone. There are both benefits and drawbacks to each colloid preparation.

Albumin

Albumin is the predominant plasma protein and is pooled from human donors. It is available in both a 4% and a 25% preparation. However, the 25% preparation is the most widely used in clinical settings. Vascular expansion depends on the amount given, not on the solution concentration. The main drawback to albumin administration is the cost. A hypersensitivity reaction can also be seen, even with the first dose administered, because it is a human product. Care should also be taken when administering albumin so as not to fluid-overload the patient, especially when using the 25% preparation.

Hetastarch

Hetastarch is a plasma volume expander and will give equivalent plasma volume expansion to that of 4% albumin, but for a lower cost. Coagulopathies have been shown with hetastarch, but they are most likely to be seen when the recommended dosages have been exceeded (DiBartola and Bateman 2006). This is thought to be caused through hemodilution. It can also interfere with factor VIII and von Willebrand's factor. Hetastarch is dosed at 10–40 mL/kg/day IV to effect in the canine. In felines the dose is 5 mL/kg IV to effect, with a maximum of 40 mL/kg/day. However, many feel that a maximum of 20 mL/kg/day should be sufficient. This is especially true in felines due to a potential risk for fluid overload and pulmonary edema (Roberts and Bratton 1998). Careful monitoring of the patient's hemodynamic parameters should be done to evaluate them during fluid resuscitation. This is especially true in shock patients or those with potential lung injury. These types of patients are more prone to fluid overload and the possibility of extravascular lung water (Roberts and Bratton 1998).

Dextran

Dextran solution preparations come as either Dextran 40, a 10% solution or Dextran 70, a 6% solution. They are made from a glucose polymer that is produced by bacteria grown on sucrose media. Both preparations produce an initial intravascular volume expansion, but the effect is temporary. Fifty percent is lost within 3 hours, and 60% is lost within 6 hours (DiBartola and Bateman 2006). Dextrans is dosed at 10–

40 mL/kg/day IV in canines. In felines the dose is 5 mL/kg IV over 5–10 minutes, and it can be redosed as needed, not to exceed 40 mL/kg (Kirby and Rudloff 2000). Dextran solutions should be used cautiously. Dextran 70 can have a more dramatic effect on coagulopathies than other colloid preparations. Dextran 40 has been shown to lead to renal failure in some patients and is not widely used.

Types of Fluid Therapy

The purpose of fluid therapy is to be supportive. This can be accomplished through three phases: resuscitation, rehydration or maintenance fluid therapy. A healthy patient undergoing general anesthesia for a routine procedure may require only maintenance fluids. These would help to maintain an open catheter in the case of an emergency while also helping to maintain hydration, blood pressure, and therefore adequate blood flow to vital organs. A patient that is dehydrated will require prolonged fluid therapy over 12–36 hours to replace fluid losses (DiBartola and Bateman 2006). An unstable patient may require resuscitation with bolus therapy by a combination of crystalloids and colloids.

Maintenance fluid therapy

Maintenance fluids are administered at a rate of 40–60 mL/kg/day (Seeler 1996). They are designed to meet the water and electrolyte requirements for patients that are not taking in enough fluids to meet their daily losses. These losses can occur as either insensible or sensible losses. Insensible losses are those that occur through the skin, fecal waste, and respiratory tract. Sensible losses occur as urine output (Plunkett 2002). Maintenance fluid solutions should be isotonic, meaning they closely match the sodium and chloride concentration and have a higher potassium concentration compared to the patient's extracellular fluid.

Hypotonic solutions, those that have a lower concentration of sodium and chloride than that of the extracellular fluid, may also be used for maintenance fluid therapy. Other uses of hypotonic solutions are in renal failure patients, those with congestive heart failure or hypernatremia, and patients on potassium bromide (KBr) therapy. Patients receiving KBr should be on a lower chloride-containing fluid because bromide will follow chloride, and a higher concentration of chloride in the blood will decrease serum bromide levels. However, these fluids should be used cautiously. They should not be administered as bolus doses and can cause electrolyte abnormalities in some patients.

Long-term fluid therapy of any kind may cause a hypokalemia by evoking a diuresis. Therefore, fluids should be supplemented with potassium chloride (KCl) at 20 mEq/L. Caution should be used to not administer bolus doses of fluids containing supplemental KCl. The maximum rate of KCl administration should not exceed 0.5 mEq/kg/hr (Seeler 1996).

Replacement fluid therapy

Replacement fluids should be isotonic and contain a balanced electrolyte solution. They then can be given as a bolus dose without causing electrolyte abnormalities in a patient with already normal electrolyte values. Isotonic fluids do not lead to fluid shifts between the intracellular and extracellular spaces, but they rapidly equilibrate across the intravascular and interstitial spaces. Therefore, only 25% of the total volume administered stays within the intravascular space. If replacing blood loss with crystalloids alone, three times the volume of blood lost must be given. When replacing losses due to dehydration,

Table 12.1. Physical findings in dehydration.

Percent Dehydration	Clinical Sign
<5	Not detectable
5–6	Subtle loss of skin elasticity
6–8	Definite delay in return of skin to normal position Slight prolongation of CRT Eyes possibly sunken in orbits Possibly dry mucous membranes
10–12	Tented skin stands in place Definite prolongation of CRT Eyes sunken in orbits Dry mucous membranes Possible signs of shock (tachycardia, cool extremities, rapid and weak pulses)
12–15	Definite signs of shock Death imminent

From Muir, WW, DiBartola, SP. 1983. Fluid therapy. In Current Veterinary Therapy VIII, edited by Kirk, RW. Philadelphia: WB Saunders, p.33.

the percent of dehydration should be calculated first (Table 12.1) (Muir and DiBartola 1983). Next, the required replacement fluids should be calculated (Figure 12.1).

The same fluids can be used for both replacement and maintenance fluid therapy. However, adequate renal function should be present to

1. Hydration deficit (replacement requirement)
   a. Body weight (lbs) × % dehydration as a decimal
      X 500* = deficit in milliliters
   b. Body weight (kg) × % dehydration as a decimal
      = deficit in liters

   *500 ml = 1 lb

Figure 12.1. Calculation of replacement requirement (hydration deficit) (From Muir, WW, DiBartola, SP. 1983. Fluid therapy. In Current Veterinary Therapy VIII, edited by Kirk, RW. Philadelphia: WB Saunders, p.35.)

ensure appropriate elimination of electrolytes in excess of daily requirements.

Isotonic saline, also known as normal saline or physiologic saline, can also be used as a replacement fluid. It is available as 0.9% NaCl and only the sodium is isotonic. It does not meet the patient's daily electrolyte requirements when used as a maintenance fluid. It is used for rapid expansion of the extracellular fluid volume and is quickly redistributed throughout the extracellular space. Isotonic saline can have an acidifying effect because of its high chloride content and should be used cautiously in patients that are already acidemic.

Resuscitation fluid therapy

The patient's clinical history and physical exam findings should determine whether the fluid resuscitation phase is needed. A patient in shock will usually present with pale mucous membranes and a prolonged to absent capillary refill time (CRT), tachycardia or severe bradycardia, cool extremities, weak to absent peripheral pulses, and hypotension. There are several different forms of shock that will be discussed more in depth later in the chapter. Hypovolemic and distributive types of shock typically respond better to rapid volume expansion. Obstructive shock responds better to moderate fluid therapy. Fluid therapy is contraindicated in most cases of cardiogenic shock (DiBartola and Bateman 2006). Shock fluid resuscitation can include crystalloids, colloids, and blood products if needed.

Electrolyte Abnormalities

Hypochloremia/hyperchloremia

Hypochloremia can result due to a lipemic blood sample, vomiting of stomach contents, chronic respiratory acidosis, hyperadrenocorticism (Cushing's disease), exercise, or sodium bicarbonate therapy. It can also be a result of thiazide (hydrochlorothiazide) or loop diuretic (furosemide) drug therapy (Autran de Morais and Biondo 2006).

Hyperchloremia can also be a result of a lipemic blood sample. Other causes are potassium bromide (KBr) therapy, which causes the analyzer to read bromide as chloride, high chloride-containing fluids, diarrhea, or an overall gain of chloride due to potassium supplementation or salt poisoning. Renal chloride retention can occur as a result of renal failure, hypoadrenocorticism (Addison's disease), diabetes mellitus, chronic respiratory alkalosis, or spironolactone drug therapy.

The treatment for both hypochloremia and hyperchloremia is accomplished through finding and treating the underlying cause (Autran de Morais and Biondo 2006), although fluid therapy should be implemented in the meantime.

Hyponatremia/hypernatremia

Sodium is a major extracellular cation. A serum sodium concentration tells the amount of sodium compared to the amount of water in the patient's extracellular fluid. A patient is considered hyponatremic if its sodium is less than 140 mEq/L for a canine and less than 149 mEq/L for a feline. Hyponatremia will result when a patient is unable to excrete ingested water or when its urinary and insensible losses have a greater osmolality than that of the ingested or administered fluids (DiBartola, 2006).

A patient is considered hypernatremic when its sodium is greater than 155 mEq/L for a canine and greater than 162 mEq/L for a feline. Hypernatremia can result due to an inadequate intake of water, an excessive amount of sodium ingested or administered, a pure water deficit, hypotonic loss, or hemorrhagic shock.

Clinical signs of hyponatremia and hypernatremia are the same, but they have very different causes. In hypernatremia neurologic effects can be seen due to a rapid decrease in brain volume caused by rupture of cerebral vessels or focal hemorrhage. Hyponatremia leads to cerebral edema, which will also cause the patient to exhibit neurological signs. The severity of signs is related to the rapidity of onset, not to the magnitude. The neurologic signs can include weakness, behavioral changes, disorientation, ataxia, seizures, coma, and death. Anorexia, lethargy, and vomiting can also be seen (DiBartola 2006).

Acute hyponatremia can be corrected with LRS, 0.9% NaCl, or even hypertonic fluid administration. Chronic hyponatremia, as well as chronic hypernatremia must be treated much more slowly. Sodium levels must not be changed any more rapidly than 10–12 mEq/L in 24 hours (0.5 mEq/L/hr) for fear of causing some of the same neurologic effects that are trying to be resolved (DiBartola 2006). See Figure 12.2 for calculating fluid rates for sodium changes. When treating chronic hyponatremic patients, be sure to keep their water intake less than their urine output in the case of psychogenic polydipsia. Also be sure to discontinue any antidiuretic medications.

In the case of a pure water deficit leading to hypernatremia, the treatment is 5% dextrose in water (D5W) or 0.45% NaCl administration. When using DW the glucose will quickly enter the cells and be metabolized, leaving only water. Be sure to replace the water deficit slowly. If a hypotonic loss has occurred and signs of volume depletion are seen, rapid extracellular volume repletion with an isotonic fluid is necessary. In the case of hemorrhagic shock, whole blood, plasma, or colloid solutions can be administered in conjunction with crystalloids (DiBartola 2006). The important thing to remember is to closely monitor the sodium levels of your patient.

Hypokalemia/hyperkalemia

Potassium is a major intracellular cation. Hypokalemia can be caused by an insulin administration or glucose-containing fluids, vomiting of stomach contents, or diarrhea. Urinary losses can also occur. They are seen in chronic renal failure patients, postobstructive diuresis, dialysis, hyperadrenocorticism (Cushing's disease), or primary hyperaldosteronism. Medications such as loop diuretics, thiazide diuretics, amphotericein B and pencillins can also lead to a hypokalemia (DiBartola and Autran de Morais 2006).

Signs of hypokalemia will vary patient to patient and also depend on the severity. Some patients will have no clinical signs. Other patients with values less than 3.0 mEq/L will exhibit signs such as polyuria/polydipsia (PU/PD), a decrease in urine-concentrating capabilities, and even muscle weakness possibly leading to respiratory paralysis. Cardiovascular signs may also be noted. These include delayed ventricular repolarization, increased duration of action potential, and an increased automaticity. Supraventricular and ventricular arrhythmias can be seen. A prolongation of the QT interval may be seen with

$$\text{Rate of Na+ Change} = \frac{(\text{Na+ of the fluid} - \text{Na+ of the patient})}{(0.6 \times \text{BW in kg}) + 1}$$

For example:
Patient's Na+ 190mEq/L
Wt. 20 kg
LRS (Na 130 mEq/L Na+)
Fluid rate 100 ml/hr

$$= \frac{130 - 190}{(0.6 \times 20) + 1} = 4.6 \text{ mEq/L}$$

This is a safe fluid choice and rate. A liter bag would last 10 hours and the Na+ can safely be adjusted by 5 mEq.

Figure 12.2.   Fluid rate calculation for sodium correction.

potassium values less than 2.0 mEq/L, and they may become unresponsive to antiarrhythmic therapy (DiBartola and Autran de Morais 2006).

The treatment for hypokalemia is potassium supplementation. To avoid adverse cardiac effects during potassium supplementation do not administer potassium any faster than 0.5 mEq/kg/hr IV. Potassium is available as KCl (2 mEq/mL) or potassium phosphates (4.36 mEq K+/mL). If the hypokalemia is due to vomiting or diuretic administration, KCl is the treatment of choice. See Table 12.2 for an estimate on the amount of KCl to add to parenteral fluids based on the patient's serum potassium value.

The effects of hyperkalemia, like hypokalemia, depend on the individual patient as well as the magnitude of the elevation. A potassium value greater than 6.5 mEq/L needs immediate treatment. Hyperkalemia is an uncommon finding in patients with normal renal function and urine output.

Hyperkalemia can have many causes. It can be due to calculation errors with constant rate infusions. It is seen in diabetic patients due to an insulin deficiency and hyperosmolality. Decreased urinary excretion from a urethral obstruction, ruptured bladder, or anuric/oliguric renal failure will also lead to an increased potassium. Hypoadrenocorticism will also cause hyperkalemia.

Table 12.2. Guidelines for routine intravenous supplementation of potassium in dogs and cats.

Serum Potassium Concentration (mEq/L)	mEq KCl to Add to 250 mL Fluid	mEq KCl to Add to 1 L Fluid	Maximal Fluid Infusion Rate (mL/kg/hr)
<2.0	20	80	6
2.1–2.5	15	60	8
2.6–3.0	10	40	12
3.1–3.5	7	28	18
3.6–5.0	5	20	25

From Greene, RW, Scott, RC. 1975. Lower urinary tract disease. In Textbook of Veterinary Internal Medicine, edited by Ettinger, SJ. Philadelphia: WB Saunders, p.1572.

Changes on an electrocardiogram (ECG) can be indicative of hyperkalemia. Shortening of the QT interval, tented T-waves, prolongation of PR interval, widening of the QRS complex, and disappearance of the P waves are all common findings on the ECG (DiBartola and Autran de Morais 2006). These arrhythmias can progress to atrial standstill and asystole.

Hyperkalemia is a life-threatening condition and needs to be treated immediately. The patient should be started on intravenous fluids. Lactated Ringer's solution and Plasma-Lyte 148 could both be used. Historically, the fluid of choice has been 0.9% NaCl because of its lack of potassium and maximal dilutional effects. Fluid therapy will improve renal perfusion and enhance urinary excretion of potassium. Ultimately, the underlying cause needs to be addressed. For example, if the hyperkalemia is caused by a urethral obstruction, the patient needs to be stabilized and then deobstructed.

If intravenous fluid therapy does not act quickly enough, calcium gluconate 10% solution should be administered at a dose of 2–10 mL total to protect the heart against the effects of hyperkalemia on electrical conduction. Its effects are short-lived, so the potassium level should still be corrected. Sodium bicarbonate can be administered at a dose of 1–2 mEq/kg IV to help move K+ ions into cells as H+ ions leave cells. Insulin can also be used to treat hyperkalemia by shifting potassium into the cells in exchange for sodium. The dose is 0.55–1.1 µ/kg IV for dogs, and for cats the dose is 1 unit per cat. There is a risk of hypoglycemia occurring; therefore, dextrose can be added to the fluids at a 5% concentration. The patient's potassium and glucose values should be closely monitored. Dextrose alone can also be used. It will stimulate endogenous insulin release.

Hypovolemic Shock

Hypovolemic shock is caused by a loss of intravascular volume. This can occur through dehydration, acute blood loss (hemorrhagic shock), or third-space loss of fluids. Patients with hypovolemic shock can present with hemoperitoneum secondary to hepatic or splenic neoplasia or trauma. They can also have hemoperitoneum or hemothorax due to anticoagulant rodenticide toxicity, thrombocytopenia, or thrombocytopathia. A patient can also be in hypovolemic shock due to gastrointestinal hemorrhage, epistaxis, or lacerations of major arteries.

Nonhemorrhagic hypovolemic shock is a loss of circulating blood volume without a loss of whole blood. This occurs as a result of a loss of plasma through either severe dehydration or third-space loss into the peritoneum, pleural space, or gastrointestinal tract.

In this type of shock, acute volume resuscitation and interstitial fluid replacement (in the case of severe dehydration) are necessary. Crystalloids (0.9% NaCl, Normosol, Plasma-Lyte) can be used. The dose for a dog is 90 mL/kg IV and 55 mL/kg IV for a cat. These doses have been traditionally given as fast as possible. They can still be given as fast as within 10–15 minutes, but many clinicians are dividing this dose into aliquots (1/4, 1/3, etc.), giving that volume over 10–15 minutes and then assessing the patient before giving the next volume. Titrating to effect to achieve certain end points should help prevent fluid overload. These end points should include a return to normal heart rate, systolic blood pressure between 90–120 mm Hg, improved capillary refill time, and mucous membrane color.

Hypertonic crystalloids can also be used. With 7% NaCl the dose is 4 mL/kg IV over 5 minutes. 23.4% hypertonic NaCl can also be diluted with 6% hetastarch to make a 7.5% solution (approximately a 1:2 ratio of 23.4% NaCl to hetastarch). When using this method, intravascular volume expansion is obtained with additional and longer lasting support of the colloid. The dosage is 4 mL/kg of the combination and can be administered at no faster than 1 mL/kg/min (Day and Bateman 2006). Another choice for fluid resuscitation is hetastarch alone. It is dosed at 20 mL/kg/day.

Cardiogenic Shock

Fluid therapy is typically contraindicated in this type of shock. The use of diuretics to help redis-tribute fluid from the lungs back into circulation, inotropic support (by way of dopamine or dobutamine), and antiarrhythmic agents are the most important means of support and stabilization for these patients (Day and Bateman 2006).

Obstructive Shock

Causes of obstructive shock are pericardial effusion causing cardiac tamponade, heartworm disease leading to caval syndrome, pulmonary thromboembolism (PTE), and aortic thromboembolism, as well as cardiac neoplasia. A patient presenting with a gastric dilatation and volvulous (GDV) can also have decreased ventricular filling due to a decrease in venous return to the heart (Day and Bateman 2006). In obstructive shock patients, initiating a moderate or maintenance fluid therapy is appropriate while attempting to find and treat the underlying cause of the obstruction. The one exception to this would be in GDV patients. They benefit from shock dose fluid therapy using crystalloids at up to 90 mL/kg IV. This will help restore vascular volume.

Blood Products

There are many different types of blood products to choose from depending on the desired effect. Blood products can be either natural or synthetic colloids. Natural colloids include whole blood, packed red blood cells (PRBC), plasma, or human immunoglobulin (IGg). Oxyglobin is an example of a synthetic colloid.

Whole blood

Whole blood, the most commonly used of all blood products is combined with an anticoagulant during the collection process. The dose can be calculated one of two ways. It can be dosed at 13–22 mL/kg or can be calculated using the desired packed cell volume (PCV), current PCV and donor PCV. This calculation is shown in

Figure 12.3. Whole blood must be used within 8 hours of collection. It is used in anemic patients for oxygen-carrying capacity and in patients with coagulation factor deficiency. However, it is not recommended to use whole blood solely for coagulation factors; this can lead to an iatrogenic polycythemia.

Packed red blood cells (PRBCs)

PRBCs are whole blood that is centrifuged into PRBC and plasma. One unit from a canine would contain around 200 mL/unit, have a hematocrit of 80%, and cost around $121.00. Packed red blood cells are used for restoring and maintaining enough of an oxygen supply to meet tissue demands. They are used to treat anemia due to blood loss, hemolysis, and bone marrow dysfunction. The decision to transfuse should not be based solely on the patient's hematocrit or hemoglobin values. It should be based on the cardiovascular status, anticipated blood loss, ability of the bone marrow to respond, and chronicity of the anemia (Hohenhaus 2000).

Fresh frozen plasma (FFP)

FFP is collected and frozen within 8 hours to maintain clotting factors V and VIII. It is whole blood that is collected and centrifuged, and then the plasma is expressed into a satellite bag. It contains electrolytes, albumin, globulins, coagulation factors, and other proteins. It is used to treat coagulation factor deficiencies due to rodenticide intoxication, vitamin K–dependent coagulopathies in Devon Rex felines, hemophilia B (factor IX deficiency), von Willebrand's disease,

and hemophilia A (factor VIII: C deficiency). The dose is 6–10 mL/kg IV over 4 hours. The cost is around $104.00 per unit with a canine unit containing 100–140 mL.

Cryoprecipitate

Cryoprecipitate is collected by thawing FFP at a temperature of 1–6 °C until a thick white precipitate is formed and centrifuges off. Cryoprecipitate contains factors VIII: C, XIII, von Willebrand's factor, and fibrinogen. The cost is around $123.00 per unit and the dose is 1 unit per 10 kg. The benefit of using this over FFP is the decreased amount being administered and therefore a decreased risk of volume overload in the patient.

Human immunoglobulin (IGg)

Human IGg is used along with immunosuppressive therapy to treat immune-mediated hemolytic anemia (Fig. 12.4). It is prepared from pooled human plasma and therefore still runs a risk of reaction with repeated doses. The dose is 0.5–1 gram/kg and is administered over 6–8 hours. The major downfall is cost. It can cost up to $300.00 to treat a 10 kg dog (Hohenhaus 2000).

Blood Typing

There are more than 13 canine blood types that have been identified. However, there are tests available for typing only 6 of them for lab use. There are typing cards available for clinic use for DEA (dog erythrocyte antigen) negative and

$$\frac{\text{Desired PCV} - \text{Actual patient PCV}}{\text{PCV anticoagulant donor blood}} \times \frac{\text{Recipient blood}}{\text{volume}}$$

$$\text{Blood volume} = 88 \text{ ml/kg in a canine}$$
$$66 \text{ ml/kg in a feline}$$

Figure 12.3. Amount of transfused blood needed. (From Muir WW, et al. 2000. Blood transfusion. In Handbook of Veterinary Anesthesia, 3rd ed., edited by Schrefer, JA. St. Louis: Mosby, Inc., pp.424–425.)

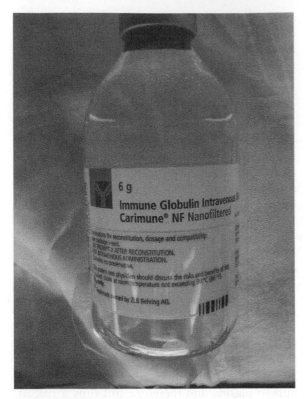

Figure 12.4.   Photo of a 6 g vial of immune globulin. (Photo taken by author.)

positive patients. Use of the typing cards is very easy. Blood is obtained from the patient and a drop is placed on the three wells: the patient sample, the DEA 1.1–, and the DEA 1.1+. A drop of diluent is also placed on each well. Each drop then needs to be stirred and mixed for 1 minute. Autoagglutination over one of the wells means that is the correct blood type. This is always going to be true except in the case of the patient autoagglutinating. In that case, the patient should be given DEA 1.1– blood for a decreased chance of a transfusion reaction (Hohenhaus 2000).

Cats historically have been thought to have only one blood group that contains the types A, B, and AB. Cats naturally have antibodies against other blood group antigens that they lack. Type A cats will have anti-B antibodies and type B cats will have anti-A antibodies. It is these antigens that are responsible for hemolytic transfusion reactions. Recently, another blood group antigen has been discovered that is clinically significant. It has been named the *Mik* antigen. In cats that

are *Mik* negative anti-*Mik* antibodies are present and could cause a hemolytic transfusion reaction. It is recommended that all cats be blood-typed prior to any blood transfusion. They should also be cross-matched with donors in their blood type to avoid a transfusion reaction (Lynel and Ewing 2009).

The majority of cats are type A, less than 1% are going to be type AB. If the wrong type of blood is administered, a transfusion reaction will occur leading to a shortened RBC survival or acute hemolysis. Blood typing is quick and easy for cats as well. After a blood sample is obtained, a drop of diluent and a drop of blood is placed on the type A and type B wells and are mixed for 1 minute; then the results can be read. Whichever agglutinates well is the correct blood type (Fig. 12.5).

Any patient that has received a transfusion in the past (greater than 4 days) needs to be cross-matched before receiving a subsequent transfusion.

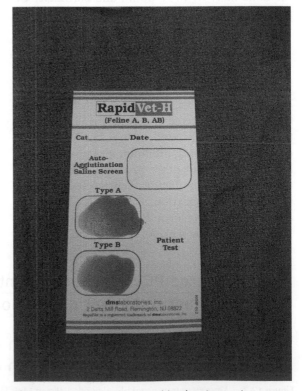

Figure 12.5.   Photo of a feline blood typing card. Patient is type A; note the agglutination in the type A box. (Photo taken by author.)

Transfusions

Caution needs to be taken with any transfusion being administered. If FFP is being used, the unit needs to be thawed first. There is no need to warm a unit of PRBC or whole blood (Fig. 12.6, 12.7). Any unit being used needs to be closely inspected for leaks or signs of contamination such as a brownish color. The label should be checked to ensure the correct species and the correct blood type or plasma type (Fig. 12.8). No medications should be added to the transfusion line after it is being administered. Normal saline is the only type of fluid compatible with a transfusion. All blood products need to be delivered through a 170 micron filter that will help remove any clots or debris. If using a syringe for smaller amounts of blood administration, an 18 micron filter can be used instead.

When starting a transfusion with any type of blood product, the full volume must be administered within 4 hours to avoid contamination. A temperature, pulse, and respiratory rate (TPR) should be obtained from the patient, and then the transfusion can be started. The first 15 minutes of the transfusion should be administered at half the rate, a TPR repeated, and if still within normal limits, the transfusion rate doubled. A TPR should then be checked every 30 minutes to continue to monitor for a reaction.

A hemolytic transfusion reaction can occur as a result of naturally occurring, preformed alloantibodies against the RBC. This is induced

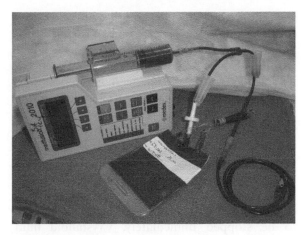

Figure 12.7. Photo of a unit of feline PRBC loaded into a syringe pump for administration. (Photo taken by author.)

when previous transfusions have been administered and is why all patients must be crossmatched if they have been previously transfused. Clinical signs can include hemoglobinuria, hemoglobinemia, icterus, and fever. A febrile, nonhemolytic reaction is classified as an increase in temperature by 1°.

All patients receiving a transfusion should be closely monitored throughout their entire transfusion. Clinical signs of a transfusion reaction differ in dogs and cats. In dogs, you can see restlessness,

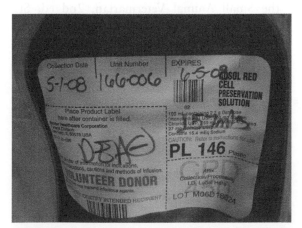

Figure 12.6. Photo of a unit of canine PRBC; note the labeling. (Photo taken by the author.)

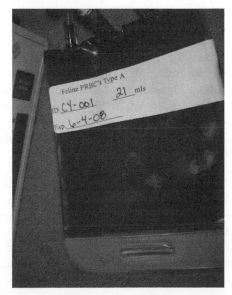

Figure 12.8. Photo of a unit of feline PRBC; note the labeling. (Photo taken by author.)

salivation, incontinence, dyspnea, hypotension, collapse, convulsions, vomiting, and acute death, which is uncommon. Note that in patients under anesthesia these reaction signs can go unnoticed. In patients under anesthesia it is important to monitor trends. Any change in trends once a transfusion is started should be investigated.

If a type B cat is given type A blood, acute death can occur. Cats having transfusion reactions will exhibit extension of limbs and apnea. An increase in respiratory rate and heart rate can be seen along with shock and hypotension.

If a transfusion reaction is suspected, it needs to be stopped immediately. Crystalloid fluid administration is recommended along with antipyretics. If the reaction is not thought to be severe, antihistamines can be administered and the transfusion started with the rate decreased by half.

Acknowledgment

The author thanks Dr. Edward Cooper, VMD, MS, DACVECC, at the Ohio State University Veterinary Teaching Hospital, for his help in reviewing this chapter.

References

Autran de Morais, H, Biondo, AW. 2006. Disorders of chloride: Hyperchloremia and hypochloremia. In Fluid, Electrolyte, and Acid-Base Disorders in Small Animal Practice, edited by DiBartola, S. St. Louis: Elsevier Inc. pp.80–90.

Blood, DC, Studdert, VP. 1999. Saunders Comprehensive Veterinary Dictionary, 2nd ed. New York: WB Saunders, pp.815.

Day, TK, Bateman, S. 2006. Shock syndromes. In Fluid, Electrolyte, and Acid-Base Disorders in Small Animal Practice, edited by DiBartola, S. St. Louis: Elsevier Inc., pp.540–564.

DiBartola, SP. 2006. Disorders of sodium and water: Hypernatremia and hyponatremia. In Fluid, Electrolyte, and Acid-Base Disorders in Small Animal Practice, edited by DiBartola, S. St. Louis: Elsevier Inc., pp.47–79.

DiBartola, SP, Autran de Morais, H. 2006. Disorders of potassium: Hypokalemia and hyperkalemia. In Fluid, Electrolyte, and Acid-Base Disorders in Small Animal Practice, edited by DiBartola, S. St. Louis: Elsevier Inc., pp.91–121.

DiBartola, SP, Bateman, S. 2006. Introduction to fluid therapy. In Fluid, Electrolyte, and Acid-Base Disorders in Small Animal Practice, edited by DiBartola, S. St. Louis: Elsevier Inc., pp.325–344.

Greene, RW, Scott, RC. 1975. Lower urinary tract disease. In Textbook of Veterinary Internal Medicine, edited by Ettringer, SJ. Philadelphia: WB Saunders, p.1572.

Hohenhaus, AE. 2000. Blood banking and transfusion medicine. In Textbook of Veterinary Internal Medicine, edited by Ettinger, SJ. St. Louis: WB Saunders Co., pp.348–356.

Kirby, R, Rudloff, E. 2000. Fluid and electrolyte therapy. In Textbook of Veterinary Internal Medicine, edited by Ettinger, SJ. Philadelphia: WB Saunders Company, pp.325–347.

Muir, WW, et al. 2000. Blood transfusion. In Handbook of Veterinary Anesthesia, 3rd ed., edited by Schrefer, JA. St. Louis: Mosby, pp. 424–425.

Muir, WW, DiBartola, SP. 1983. Fluid therapy. In Current Veterinary Therapy VIII, edited by Kirk, RW. Philadelphia: WB Saunders, p.33.

Plunkett, SJ. 2002. Emergency Procedures for the Small Animal Veterinarian, 2nd ed. St. Louis: WB Saunders, pp.475.

Roberts, JS, Bratton, SL. 1998. Colloid volume expanders: Problems, pitfalls and possibilities. Drugs 55(5):621–630.

Seeler, DC. 1996. Fluid and electrolyte therapy. In Lumb & Jones' Veterinary Anesthesia, 3rd ed., edited by Thurmon, JC. Philadelphia: Lippincott Williams & Wilkins. pp.572–589.

Tocci, LJ, Ewing, PJ. 2009. Increasing patient safety in veterinary transfusion medicine: An overview of pretransfusion testing. J Vet Emerg Crit Care 19(1):66–73.

13

Premedication and Sedation Drugs

Sandra Robbins

Premedication drugs, also known as preanesthetic drugs, are by definition drugs given before anesthesia begins. The different categories of premedication drugs are: anticholinergics, tranquilizers, alpha-2 agonists, dissociative drugs, and opioids (Muir et al. 2000). There are many different reasons to use premedications and many different useful combinations of drugs. A common question people will ask is, "Does my animal really need a premed?" While premedication drugs are not always necessary, they can be helpful and are usually incorporated into a safe, controlled, and well-balanced anesthetic plan. Preanesthetic drugs are helpful in that they decrease anxiety, provide analgesia, and cause sedation and muscle relaxation. When given appropriately, premedication drugs can decrease anesthetic induction and maintenance drug requirements, aid in restraint, reduce apprehension, provide analgesia and also promote a smooth induction and recovery from anesthesia (Bednarski 2007).

The perianesthetic period can be stressful for veterinary patients as a result of physical restraint, medication administration, and induction technique. Premedication drugs can have an anxiolytic effect and can therefore limit stress. When patients are calm and more relaxed, the premedication drugs tend to work better than when they are nervous or excited. A calm, quiet environment is recommended to assist with the anxiolytic effects of the drugs. Along with anxiolytic effects, sedation and muscle relaxation are expected from premedication drugs. All of these effects help to facilitate restraint and intravenous catheter placement, and to reduce patient stress and maintenance drug requirements.

Depending on the procedure requiring anesthesia, the premedication may warrant some analgesia. If the procedure is painful, or if the positioning required for the procedure may cause discomfort (old dogs with arthritis or hip dysplasia), a good premedication can reduce pain and the patient's requirements for induction and maintenance anesthesia. Certain drugs, while providing analgesia, also result in some sedation.

Salivation during the perianesthetic period is commonly encountered due to anxiety or from drug administration. During intubation, excessive salivation can make it difficult to properly visualize the arytenoids and prevent a smooth and timely induction. Excessive salivation can be due to a particularly nervous or anxious animal or from nausea. In addition to being a nuisance, excessive amounts of salivation can be dangerous. The endotracheal tube can be occluded by a mucous plug blocking the patient's only airway. Premedicating with drugs to prevent excessive salivation is sometimes helpful if not contraindicated.

By providing a calm, pain-free, sedate patient, in a stress-free environment, a smooth induction is easier to achieve. Typically, a sedate animal will struggle less and not achieve as profound an excitement phase at induction. The patient will also require less induction drug and maintenance anesthetic. Less induction and maintenance drug means lower potential for depressive cardiovascular effects. Premedications can also aid in smoothing recoveries depending upon the length of the procedure.

Deciding on a particular drug protocol can be overwhelming at first due to the vast number of drugs available. However, the task of choosing a drug protocol can be made much more manageable by breaking the drugs down by their categories and deciding which drug(s) best suit the individual patient's needs. Anticholinergics are drugs that block acetylcholine, the primary neurotransmitter of the parasympathetic nervous system. Increased heart rate and decreased salivation are two of the most commonly desired effects of anticholinergic administration. Bradycardia is commonly encountered in the perianesthetic period due to the cardiovascular effects of several anesthetic medications. Anticholinergics are effective at maintaining heart rate and preventing bradycardic decreases in cardiac output.

Secondary atrioventricular blockade is an arrhythmia commonly seen after anticholinergic administration, but it usually subsides within a couple of minutes of onset. Anticholinergics are contraindicated for animals with high heart rates or some cardiac diseases. Anticholinergics are not always considered necessary, but may be particularly useful in neonates who have underdeveloped sympathetic nervous systems and rely heavily on heart rate to maintain cardiac output (Pettifer and Grubb 2007).

The two most common anticholinergics encountered in veterinary medicine are atropine and glycopyrrolate. Both drugs can be administered subcutaneously, intramuscularly, or intravenously. Glycopyrrolate has a longer duration of action and a "gentler" onset of action. Atropine has greater lipid solubility than glycopyrrolate; therefore, atropine can cross the placenta as well as the blood-brain barrier (Stoelting and Miller 2007; Lemke 2007). Atropine may be the preferred anticholinergic during cesarean sections if fetal heart rate is of concern. It is also the anticholinergic of choice in an emergency because of its rapid onset of action.

Tranquilizers are comprised of several different groups: phenothiazines, butyrophenones, and benzodiazepines. These drugs can provide good sedation and muscle relaxation when included in the premedication. One phenothiazine derivative, acepromazine, is widely used in veterinary medicine. Acepromazine can be used in young, healthy anesthetic candidates. Its effects include sedation and muscle relaxation, and it can decrease the amount of inhalant anesthetic needed. It is an excellent anxiolytic. It also has some antiemetic and antiarrhythmic properties (Lemke 2007). Some less desirable effects are hypotension due to vasodilation and subsequent hypothermia from the vasodilation (Muir et al. 2000). The drug and its effects are not reversible. It should be used with caution or not at all in critical patients. Acepromazine also causes splenic engorgement, decreasing the circulating blood volume, and it inhibits platelet aggregation (Muir et al. 2000). Acepromazine alone is not a sufficient premedication for a painful procedure because it has no analgesic effects. Bottle doses are much higher than is often required to achieve the desired effect (Table 13.1).

Droperidol, a butyrophenone, is not commonly used in veterinary medicine in the U.S. Effects of this type of drug are similar to those of phenothiazines. Both have some antiemetic, antiarrhythmic, and sedative effects, and they decrease the amount of inhalant anesthetic needed.

Benzodiazepines are tranquilizers that cause muscle relaxation but may also cause excitement in healthy animals. Calming effects tend to be more profound in sick, debilitated, or depressed animals. There are three different benzodiazepine drugs used in veterinary medicine: diazepam, midazolam, and zolazepam. Benzodiazepines work with GABA receptors

Table 13.1. Anesthesia doses.

Drug	Conc. mg/mL	Dose Range mg/kg	Standard Dose mg/kg IM	Standard Dose mg/kg IV
Acepromazine	10	0.1–0.05	0.05[*]	0.025
Atropine	0.4	0.02–0.04	0.02	0.02
Buprenorphine	0.3	0.01–0.015	0.01	0.01
Butorphanol	10	0.1–0.3	0.1–0.2	0.1–0.2
Diazepam	5	0.1–0.5	0.2	0.2
Dexmedetomidine	0.5	0.002–0.02	0.005–0.01	0.005
Fentanyl	50[**]	2–10[**]	3–5[**]	3–5[**]
Glycopyrrolate	0.2	0.01–0.02	0.01	0.005–0.01
Hydromorphone	2	0.1–0.3	0.1	0.05–0.1
Ketamine[+]	100	2–10	2–4 Dogs 7–10 Cats	2–4 Dogs 4 Cats
Medetomidine	1	0.005–0.04	0.01–0.02	0.005–0.007
Methadone	10	0.1–2.2	0.5–1.0	0.1–0.2
Midazolam	5	0.1–0.2	0.2	0.1–0.2
Morphine	15	0.5–1.0	1.0	n/a
Oxymorphone	1	0.05–0.2	0.1	0.5–0.1
Xylazine	20 (SA)	0.1–0.5	0.2	n/a

[*]This dose of acepromazine should be reduced for older or compromised patients.

[**]Fentanyl concentration is μ/mL and dosed in μ/kg.

[+]Ketamine is not a sufficient premedication alone.

Source: Drug doses are those used at Tufts University Cummings School of Veterinary Medicine, Anesthesia Section, 2009.

(Lemke 2007). Diazepam has anticonvulsant properties, and is often used for the emergency treatment of seizures (Lemke 2007). Unlike the other benzodiazepines, diazepam is not water soluble and is in a carrier solution of propylene glycol (Muir et al. 2000). Its insoluble nature makes it a poor choice to mix with other drugs and it should not be administered intramuscularly due to pain on injection. Recommended routes of administration include oral and intravenous. Diazepam is highly protein-bound (approximately 90%) (Lemke 2007). Care should be used when administering diazepam to animals with low total protein levels. Midazolam and zolazepam are very similar to diazepam but are water soluble, and thus can be combined with other drugs, and are less irritating when administered intramuscularly (Muir et al. 2000). Telazol is a combination of zolazepam and a dissociative drug, tiletamine; this is the only form of zolazepam available. Full reversal of benzodiazepines can be accomplished with flumazenil.

Alpha-2 (α_2) agonists can cause profound sedation and due to their rapid effectiveness following intramuscular administration can be convenient in animals that are difficult to restrain. Due to the profound sedation, usually less inhalant anesthetic is necessary, and induction drug doses can be markedly decreased. Occasionally, animals will respond in less desirable ways from the α_2 agonists, such as extreme aggression when touched, or they can become very ataxic (Muir et al. 2000).

Dexmedetomidine, medetomidine, and xylazine are the three most commonly used α_2 agonists in small animal medicine. Medetomidine and dexmedetomidine have largely replaced xylazine in small animal medicine due to their higher specificity for the alpha-2 receptor and decreased side effects. All three drugs are listed with much higher doses on the bottle in comparison with what is commonly used in practice (see Table 13.1). Cardiovascular effects include an initial spike in arterial blood pressure due to intense vasoconstriction and increased systemic vascular resistance (SVR) and a reflexive bradycardia. These effects are usually transient, and the arterial blood pressure, in most cases, normalizes. Due to a decrease in the release of norepinephrine, there is usually a decrease in arterial blood pressure over time (Tranquilli 2002).

Dysrhythmias from α_2 agonists can include 1st, 2nd, and even 3rd degree atrioventricular block (Muir et al. 2000). Pale mucous membranes may be noted due to the profound peripheral vasoconstriction. Heart rates in the 40s and 50s are commonly encountered after the administration of an α_2 agonist. The bradycardia should be tolerated as long as evidence of tissue perfusion is maintained. This is noted by observing the waveform on the pulse oximeter and by monitoring arterial blood pressure. If tissue perfusion is in doubt, the α_2 agonists can be antagonized with yohimbine or antipamazole. Treating α_2 agonist–induced bradycardia with anticholinergics is controversial because of the added myocardial work induced with anticholinergic administration. If reducing doses of anesthetic concentrations does not improve heart rate and blood pressure, reversal of the drugs may be the next best step.

Dose-dependent respiratory depression is a common side effect of α_2 agonists, and in larger doses apnea and cyanosis may occur. However, ventilation is usually well maintained with therapeutic doses. Due to the vasoconstriction, decrease in cardiac output, and respiratory depression, oxygen transport is reduced. Because of the depressive effects on the cardiovascular system, α_2 agonists should be avoided in cardio-

vascularly compromised patients or patients with a systemic illness. An increase in urine production is typically noted after administration of these drugs, so care should be used when administering to animals in renal failure or with obstructed urinary tracts (Blaze et al. 2004). Care should also be used with laryngeal paralysis patients because α_2 agonists can depress swallowing reflexes. Hyperglycemia may be induced after α_2 agonist administration; this results from a suppression of insulin release (Muir et al. 2000). Unlike tranquilizers, α_2 agonists have potent analgesic effects by stimulating the central nervous system α_2 receptors (Muir et al. 2000). Most of the positive effects of α_2 agonists are enhanced when combined with other drugs such as dissociative drugs or opioids.

Dissociative drugs include ketamine and tiletamine. These drugs are categorized by the cataleptic-like state they cause. Ketamine should be avoided in epileptic animals because it has been found to cause seizures in those patients (Lin 2007). Increased heart rate and blood pressure are due to an indirect stimulation of the cardiovascular system by ketamine. Other effects are an increase in cerebral blood flow, intracranial pressure, and cerebrospinal fluid because of cerebral vasodilation and an increase in blood pressure (Lin 2007). Cats tend to have poor or sometimes even violent recoveries from ketamine alone. Symptoms include an increased sensitivity to touch, ataxia, possible hallucinations (cats may seem extremely jumpy as though they are avoiding something invisible), increased motor activity (as if they can't sit still), and even hyperreflexia (stiffness) (Lin 2007). When ketamine is combined with other drugs such as tranquilizers, these effects tend to be less extreme, and the cardiovascular effects of ketamine are lessened or negated (Lin 2007).

Historically, it was believed that ketamine provided good somatic analgesia but poor visceral analgesia in most patients. Recently evidence has been brought to light that ketamine may have some additional analgesic qualities when used in the perioperative period such as decreasing opiate requirements (Bilgin et al. 2005). Ketamine works as an NMDA receptor antagonist, blocking the effects of glutamate, which is an excitatory neurotransmitter. In this way, ketamine helps prevent windup pain. Cats receive visceral analgesia similar to the analgesic effects of butorphanol, but it does not last very long and is not sufficient for abdominal surgeries (Lin 2007). Hypersalivation is common following ketamine, especially with oral administration.

Finally, opioid drugs are commonly a key component in preanesthetic protocols. All opioids provide analgesia; however, there are several different receptors on which opioids work and several different categories into which they fall. Most opioids will cause sedation, but the extent is dependent upon the drug, the dosage, and the health of the animal. Nonpainful animals may become nauseous or vomit; an example would be a healthy animal undergoing an ovariohysterectomy. Panting is another common side effect of opioids in many animals. Cats tend to get mydriasis and dogs miosis after opioid administration. Most opioid drugs are reversible, either by an agonist-antagonist opioid (butorphanol) or by an opioid antagonist (naloxone). The different categories of opioids are: partial agonists, agonists, agonist-antagonists, and antagonists.

Buprenorphine is a partial agonist. Buprenorphine works at the mu receptor to provide moderate analgesia and minimal sedation. Because of its strong affinity for the mu receptor, buprenorphine is difficult to antagonize; yet it can partially antagonize some of the effects of pure agonists. The full onset of action for buprenorphine is about 30–45 minutes, so it cannot be titrated to effect (Blaze et al. 2004). Buprenorphine is not commonly used as a premedication drug except perhaps in routine cases such as ovariohysterectomy and neuter patients. It is commonly used for postoperative pain management. Buprenorphine's duration of action when given intravenously can be up to 6–8 hours.

Agonist opioids include morphine, hydromorphone, oxymorphone, fentanyl, and methadone. These drugs work at the mu and kappa receptors; they provide analgesia that is more profound than buprenorphine for painful procedures and they can provide profound sedation as well.

Nonpainful patients often vomit after being given an opioid premedication. Opioid agonists can be partially reversed with an opioid agonist-antagonist or fully reversed with an opioid antagonist. Fentanyl and its derivatives (sufentanil, alfentanil, and remifentanil) can cause profound bradycardia and respiratory depression.

Animals, like humans, can be allergic to morphine. When given intravenously, morphine can cause a release of histamine, which results in profound hypotension (Muir et al. 2000). Typically, depending on how they are administered, these drugs will last from 2–6 hours. Duramorph is a preservative-free morphine that is commonly administered epidurally.

Opioid agonist-antagonists are drugs that can provide some analgesia but can also reverse some of the effects of opioid agonist drugs. One example of this category is butorphanol. Butorphanol alone is not a sufficient opioid for painful procedures such as abdominal surgeries. Butorphanol can be a great choice alone or in combination with other drugs as a premedication for a simple procedure requiring little to no analgesia. Butorphanol provides good sedation in most cats and in pediatric and geriatric dogs. It also works well when trying to partially reverse opioid agonists so that the patient will wake up and extubate, and yet some of the analgesic properties will remain. When reversing an opioid agonist with butorphanol, the level of analgesia that the patient is left with depends upon how much butorphanol the patient receives. To completely reverse an opioid agonist in an emergency, an opioid antagonist should be given, because an opioid agonist-antagonist will leave some level of analgesia and sedation with the patient (which is usually beneficial in a nonemergency situation).

Pure antagonists, such as naloxone, completely reverse opioid agonists and agonist-antagonists. There is no analgesia remaining and so it should be used only when absolutely necessary. After giving naloxone, administration of an opioid agonist will not be effective until the antagonist has fully detached from the receptors.

A balanced preanesthetic protocol typically includes a number of drugs. Often, it is because several different effects are desired that cannot be accomplished with only one drug. Neuroleptanalgesia is the combination of an opioid with a tranquilizer or sedative (Muir et al. 2000). This combination results in better sedation than could be achieved with either of the drugs alone and allows for lesser doses of each of the drugs to be used. Often with higher doses, unconsciousness can be achieved, especially in critical patients. Neuroleptanalgesia is beneficial for certain procedures that do not require general anesthesia, such as bandage changes, cat castrations, and most radiographs. Drug doses for combinations of drugs can be found in Tables 13.2 through 13.6.

The following are some examples of specific combinations of drugs and different procedures in which they can be used. The combinations below are not a complete list; they are simply a few examples to demonstrate the possibilities of drug combinations. In sick or compromised patients, a phenothiazine can be substituted with a benzodiazepine to provide a more "cardiovascular friendly" preanesthetic protocol. Butorphanol, acepromazine, and glycopyrrolate (BAG) can be a good premedication combination for healthy animals undergoing minor surgical procedures and other procedures such as dentals, x-rays, and difficult ear cleanings. Because butor-

Table 13.2. Drug combination doses.

Drug Combination	Dose Rate IM or SC (Give ½ dose IV)
BAG	Butorphanol 0.2 mg/kg Acepromazine 0.05 mg/kg Glycopyrrolate 0.01 mg/kg
O'BAG	Butorphanol 0.2 mg/kg Acepromazine 0.025 mg/kg Glycopyrrolate 0.01 mg/kg
BMG	Butorphanol 0.2 mg/kg Midazolam 0.2 mg/kg Glycopyrrolate 0.01 mg/kg

Source: Drug doses are those used at Tufts University Cummings School of Veterinary Medicine, Anesthesia Section, 2009.

Table 13.3. Drug combination doses.

Drug Combination	Dose Rate (mg/kg) IM
Acepromazine	0.05
Glycopyrrolate	0.01
+ **ONE** of the following for painful procedures:	
Hydromorphone	0.1
Morphine	1.0
Oxymorphone	0.05–0.1

Source: Drug doses are those used at Tufts University Cummings School of Veterinary Medicine, Anesthesia Section, 2009.

Table 13.4. Drug combination doses.

Drug Combination	Dose Rate (mg/kg) IM
Midazolam	0.2
Glycopyrrolate	0.01
+ **ONE** of the following for painful procedures:	
Hydromorphone	0.1
Oxymorphone	0.5–0.1

Source: Drug doses are those used at Tufts University Cummings School of Veterinary Medicine, Anesthesia Section, 2009.

phanol provides little analgesia and it does not last very long, a dose of buprenorphine can be given shortly after anesthetic induction and before the procedure to treat pain during minor procedures with BAG. "Old dog BAG" (O'BAG) is used for the same purposes as BAG, but it is 1/2 the dose of acepromazine. This combination is appropriate for older animals because sensitivity to acepromazine seems to increase with age. Both of these combinations may be made into a mixture in one bottle (see Table 13.2 for doses). When performing more painful proce-

Table 13.5. Drug combination doses.

Drug Combination	Dose Rate (mg/kg) IM
Ketamine	2–4, Dogs 7–8, Cats
Acepromazine	0.05
Glycopyrrolate	0.01
+ **ONE** of the following for painful procedures:	
Butorphanol	0.2
Hydromorphone	0.1
Morphine	1.0
Oxymorphone	0.1

Source: Drug doses are those used at Tufts University Cummings School of Veterinary Medicine, Anesthesia Section, 2009.

Table 13.6. Drug combination doses.

Drug Combination	Dose Rate (mg/kg) IM
Ketamine	2–7
EITHER:	
Dexmedetomidine	0.006–0.012
OR Medetomidine	0.01–0.02
+ **ONE** of the following for painful procedures	
Butorphanol	0.2
Buprenorphine	0.01

Source: Drug doses are those used at Tufts University Cummings School of Veterinary Medicine, Anesthesia Section, 2009.

dures or major surgeries, additional analgesia should be provided.

Orthopedic and abdominal surgeries, or dentals with root canals, typically need more analgesia than butorphanol and buprenorphine. Hydromorphone, acepromazine, and glycopyr-

rolate (HAG) is a combination that is similar to BAG, but has much greater analgesia. This combination should never be found premixed in a bottle. Hydromorphone is a class II controlled drug and its use needs to be very strictly regulated. Similarly to O'BAG, a combination of HAG with half the acepromazine would be more appropriate for older or quiet animals.

Aggressive animals tend to need more drugs to sedate them than an older quiet patient. One good combination for aggressive dogs may be ketamine, hydromorphone, acepromazine, and glycopyrrolate (KHAG). The acepromazine dose is not usually decreased for these animals, but the ketamine dose is changed depending on how aggressive the animal is (see Table 13.6 for doses). Another good combination for aggressive dogs is dexmedetomidine and hydromorphone. The idea behind combinations for aggressive animals is to have them not just sedated but immobilized.

There are good combinations for cats as well. Ketamine and BAG (KBAG) is for cats that are mildly aggressive to very aggressive and need some sedation for intravenous catheter placement before surgery. The dose of ketamine is variable, and this combination should be followed up with a dose of buprenorphine to provide adequate analgesia (see Tables 13.6 and 13.1 for doses). Another combination that is very effective for healthy cats, is what is referred to as "Kitty Magic." This combination includes an α_2 agonist (either dexmedetomidine or medetomidine) and ketamine at variable doses, and an opioid (either butorphanol or buprenorphine) (see Table 13.6 for doses). Kitty Magic can be used when a cocktail of drugs is needed that will completely immobilize a cat for an examination, radiographs, or even a castration. Typically, this combination does not require any inhalant anesthetic, depending on the doses used and the duration of the procedure. The drugs tend to work very fast, and full effect may occur in as little as 10 minutes when given intramuscularly. It's best to have all supplies ready for quick surgical procedures to be performed. It is handy to have an anesthesia machine and small cat mask nearby in case procedures are prolonged and the cat begins waking up. Kitty

Magic should be reserved for young, healthy animals.

A multimodal analgesic approach is thought to more adequately control pain. Using several different drugs to treat pain can decrease the doses needed of each drug and may better treat and control the pain. Administering analgesic drugs before painful stimuli can make controlling and treating the pain easier. Each drug has its own individual applications, but when used in careful combinations these drugs can serve to create greater anesthetic protocols.

References

Bednarski, RM. 2007. Anesthesia, analgesia, and immobilization of selected species and classes of animals: Dogs and cats. In Lumb & Jones' Veterinary Anesthesia and Analgesia, 4th ed. Ames, IA: Blackwell Publishing.

Bilgin, H, et al. 2005. The influence of timing of systemic ketamine administration on postoperative morphine consumption. J Clin Anesth 17:592–597.

Blaze, CA, Glowaski, MM. 2004. Individual drugs. In Veterinary Anesthesia Drug Quick Reference. St Louis: Elsevier Saunders.

Lemke, KA. 2007. Pharmacology: Anticholinergics and sedatives. In Lumb & Jones' Veterinary Anesthesia and Analgesia, 4th ed. Ames, IA: Blackwell Publishing.

Lin, HC. 2007. Pharmacology: Dissociative anesthetics. In Lumb & Jones' Veterinary Anesthesia and Analgesia, 4th ed. Ames, IA: Blackwell Publishing.

Muir, WW, Hubbell, JAE, Skarda, RT, Bednarski, RM. 2000. Drugs used for preanesthetic medication. In Handbook of Veterinary Anesthesia, 3rd ed. St. Louis: Mosby.

Pettifer, GR, Grubb, TL. 2007. Anesthesia and analgesia for selected patients and procedures: neonatal and geriatric patients. In Lumb & Jones' Veterinary Anesthesia and Analgesia, 4th ed. Ames, IA: Blackwell Publishing.

Stoelting, RK, Miller. 2007. Autonomic nervous system. In Basics of Anesthesia, 5th ed. Philadelphia: Churchill Livingston.

Tranquilli, WJ. 2002. α_2 agonists. In Veterinary Anesthesia and Pain Management Secrets. Philadelphia: Hanley & Belfus.

14

Induction Drugs

Lori Fuehrer

Induction of anesthesia occurs when a patient transitions from a conscious state to an unconscious state. Induction can be achieved by inhalant or injectable anesthetic agents, and routes of administration can include mask, chamber, IV, or IM injection or oral administration. Temperament of the patient may dictate the use of inhalant (chamber induction) or IM administration rather than IV routes. Although it's easy to get into a routine of what agents are used for induction, it is vital to treat each patient individually to ensure safety. It is important to know each patient's disposition and history, overall health, and any underlying disease processes prior to choosing an anesthetic protocol. The reason for anesthesia (procedure to be performed) will play a role as well.

Inhalant Induction Procedures

Anesthesia induction can be accomplished with the use of inhalant anesthetics being administered via a mask or chamber. Because of the delay in capturing the airway during inhalant inductions as well as the potential for excessive stress and anxiety placed on patients, these methods should be reserved for use in animals that will not

tolerate injectable induction protocols. Higher oxygen flow rates of 3–5 liters per minute and higher gas concentrations of 3–4% for isoflurane and 4–5% for sevoflurane are used to help speed induction (McKelvey and Hollingshead 2000).

Patients may go through an excitement phase (particularly if they haven't received adequate premedication) prior to being anesthetized enough to allow for endotracheal intubation. A muzzle can be placed over the mask and secured behind the patients' ears to help maintain a proper seal and free up the technicians' hands (Fig. 14.1).

Mask inductions are preferable to chamber inductions because they can be faster and there may be less exposure of waste gases to personnel. When mask induction is used, be sure to use an appropriate size mask for each patient to reduce the amount of dead space and leakage. A gradual increase in the level of anesthetic being delivered is recommended to reduce stress. Start with the vaporizer setting at 0.5% and increase in 0.5% increments every 15–30 seconds (McKelvey and Hollingshead 2000). The patient can also be wrapped in a towel or blanket to help reduce stress and possible injury to the patient and staff members.

When chamber induction is chosen, the patient is placed in a closed container, which is then

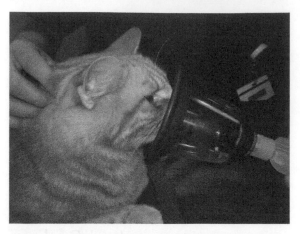

Figure 14.1. The muzzle over mask technique.

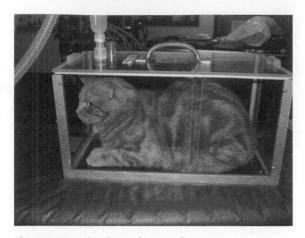

Figure 14.2. Chamber induction of a cat.

filled with oxygen and an anesthetic agent. The chamber should be small, but large enough for the patient to lie down with its neck extended (Fig. 14.2). The patient is removed when it is no longer able to stand. If the patient, once removed from the chamber, is still not sedate enough to intubate, a mask can be used until it is more deeply anesthetized (see Fig. 14.1) (McKelvey and Hollingshead 2000).

Injectable Induction Agents

Injectable induction can be attained with the use of one or multiple agents given IV or IM. The duration of anesthesia is usually less than 20 minutes, but it varies based on the drug(s) and route of administration used (McKelvey and Hollingshead 2000). Induction via IM routes is beneficial in animals that cannot be handled. The most common IM induction drugs are ketamine, tiletamine and zolazepam (Telazol), xylazine, neuroleptanalgesics, and opioids. The use of premedications will commonly reduce the amount of induction agents needed.

Benzodiazepines

Benzodiazepines include diazepam, midazolam, and zolazepam (Greene 2002). They decrease anxiety and produce calming effects and pro-

found skeletal muscle relaxation in most patients. The benzodiazepines are metabolized in the liver and excreted in the urine and feces. They do not produce much sedation (except possibly in pediatric or critically ill patients) because most animals are still alert and aware of their surroundings. These drugs can cause excitement more often in young healthy animals and cats, so they are not commonly used as sole agents. They are more effective when combined with cyclohexamines, tranquilizers, or opioids that will help decrease the occurrence of excitement.

Benzodiazepines are also used for anticonvulsant therapy, making them a good adjunctive induction agent in patients that have a history of seizures or other intracranial disease (McKelvey and Hollingshead 2000). They can also be used with other anesthetics that may lower the seizure threshold and during procedures that may cause seizure activity, such as myelogram, cerebrospinal fluid centesis, or brain surgery.

Diazepam (valium)

Diazepam is one of the most commonly used benzodiazepines. It is not water soluble and cannot be mixed in the same syringe with other medications, with the exception of ketamine. It can be irritating to tissues when injected IM because it contains propylene glycol; when used in this manner, its absorption rate is somewhat unreliable and IV dosing is the preferred route.

It has very little depressant effects on the cardiovascular and respiratory systems, making it a safe choice for most patients. The propylene glycol component in diazepam may cause hypotension, bradycardia, or apnea after rapid IV administration; therefore, care should be taken to administer it slowly (Paddleford 1999).

Midazolam (versed)

Midazolam is the second most commonly used benzodiazepine; it is water soluble and can be mixed with other anesthetic agents. Midazolam is not as irritating to tissues and can be administered IM; absorption after IM injection is more reliable than it is with diazepam. The cardiovascular effects are similar to diazepam with rapid IV administration. Midazolam can, however, cause more respiratory depression than is seen with diazepam (Paddleford 1999).

Zolazepam

Zolazepam is the benzodiazepine mixed with tiletamine, a cyclohexamine, and the mixture is sold as Telazol. As a sole agent, it produces little sedation but provides excellent skeletal muscle relaxation, as does diazepam.

Cyclohexamines (ketamine, tiletamine)

Cyclohexamines work in a different manner than most other agents by stimulating the CNS rather than depressing it. This stimulation results in what is termed *dissociative anesthesia* or *catalepsy*, in which animals are in a trancelike state unaware of their surroundings. Stimulation of the CNS produces muscle rigidity characterized by extension of the front limbs and head and neck flexed back, increased reflexes such as the palpebral and pharyngeal, and sensitivity to light, sound, and touch. These effects can be diminished by using a benzodiazepine, opiate, or tranquilizer in combination with the cyclohexamine. Cyclohexamines typically do not cause cardiovascular depression. More often, tachycardia and increased blood pressure are seen after administration of a cyclohexamine due to indirect sympathetic stimulation. Because of this, they are not recommended for use in animals with known cardiac disease. Apneustic respirations are commonly seen. This is a particular type of breathing pattern in which inspiration is followed by a long pause and short expiration; some animals may hold their breath but can usually be easily stimulated to breathe by stroking their chest. The apneustic breathing pattern is not detrimental, and oxygen levels typically stay within normal limits. Cyclohexamines can also produce an increase in intraocular pressure and are not recommended for use in animals with ocular disease (Lin 1996). The eyes do not rotate as they do with other anesthetic agents, and nystagmus is commonly seen. Cyclohexamines also cause an increase in intracranial pressure and should not be used in animals with known head trauma or other intracranial disease (Lin 1996).

Recovery of cyclohexamine anesthesia can be rough because of the hypersensitivity to sound, light, and touch. Some animals will paw at their face or experience bizarre behavior. It is recommended that patients recover in a quiet dark environment to reduce stress, and occasionally additional sedatives are needed to smooth out the recovery.

Ketamine (ketaset, vetalar, ketalean)

Ketamine is a highly lipid soluble and has a fast onset of action. After IV administration, an endotracheal tube can usually be placed very quickly. After IM injection, intubation can be performed in 2–4 minutes. Recovery after IM administration can be prolonged and may take 3–5 hours (McCurnin 1994).

Ketamine in the dog is primarily excreted by hepatic metabolism and is not recommended for use in dogs with known liver problems. In the cat, it's primarily excreted via the kidneys and should not be used in cats with renal disease or urinary obstruction (Lin 1996).

Tiletamine

Tiletamine is purchased as a mixture with zolazepam; it is sold as Telazol and comes as a powder that must be reconstituted. Once in solution, it remains stable for 4 days at room temperature and 14 days when refrigerated (Paddleford 1999). After IV injection, intubation can be performed within 1–2 minutes, and after IM injection, intubation can be performed within 2–4 minutes. Recovery after IM administration can take 3–5 hours. It can also be given SQ or orally.

Tiletamine has similar effects as ketamine, but because it's mixed with zolazepam, it is more like a ketamine-diazepam combination. It produces good muscle relaxation and less apneustic breathing patterns; however, respiratory depression is more commonly seen, especially when administered in conjunction with other tranquilizers or sedatives (Lin 1996).

Tiletamine is excreted via the kidneys in both dogs and cats and is not recommended for use in patients with known renal disease or urinary obstruction (Lin 1996).

Propofol (diprivan, rapinovet)

Propofol is unlike any other anesthetic agent. It's an oil-in-water emulsion, and although it has a milky appearance, it is to be administered IV only (McKelvey et al. 2000). It is metabolized quickly, has a fast onset of action, and has short duration of effect, making it a relatively safe induction agent when administered correctly. It can also be used as a CRI or redosed through multiple low-dose injections given for a short procedure.

Propofol is not without negative side effects, including a transient decrease in cardiac contractility and hypotension due to vasodilation. Propofol is a potent respiratory depressant and if given too rapidly it can cause apnea following induction. This can be greatly diminished by slow injection (dose given over 90 seconds), titrating to effect, and the use of premedications that lower the dose of propofol required (Paddleford 1999). Transient tachycardia and bradycardia have also been noted but are typically not detrimental if the patient is healthy. Repeated doses of propofol over a short period of time in cats may cause oxidative injury to the red blood cells called *Heinz body formations*

(Paddleford 1999). The clinical side effects of this are lethargy, vomiting, diarrhea, and anorexia.

Excitement may be seen during administration and is more common in younger healthy animals. The use of premedications or combining the induction dose with a benzodiazepine will decrease the excitement phase. Recovery is quick and usually smooth, especially when premedications have been used (Paddleford 1999).

Propofol also causes a decrease of intracranial and intraocular pressure, making it a good choice for animals with known intracranial disease, head trauma, or ocular disease (Branson 2007). It can also be safely used as an induction agent for cesarean sections as it has minimal depressant effects on the fetus, increasing survival rates (Paddleford 1999).

Propofol contains soybean oil, egg lichen, and glycerol, making it an easy environment for microbes to grow in. Left unopened the shelf life may be several years. The exact shelf life of an opened bottle is under debate; some studies suggest that keeping an opened bottle refrigerated will allow for a shelf life of 5–7 days, while others recommend that an opened bottle be discarded at the end of each day. Regardless of the debate over shelf life, everyone agrees that strict sterile technique should be used to prevent possible contamination of the bottle or ampule. Because of the potential for contamination there is some debate over this drug's safe use in septic patients.

The induction dose for patients that have not received premedications is 8–10 mg/kg IV, if premedications have been given, the dose is 4–6 mg/kg IV (Thurmon et al. 1996). There are several techniques for the administration of propofol to reduce the occurrence of respiratory depression, apnea, and hypotension. The commonality of all techniques is slow administration and titrating to effect. Some techniques include the following:

1. As a sole agent, administer 1/3–1/2 of the calculated dose over 35–45 seconds, wait a few seconds, and then slowly titrate the remainder of the dose over the next 35–45 seconds.

2. When using diazepam in conjunction: Administer diazepam dose first, and then give the propofol as described above. This may result in less propofol required to produce anesthesia.
3. Another technique when using diazepam in conjunction: Administer 1/3–1/2 the calculated propofol dose over 35–45 seconds, administer the diazepam dose, and then give the remainder of the propofol dose titrated to effect. This may decrease the occurrence of respiratory depression or apnea.
4. The same techniques above can be accomplished with opioids or tranquilizers other than diazepam in the methods as described.

The goal is to use a smaller dose of propofol and ensure that it is being given very slowly to prevent respiratory depression.

Etomidate (amidate)

Etomidate is a sedative hypnotic imidazole induction agent. It can be used as a sole agent or in combination, most commonly with diazepam or midazolam. Metabolism is rapid and so it can be administered as a single bolus titrated to effect, repeated injections, or CRI. Etomidate has little to no effect on the cardiovascular or respiratory systems. When used as the sole agent it causes no change to heart rate, blood pressure or cardiac output (Branson 2007). For these reasons it can be a good choice in critical patients. Etomidate maintains cerebral perfusion and is therefore a good induction choice for patients with suspected intracranial disease. It is also safe for use in cesarean sections because it has very little fetal depressant effects. It may cause agitation or excitement, especially in patients that have not been premedicated. This is why it's commonly combined with diazepam or similar drugs. It can be irritating to vessels due to its carrier agent, propylene glycol, and may cause phlebitis.

The dose of etomidate is 1.5–3 mg/kg IV (Thurmon et al. 1999). Etomidate has become a great drug of choice for cesarean sections and for patients with known cardiac disease or cardio-

Table 14.1. Combinations of induction agents.

Diazepam or midazolam	Ketamine
	Propofol
	Etomidate
	Acepromazine
	Butorphanol
	Xylazine
	Medetomidine
	Thiopental
	Methohexital
Ketamine	Diazepam
	Midazolam
	Acepromazine
	Butorphanol
	Xylazine
	Medetomidine
Telazol (zolazepam and tiletamine)	Propofol
	Butorphanol
	Acepromazine
Propofol	Diazepam
	Midazolam
	Telazol
	Etomidate
	Xylazine
	Medetomidine
Etomidate	Diazepam
	Midazolam
	Propofol

vascular instability due to trauma or shock, although it may be cost prohibitive because it is expensive (Branson 2007).

Table 14.1 lists anesthetic agents that can be used for induction. An agent can be chosen from the left column and combined with one or more of the agents from the right column. Not all agents in this table are discussed in depth within this chapter.

Barbiturates as Induction Agents

Barbiturates are classified into different categories based upon their duration of action. This chapter discusses only the thiobarbiturate (thiopental) and methylated oxybarbiturate (methohexital), which are both ultra–short-acting. Their rapid onset of action and short duration of effect makes them useful for anesthetic inductions.

Because of the contraindications of barbiturates, proper patient selection and close monitoring is necessary. They are not recommended for use for cesarean sections or in patients with cardiac or respiratory disease, hypoproteinemia, acidosis, hepatic insufficiency, or hypothermia. Although they have their place, the availability of other induction agents with fewer side effects has lessened the use of barbiturates. Barbiturates flow first to the brain, resulting in depression of the CNS, which produces a state of unconsciousness. Redistribution of thiopental and methohexital starts to occur 10–20 minutes after IV injection as the barbiturates move from the brain toward muscle and fat tissue. As redistribution occurs, the concentration within the brain starts to decrease, the state of unconsciousness begins to wear off, and the patient may start to recover. It's important to recognize that as redistribution starts to occur and consciousness begins to return, the barbiturates have not been eliminated from the body. They are highly lipid soluble and tend to stay within fat tissue for several hours before elimination from the body (McKelvey and Hollingshead 2000).

Thiobarbiturate (thiopental)

Thiopental's onset of action is 30–60 seconds, and the duration of effect is 10–20 minutes (McKelvey et al. 2000). Recovery is usually seen within 1–2 hours even though redistribution occurs 4–6 hours after administration and complete elimination from these tissues may take up to 10–12 hours. Because of this, it is not recommended that repeat doses be administered because overdose or prolonged recovery periods may result (McKelvey and Hollingshead 2000). Final elimination of thiopental from the body occurs mainly through hepatic metabolism, although some metabolism occurs within the brain and kidneys.

The induction dose of thiopental is 10–12 mg/kg IV (Branson 2007). Administration is much like that of propofol, giving 1/3–1/2 the calculated dose over 15–20 seconds and the remainder

of the dose slowly titrated to effect. It is purchased in a powder form and must be reconstituted. Once reconstituted, it will remain stable for only 2 weeks when refrigerated and for a shorter time when stored at room temperature.

Sight hounds and patients with low body fat can be particularly susceptible to the effects of thiopental because of its affinity to redistribute to highly lipid areas of the body. Animals with little fat tissue will require greater metabolism by the brain, liver, and kidneys, which produces more pronounced CNS depression. Thiopental should be used with extreme caution in lean animals because overdose can occur and recovery time may be dramatically delayed 6–24 hours longer than with other patients (Greene 2002).

Thiopental may cause tissue irritation and necrosis when injected perivascularly. If this occurs, the area should be infiltrated with saline to reduce the chance for tissue necrosis (McKelvey et al. 2000). Lidocaine or bupivicaine can also be infiltrated into the area to prevent the animal from excessively licking at an irritated area and causing more damage.

Methylated oxybarbiturate (methohexital)

Methohexital's onset of action is 15–60 seconds and the duration of effect is 5–10 minutes (McKelvey et al. 2000). It has several advantages over thiopental, including a shorter duration of effect and faster recovery because it is not as lipid soluble and does not redistribute to other tissues as much as thiopental. Complete elimination from the body occurs within 3–5 hours, making it safer to administer multiple doses if needed. It also relies more on hepatic metabolism and renal excretion, making it a better choice for use in sight hounds (McKelvey et al. 2000). It does, however, have more profound respiratory depressant effects than thiopental; the lethal dose is only 2–3 times the induction dose, so proper calculation and careful monitoring should be used (McKelvey et al. 2000).

The induction dose of methohexital is 6–10 mg/kg IV (Branson 2007). The method of administration is the same as thiopental, giving

1/3–1/2 the dose over 15–20 seconds followed by titrating the remainder of the dose to effect. It does not cause tissue irritation if accidentally injected perivascularly. Methohexital is also purchased in a powder form that must be reconstituted, which is similar to thiopental, but once reconstituted it can be stored safely at room temperature for up to 6 weeks.

Neuroleptanalgesia

Neuroleptanalgesia is the term used when opioids are combined with a tranquilizing agent to produce profound sedation. They are not commonly used in cats because IV administration of some opioids can cause excitement. They are also not commonly used for induction of young or healthy patients because they may not produce enough sedation to allow for intubation. Neuroleptanalgesia is more commonly used in geriatric or high-risk patients.

The opioids commonly used in neuroleptanalgesia include oxymorphone, hydromorphone, fentanyl, morphine, and meperidine. The tranquilizers commonly used are diazepam, midazolam, and acepromazine (McKelvey and Hollingshead 2000).

Oxymorphone (Numorphan) is one of the more commonly used opioids for use in neuroleptanalgesia. It is recommended that IV injection be given slowly, but it does not have to be given as slowly as morphine or meperidine and can be given IV to cats. Cardiovascular effects are minimal, and it produces less respiratory depressant effects than other opioids. *Hydromorphone* is closely related to oxymorphone. Slow IV administration is recommended, but it can be given safely to cats. Cardiovascular and respiratory effects are similar to oxymorphone.

Fentanyl may cause bradycardia that is usually responsive or preventable by administration of an anticholinergic, but it has minimal effects on blood pressure and cardiac output, making it a safer choice for high-risk patients.

Morphine, when administered IV, can cause bradycardia, profound hypotension, and respiratory depression caused by the release of histamine, making it less commonly used as a neuroleptanalgesic. When given IV to cats, it may cause mania or convulsions; therefore, it is not recommended for use in the cat as an induction agent.

Meperidine (Demerol) is similar to morphine, not as commonly used because it can also cause profound hypotension and excitement with rapid IV administration. It has a slight advantage over morphine because it causes less respiratory depression.

Diazepam (Valium) is one of the safest tranquilizers to use in critical patients. It has a wide margin of safety and causes very little effect on the cardiovascular and respiratory systems.

Midazolam (Versed) is similar to diazepam and also has a wide margin of safety, making it a safe choice in high-risk patients. Midazolam may cause more respiratory depression than what may be seen with diazepam.

Acepromazine is a commonly used tranquilizer and anxiolytic that can be administered SQ, IM, or IV. Because of its hypotensive effects due to vasodilation and its inability to be antagonized it should be used cautiously in the sick or debilitated patient.

Rapid IV administration of opioids may result in CNS stimulation; therefore, they should be administered slowly and can be titrated to effect. There are multiple methods of administration including the following:

1. Anticholinergic and tranquilizer premedication given SQ or IM 15–20 minutes prior to slow IV administration of an opioid.
2. No premedication. Slow IV administration of an opioid first, and wait a few seconds, and then titrate to effect. In some cases, the opioid may produce enough sedation to allow for intubation without the need for use of the tranquilizer.

   Note: This method may be more effective than giving the tranquilizer first because diazepam and midazolam can cause CNS stimulation and excitement.
3. No premedication. IV injection of a tranquilizer followed by slow injection of the opioid titrated to effect. This method may

also produce enough sedation after injection of the tranquilizer to allow for intubation without the need for the opioid.

4. No premedication. Administration of a combination of medications in one syringe titrated to effect to allow for intubation. Although this method is useful, separating the agents in different syringes may be a safer choice in high-risk patients.

Table 14.2. Brief overview of situations in which induction agents are *not* recommended.

Inhalant inductions	Brachycephalic breeds Respiratory distress Cardiovascular disease Patients that have not been fasted Lack of proper scavenge system, etc.
Ketamine	Cardiac disease Canines with hepatic disease Felines with renal disease Felines with urinary obstruction
Telazol tiletamine and zolazepam	Cardiac disease Renal disease (canines and felines) Felines with urinary obstruction
Propofol	Shock Known hypotension Repeated doses over several subsequent days in cats
Thiopental	Cardiac disease Respiratory disease Hepatic insufficiency (neonates, geriatrics) Liver disease Hypoproteinemia Acidosis Hypothermia Cesarean section Sight hounds
Methohexital	Cardiac disease Respiratory disease Hepatic insufficiency (neonates, geriatrics) Liver disease Hypoproteinemia Acidosis Hypothermia Cesarean section

Table 14.3. Brief overview of situations in which certain induction agents *should be* considered.

Diazepam or midazolam (as an adjunct to an opioid or some other induction agent, not as sole agent)	History of seizures Head trauma Myelogram Cerebral spinal fluid centesis (CSF Tap) Brain surgery Cardiac disease Respiratory disease Renal disease

Propofol	Ocular disease
	Intracranial disease
	Head trauma
	Sight hounds
	Cesarean section
	High-risk patients (without
	  hypotension)
	Cardiac disease (without
	  hypotension)

Etomidate	Cardiac disease Respiratory disease Cesarean section Trauma or shock High-risk patients
Oxymorphone and hydromorphone and fentanyl (with euroleptic)	Trauma or shock High-risk patients Can be given IV in cats

Summary

Tables 14.2 and 14.3 can be used as a general guideline for choosing appropriate induction agents. Table 14.2 has a brief list of some, but not all, situations or disease processes in which an induction agent should not be chosen. Table 14.3 has a brief list of induction agents that are commonly used in certain situations or in patients with certain disease processes.

References

Branson, Keith. 2007. Injectable and alternative anesthetic techniques. In Lumb & Jones' Veterinary Anesthesia, 4th ed., edited by

Tranquilli, WJ, Thurmon, JV, Grimm, KA. Ames, IA: Blackwell Publishing, pp.290, 291.

Greene, SA. 2002. Veterinary Anesthesia and Pain Management Secrets. Philadelphia: Hanley & Belfus, Inc.

Lin, HC. 1996. Dissociative anesthetics. In Lumb & Jones' Veterinary Anesthesia, 3rd ed., edited by Tranquilli, WJ, Benson, GJ. Ames, IA: Blackwell Publishing, pp.242, 243, 257.

McCurnin, DM. 1994. Clinical Textbook for Veterinary Technicians, 3rd ed. Philadelphia: WB Saunders Company.

McKelvey, D, Hollingshead, KW. 2000. Small Animal Anesthesia and Analgesia, 2nd ed. St. Louis: Mosby.

Paddleford, RR. 1999. Manual of Small Animal Anesthesia, 2nd ed. Philadelphia: WB Saunders Company.

Thurmon, JC, Tranquilli, WJ, Benson, GJ. 1999. Essentials of Small Animal Anesthesia and Analgesia. Philadelphia: Lippincott Williams & Wilkins.

Thurmon, JC, Tranquilli, WJ, Benson, GJ. 1996. Lumb & Jones' Veterinary Anesthesia, 3rd ed. Philadelphia: Lippincott Williams & Wilkins.

15 Inhalant Anesthetics

Sharon Fornes

History

There has been a large rise of inhalant anesthetics in the past 50 years. Many of those inhalants discovered during this time are still being used today. Some of them have been abandoned for better, safer anesthetics, which have many of the properties of the ideal anesthetic (Eger et al. 2003).

Inhalant anesthetics were around long before their use in surgical procedures. Before inhalant use in medicine, most surgeries were performed with the patient completely awake. The only method utilized for immobilization of the patient while these painful procedures were being performed was physical restraint. Meanwhile, inhalant anesthetics were used for parties. Guests were entertained as volumes of ether or nitrous oxide were pumped into the audience or given to people on stage to enhance the performances (Fenster 2002).

The 1840s brought inhalant anesthetics into the world of medicine for use in surgical procedures. Ether was first utilized in 1842, but was not documented correctly, so proper credit for use of anesthesia was not given until later. In 1844, nitrous oxide in a dental procedure was documented for the first time. The first documented case of ether was in 1846 and of chloroform in 1847. The 1950s brought us halothane and then methoxyflurane. Isoflurane, sevoflurane, and desflurane were discovered earlier but were not utilized in clinical practice until the 1980s (Eger et al. 2003).

The development of the perfect inhalant anesthetic is an ongoing process. Although there is no perfect inhalant, knowing what each agent does and balancing that with other anesthetic drugs can provide what is needed for a safe anesthetic procedure.

The Ideal Anesthetic

The ideal anesthetic should have the following characteristics:

- Sufficient (potency) anesthesia with lowest toxicity
- Minimal side effects on the nervous, cardiovascular, and respiratory systems
- Able to be metabolized and excreted with little effect on the hepatic or renal system

153

- Enough muscle relaxation with proper analgesia and immobilization to perform procedures
- Minimal exposure of waste gas to clinical personnel
- Agreeable smell, not irritating to respiratory mucosa
- Swift and tranquil anesthetic induction and recovery
- Ability to change anesthetic depth quickly and smoothly
- Inexpensive (both agent and equipment)
- Minimal safety of storage or handling concerns (nonflammable, chemically stable)
- No reactions with components of the anesthetic equipment (CO_2 absorbent, metal, rubber or plastic) (Muir et al. 2000)

Mechanism of Action

The mechanism of action for inhalant anesthetics is constantly debated, and it is still not fully understood. There is central nervous system (CNS) activity but the location of the activity has not been established. There are many possible sites of action. Research regarding the mechanism of action in the inhalant anesthetic is still being explored (Eger et al. 2003; McKelvey et al. 2003; Eger 1984).

Pharmacokinetics

The pharmacokinetics of an inhaled anesthetic is as follows: The anesthetic is inhaled into the lungs where it passes into the alveoli and is absorbed in the pulmonary capillaries, thus achieving blood levels of anesthetic. The inhalant anesthesia is distributed to the central nervous system. The metabolism and elimination vary between agents (Eger et al. 2003; Eger 1984; Stoelting 1999).

Minimum Alveolar Concentration (MAC)

There are many ways to measure the anesthetic potency. MAC is most often used clinically for measurement of anesthetic potency. The lower the MAC, the higher the potency of the anesthetic gas. Physiologic response to anesthetic can vary and is unreliable, particularly in comparing the different anesthetic agents available. MAC is not vaporizer settings.

MAC is the concentration of anesthetic that produces anesthesia in 50% of patients that are given a noxious stimulant. MAC is influenced by temperature (hyperthermia and hypothermia), disease processes (lung disease, thyroid disease), some drugs, some species variance, circadian

Table 15.1.　MAC of anesthetics by species.

Agent	Man	Dog	Cat	Rat	Swine	Horse
Methoxyflurane	0.16	0.23	0.23	0.22	0.91	0.28
Halothane	0.75	0.87	0.82	0.95	1.45	0.88
Isoflurane	1.15	1.28	1.63	1.17	1.45	1.28
Sevoflurane	1.58	2.1	2.6	2.29	2.4	2.3
Desflurane	6.0	7.2	9.79	7.1	10.0	7.6
Nitrous oxide	105	188	255	150	162	233

Source: Eger et al. 2003.

rhythm, stress, and age (Table 15.1) (Eger et al. 2003; Eger 1984). MAC is not influenced by the application of different noxious stimuli being applied or by the intensity of the stimulation. There is no effect of MAC in different sexes. Duration of anesthetic procedure also does not have an affect on MAC (Eger et al. 2003).

From most potent to least potent, inhalant anesthetics rank as follows: methoxyflurane, halothane, isoflurane, sevoflurane, desflurane, and nitrous oxide.

Vaporization Pressure

Concentration of inhalant anesthesia is determined by the vapor pressure. Vapor pressure is the rate at which a liquid will turn into a gas at a given temperature. Methoxyflurane has a low vaporization pressure of approximately 3% at room temperature. This allows methoxyflurane to be used in both nonprecision and precision vaporizers. Halothane, isoflurane, sevoflurane, and desflurane have vapor pressures that are over 30% at room temperature and need a precision vaporizer to deliver anesthetic to the patient (Paddleford 1999). Desflurane has a high vapor pressure and low boiling point, and it needs to have a special vaporizer to evaporate in order to be delivered to the patient (Table 15.2) (Eger et al.; Eger 1984; Paddleford, 1999).

Table 15.2 Vapor pressures of inhalant anesthetics.

Agent	Vapor Pressure at 20 °C (mm Hg)
Methoxyflurane	22.8
Halothane	244
Isoflurane	239.5–240
Sevoflurane	157–160
Desflurane	664–700

Source: Eger et al. 2003.

Solubility Coefficient

The lower the solubility of the anesthetic, the more rapid gas anesthetics will go from the alveoli into the blood (i.e., gas dissolves into a liquid). If there is low solubility, this means there will be rapid induction because the gas will quickly distribute from the alveoli into the blood. During recovery from anesthesia, the anesthetic gas will be excreted out of the body. From fastest to the slowest rate of alveolar concentration anesthetics are ranked as follows: desflurane, sevoflurane, isoflurane, and halothane. Sevoflurane is twice as soluble as desflurane and nitrous oxide. Halothane is twice as soluble as isoflurane. Isoflurane is twice as soluble as sevoflurane. If delivery of the anesthetic is somehow limited, increased induction time may be seen. This can be the case in inhalant anesthetics, which are irritating and cause the patient to produce excessive saliva, hold its breath, or experience laryngospasm (Eger et al. 2003; Eger 1984). The solubility coefficient of an anesthetic is affected by increases and decreases in body temperature. When patients become hypothermic, the inhalant anesthetics become more soluble in the cooled blood, and less inhalant anesthetic is required to maintain the patient. The opposite is true for hyperthermic patients.

Inhalant anesthetic agents have the following characteristics:

- Inhalant anesthetics affect the CNS.
- The primary method of excretion of inhalant anesthesia is via respiration.
- Most inhalants decrease the rate and volume of respiration.
- Inhalants cause vasodilation in a dose-dependent manner, thereby decreasing peripheral vascular resistance (PVR) and cardiac output.
- Low blood pressure and hypothermia will result due to the vasodilation.
- The effects on heart rate and contractility are variable between agents.
- Renal and cerebral perfusion could be compromised due to vasodilation effects of inhalant anesthetics.

- Malignant hyperthermia can occur in all modern inhalants; however, it is more prevalent in halothane.
- Because some inhalant anesthetics provide only very slight analgesia, additional analgesia should be provided.
- The National Institute for Occupational Safety and Health (NIOSH) states that the principal exposure to waste gas comes from leaks in the anesthetic machine. NIOSH recommends that exposure limits for halogenated inhalant anesthetics should be less than 2 parts per million (ppm). Nitrous oxide concentration should not exceed 25 ppm, and halogenated inhalant anesthetics should not exceed 0.5 ppm if used in combination with nitrous oxide (Paddleford 1999).
- Safety concerns with the reproduction organs, liver, and kidney, and incidences of cancer need to be considered.
- Exposure of pregnant females to inhalants should be avoided, particularly in the first trimester (Thurmon et al. 1996; Paddleford 1999).
- Monitoring for exposure to waste gas should be performed periodically, and adequate scavenging of waste gas should be utilized to decrease waste gas in the areas where inhalant anesthetics are being used.

Specific Inhalants

Nitrous Oxide (N_2O)

N_2O is supplied in compressed gas cylinders. It does not need to be vaporized to be delivered to a patient. N_2O will decrease the availability of oxygen to a patient and this can cause hypoxemia. N_2O must be delivered to the patient with oxygen. The amount of N_2O should not be delivered in excess of 66% so that a minimum of 33% oxygen (O_2) is available to the patient (Eger et al. 2003; McKelvey et al. 2003; Thurmon et al. 1996; Paddleford 1999). Typically, N_2O is used for general anesthesia by combining it with another inhalant anesthetic. This will reduce the amount of the more potent and potentially toxic inhalant anesthetics to be used (Thurmon et al. 1996).

The "second gas effect" allows for a concurrently delivered (along with the N_2O) inhalant anesthetic to be delivered to the blood and tissues faster, using less of it because the N_2O, in a sense, forces the concentration of the second gas. Because N_2O is administered in high concentrations and taken up quickly, the second gas's alveolar concentration increases more rapidly than when given as the sole inhalant (Thurmon et al. 1996).

At the end of anesthesia there is rapid movement of N_2O out of the blood and into the lungs. This will displace oxygen and cause diffusion hypoxia. The patient must be left on 100% oxygen for at least 5 to 10 minutes to prevent diffusion hypoxia (Thurmon et al. 1996; Paddleford 1999).

Closed gas pocket disease can occur with the use of N_2O in the case of a closed anatomic structure that can expand but have no escape for the gas to release if it builds up. Examples of this include GDV, colic, GI obstruction, and pneumothorax. High concentrations of N_2O will continue to diffuse into those confined areas faster than N_2 can diffuse out. Because there is no significant amount of N_2O in the body before delivering the N_2O, it will dissipate into the closed structures and could potentially double in that space, causing a great deal of pressure on the structures of the organ or the surrounding tissues (compromising respiration or cardiovascular circulation). The cuff on the endotracheal tube could also increase causing pressure on the tracheal wall (Eger et al. 2003; Eger 1974).

It's important to remember that when utilizing N_2O gas, the monitoring of CO_2 could be inaccurate (Thurmon et al. 1996). There should also be some concern that nitrous oxide could be used for recreational abuse. Precautions should be taken to avoid misuse (NIDA 2009).

Halothane (classification: halogenated hydrocarbon)

The following are characteristics of halothane:

- Vapor pressure is high.
- It utilizes precision vaporizer.

- Solubility coefficient is low; fat solubility is high.
- There is rapid induction of anesthesia, but recovery is longer because of retention in the fat tissues.
- Approximately 20% metabolism of halothane occurs in the liver.
- Cardiovascular: The heart is sensitized to catecholamines, which can cause arrhythmias. Halothane depresses the myocardium, causing decreased cardiac output and cardiac contractility.
- It causes vasodilation and subsequent hypotension.
- There is increased vagal tone, resulting in bradycardia.
- It is not as irritating to the respiratory tract as isoflurane.
- Reproduction: Halothane crosses the blood placental barrier, and it may be harmful to the fetus in pregnant animals.
- It increases cerebral blood flow, which increases intracranial pressure. It is not for use in patients with head trauma or brain disease.
- Preservative thymol is used in halothane as an antioxidant. Thymol can cause halothane to become sticky and increases the need for vaporizers to be cleaned and calibrated.
- Halothane is no longer manufactured in the U.S.

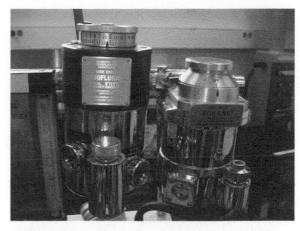

Figure 15.1. Sevoflurane and isoflurane vaporizers mounted side by side on an anesthesia machine.

- There is less cardiac depression than with halothane.
- It is absorbed and eliminated mainly by the lungs.
- Patients may hold their breath or resist during mask induction or anesthetic chamber induction due to the intense odor.
- It is irritating to the respiratory tract.

Isoflurane (classification: halogenated ether)

The following are characteristics of isoflurane:

- As a result of isoflurane having a similar vapor pressure to halothane, halothane vaporizers can be professionally converted to isoflurane vaporizors (Fig. 15.1).
- Solubility coefficient is low in the tissue and the blood, which increases induction and recovery times.
- Isoflurane does not increase cerebral blood flow as long as ventilation is maintained (McKelvey et al. 2003).
- It causes dose-dependent vasodilation and subsequent hypotension.

Sevoflurane (classification: fluorinated methyl isopropyl ether)

The following are characteristics of sevoflurane:

- Vapor pressure is lower than isoflurane. It needs to have a vaporizer that can deliver up to 8% sevoflurane (Plumb 2002).
- Sevoflurane has a low solubility coefficient. Induction and recovery of sevoflurane anesthesia is faster than with isoflurane.
- Sevoflurane is more pleasant-smelling than isoflurane. Mask induction is more favorable and rapid with sevoflurane as compared to isoflurane.
- Sevoflurane is less potent than isoflurane, but more potent than desflurane.
- 2.5–4% is necessary for maintenance of anesthesia.
- A reaction with sodalime produces compound A, which has been shown to cause

renal damage in rats. Renal damage has not been reported in dogs and cats.

Desflurane (classification: fluorinated methyl ethyl ether)

The following are characteristics of desflurane:

- Vapor pressure is very high.
- At room temperature desflurane is nearly at its boiling point.
- A special vaporizer is needed that is pressurized and heated to control the temperature of desflurane before delivery of the anesthetic to the patient. This special vaporizer is vastly more expensive than others. It requires electrical power for heating.
- It has the lowest solubility coefficient and is least potent of any of the anesthetics discussed in this chapter.
- It has extremely rapid induction and recovery.
- Cardiovascular effects are similar to isoflurane.
- Dose-dependent respiratory depression and irritation to the respiratory tract occur.
- It is absorbed and eliminated by the lung.

References

Eger, EI. 1984. Anesthetic Uptake and Action. Baltimore: Waverly Press, pp.1, 45–96, 181, 302–303.

Eger, EI, Eisenkraft, JB, Weiskopf, RB. 2003. The Pharmacology of Inhaled Anesthetics, 2nd ed. n.p. Edmond I. Eger II, M.D., pp.1–5, 8, 22–26, 33–67.

Fenster, JM. 2002. Ether Day. New York: Harper Collins Publisher, pp.1–3.

McKelvey, D, Hollingshead, KW. 2003. Small Animal Anesthesia, Canine and Feline Practice, 3rd ed. St. Louis: Mosby, pp.7, 52, 55, 145, 157.

Muir, WW, Hubbell, JAE, Skarda, RT, Bednarski, RM. 2000. Handbook of Veterinary Anesthesia, 3rd ed. St. Louis: Mosby, pp.142, 143, 155.

Paddleford, RR. 1999. Manual of Small Animal Anesthesia, 2nd ed. Philadelphia: WB Saunders Company, pp.11, 12, 62, 68, 72–74.

Plumb, DC. 2002. Veterinary Drug Handbook, 4th ed. Ames, IA: Iowa State Press, p.153.

Stoelting, RK. 1999. Pharmacology and Physiology in Anesthetic Practice, 3rd ed. Philadelphia: Lippincott-Raven, pp.20, 21.

Thurmon, JC, Tranquilli, WJ, Benson, GJ. 1996. Lumb and Jones' Veterinary Anesthesia, 3rd ed. Baltimore: Williams and Wilkins, 9, 11, 320–321.

Web Resources

Guidelines for Protecting Safety and Health of Health Care Workers, 5. Recommended Guidelines for Controlling Non-infectious Health Hazards in Hospitals continued, 5.1.12.3 Standards and Recommendations, 04/98, National Institute for Occupational Health and Safety, 01 March 2009, http://www.cdc.gov/niosh/hcwold5b.html

NIDA InfoFacts: Inhalants, 06/08, National Information on Drug Abuse, 28 February 2009, http://www.nida.nih.gov/Infofacts/Inhalants.html

NIOSH Publication No. 2007-151: Waste Anesthetic Gases—Occupational Hazards in Hospitals, 09/07, National Institute for Occupational Health and Safety, 01 March 2009, http://www.cdc.gov/niosh/docs/2007-151/

Recovery of the Anesthetic Patient

16

Michelle Cheyne

Recovery is an important part and the very last period of an anesthetic episode. Recovery begins when the anesthetic agent or agents are discontinued and the animal is allowed to return to a normal state. Recovery is often overlooked, and many complications can arise in this period even in the young and healthy patient. Many unsupervised patients suffer respiratory arrest in recovery, either because their airways are obstructed due to positioning or they aren't watched closely following extubation. All attempts should be made to plan ahead and be prepared for possible complications. There should be at least one technician assigned to the recovery area to keep an eye on postoperative patients and monitor them until they are stable enough to be released to the wards/kennels. It is important to have an anesthesia recovery protocol for all staff to follow. Planning ahead for recovery is good practice. The recovery area should be prepared to receive the patient before it gets there. Some patients will need ongoing supportive care, which should be arranged ahead of time. Many patients will need ongoing heat support, and the heating units may need to be warmed ahead of time. If the patient needs to be moved to another area of the hospital (for postop radiographs for instance), that area should be set up and ready to receive the patient.

The following is a quick overview of recovery procedures (further discussion of each of the steps follows later in the chapter):

1. Turn off or discontinue anesthetic agent/ agents. If the patient is intubated and on inhalant anesthetic, provide the patient with 100% oxygen for 5 minutes to help "wash out" some of the inhalant. Keeping the patient hooked to the anesthesia machine allows for ongoing delivery of oxygen and also allows for the removal of much of the exhaled waste gas out of the scavenge system. At this time, it is best to remove any "oral" monitors, such as esophageal temperature probes and esophageal stethoscope probes in case of sudden return to consciousness. Mechanical and physical monitoring can and should continue during this time. Some patients may need to be weaned from mechanical ventilation. Except in the most critical patients, this can usually be safely accomplished while the surgeon is closing the incision. Neuromuscular blockade must be reversed prior to weaning from the ventilator.

2. Any procedures that can be completed while the patient is still in the OR or at the

procedure site should be done before the patient is completely awake. The nature of the recovery can never be accurately determined and sometimes conscious patients won't allow the final procedures to be performed without further sedation. The application of bandages, rinsing and suctioning potential regurgitation, placement of nasal lines, and further exams (oral, ear cleaning, etc.) are best completed under the cover of anesthesia if the patient is deemed stable.

3. After the oxygen is discontinued (the oxygen flow meter should be turned off, the reservoir bag squeezed empty, and *then* the patient should be disconnected from the wye) and the patient is stable without it, the monitoring equipment can be removed and the patient moved to the recovery area or ICU. Use of a wheeled gurney or soft Quick Carry gurney is recommended for the safety of larger patients.

4. The patient should be placed in a warm, dry kennel with adequate bedding for recovery. Positioning will depend on the procedure. Patients should not be laid on incision sites if at all possible. For many patients, sternal recumbency is best for maintaining a patent airway and allowing positional atelectasis to be reversed. Usually the head can be supported with a pillow or rolled towel to help prevent airway obstruction.

5. Not until the patient has reached the final recovery spot should endotracheal ties be released. Patients can become inadvertently extubated during the move. The endotracheal tube cuff should not be deflated until just before extubation.

6. Begin postanesthetic monitoring at regular intervals. The anesthesia record should reflect recovery procedures, pulse strength and quality, heart rate, respiratory rate, temperature, mucus membrane color, capillary refill time, and if possible SpO_2. Obviously some patients will require more intensive monitoring. Patients that have experienced cardiac arrhythmias intraop (splenectomy, GDV perhaps?) should have

ongoing ECG monitoring. Thoracic surgery patients may need oxygen supplementation, so pulse oximetry can be very helpful in determining the need for that. Chest tubes may need to be evacuated if desaturation occurs. Continue to monitor the patient's temperature until it returns to near normal and the patient is alert and responsive. Heat should be removed from patients *before* they reach normal so that hyperthermia can be avoided. Be aware that patients cannot always remove themselves from heat sources when they begin to overheat.

7. Once the patient's gag reflex returns, remove the tube insuring that the pilot balloon is deflated. Cats need to be extubated a bit sooner than dogs because of the potential for laryngospasm. In brachycephalic breeds, extubation should be delayed as long as possible (Fig. 16.1).

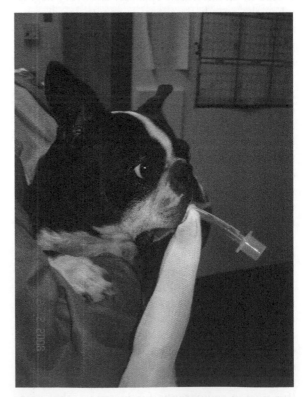

Figure 16.1. The brachycephalic breeds are often quite content to remain intubated well into the recovery process.

Not until the patient is actively trying to expel the tube or begins chewing should it be extubated. These breeds have excessively long soft palates, large tongues, and tiny tracheas in contrast to body size and other anomalies that make airway obstruction a very common event. Often these patients are perfectly content to remain intubated even though they appear very alert and awake. In some cases, with certain oral surgeries or if the patient has regurgitated, it is wise to extubate the patient with the cuff partially inflated to help prevent aspiration of blood or regurge. Following extubation, monitor the patient's chest excursions and be sure that the patient continues to move air without noise or excessive effort. Mucous membrane color should be monitored as well. In cases of suspected nasal edema, the application of dilute phenylephrine to the nasal passages via a large-bore catheter can help reduce obstruction by causing vasoconstriction of the mucous membranes.

8. Continuously monitor the patient for signs of pain, discomfort, excitement, or dysphoria. For patients that were extremely anxious in the preoperative period, it may be wise to have a dose of sedative available. Low-dose acepromazine (0.01–0.025 mg/kg) can be an excellent anxiolytic drug to have nearby for stable postop patients. It can often be enough to just "take the edge off" and allow patients to recover peacefully. Causes of anxiety can include full bladders, hunger (especially in young pets and Labradors!), and fear. Pain should be ruled out through careful patient assessment. Additional doses of analgesics should be given if pain is suspected.

9. Treatment regimens should begin in recovery. Temperature and vital sign monitoring should be done at regular intervals according to your hospital's protocol. More critical patients will require more intensive monitoring. This may include laboratory testing, such as packed cell volume and total solids or intermittent blood gas analysis. The anesthetic record should be updated accordingly, and an overall assessment of the patient's recovery should be recorded on the record. These notes can be helpful to refer to if the patient ever needs to be anesthetized again.

10. The IV catheter should be removed only after the patient is alert and, ideally, ambulatory. It is a good idea to wait several hours before pulling the catheter in case of a crisis. It can be very difficult to gain IV access in an emergency. Be sure that ongoing IV treatments are not planned prior to pulling the catheter. For difficult or "caution" dogs and cats, a long extension set can be secured to the catheter prior to recovery. This allows for additional medications to be given once the pet is awake without having to handle it. It is important to know the volume of the extension set so that sufficient flush is given to ensure that the medications reach the circulation and don't remain in the line. Low-volume (0.5–1.0 mL) extension sets are available for smaller patients. If the patient is particularly fractious, low-dose, "conscious sedation" from propofol or other sedatives can be given through the IV to facilitate catheter removal (or bandage changes) prior to going home.

The Recovery Room

The recovery room should be a quiet place away from kennels or other noisy areas. The area should have adequate but dim light to further facilitate a smooth recovery. People in the area should also maintain a quiet atmosphere, being careful not to make any loud noises or sudden movements. Cages should be available for every recovering patient. Patients should be kept in separate cages or areas away from other recovering patients (Fig. 16.2).

The cage should be large enough for the animal to turn around but not large enough to allow the patient to walk and cause injuries from being ataxic. The recovery room should be well stocked with various supplies needed to aid in

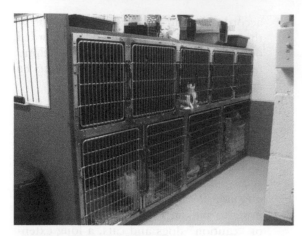

Figure 16.2.   Recovery cages.

recovery and to successfully handle any emergencies that might arise. The following is a guideline of supplies that are handy to have stocked in the recovery room:

- Various sizes of endotracheal tubes, sterile lubricant, ties, cuff inflation syringe
- Laryngoscope
- Oxygen delivery system, including oxygen lines, mask, nasal oxygen delivery setup
- Suction, suction tips, saline
- Intravenous lines, fluids, and pumps
- Intravenous catheters, T-ports, caps, saline flush
- Various sizes of needles and syringes
- Bandage materials
- Gloves, paper towels, cleaning supplies
- Thermometer
- Heat sources
- Pulse oximeter
- Blood pressure measuring device
- EKG monitor
- Emergency drugs

Transferring the Recovering Patient

Patients should be transferred on gurneys from surgery/procedure rooms to recovery or ICU. Transferring the patient on a gurney prevents spinal cord injury, airway obstruction, and regurgitation that can occur during carrying of patients. The patient should be gently lifted with the spine supported and gently placed to lie comfortably in the cage.

Removing Monitoring Equipment from the Recovering Patient

All unused monitoring equipment should be removed from the patient. Intravenous catheters should remain in place in case of an emergency. Arterial catheters should be removed at this time. A pressure bandage should be applied over the area where the arterial catheter was removed. If the arterial catheter was placed in the lingual artery, digital pressure must be applied for 5–15 minutes to inhibit the formation of hematomas. If the patient is transferred to a well-attended intensive care unit, arterial catheters can stay in place throughout the recovery period. Arterial catheters should be flushed every 2 hours to maintain patency. Patients may also need to recover with a continuous EKG monitor in place. EKG conduction patches should be placed if the patient is to be monitored. Alligator clips that are placed during anesthesia can become painful and/or uncomfortable to the recovering patient.

Monitoring the Patient during Recovery

Monitoring should continue until the animal returns to an alert and conscious state (Fig. 16.3). All monitored values should be well documented in the anesthetic record.

Observations should include, but need not be limited to, the following: heart rate, respiratory rate and ventilation, capillary refill time, and mucus membrane color. Temperature should be monitored until the return of normal values. The patient should have vital signs checked every 15 to 20 minutes or more often if the patient is critical. A patient should never be left alone to recover.

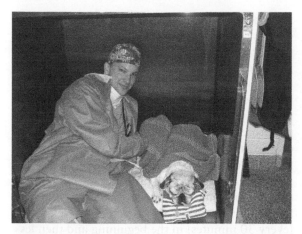

Figure 16.3. The patient must be monitored carefully throughout recovery.

Temperature

It is important to monitor the patient's temperature until it returns to normal. Patients that suffer from hypothermia will suffer from a prolonged recovery period. Smaller patients or geriatric patients are more susceptible to suffering from hypothermia, and all attempts should be made to return the patient to normal temperature. Patients' temperatures are most easily taken rectally. Temperatures may also be taken axially or aurally. Temperatures should be obtained axially or aurally if rectal temperatures are not tolerated by the patient or if perirectal surgery has been performed. Normal rectal temperature in dogs and cats is 101.5 ± 1 °F. Normal axial and aural temperature is 100.5 ± 1 °F.

Heating elements

Heating elements may be used to decrease rewarming time. Any heating element must be used with caution. Patients that are recovering from anesthesia are unable to move away from heating elements and may suffer from thermal skin burns, which are often a serious complication (Welsh 2003). Blood flow through the skin moderates temperature by warming cool areas and cooling warm areas of the body. During anesthesia and periods of hypothermia, blood flow is shunted away from the skin and concen-

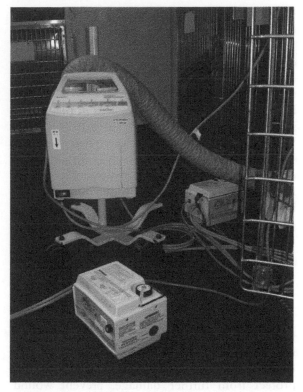

Figure 16.4. Examples of available heating units. A forced hot air blower unit and a circulating warm water pump.

trated in the body's vital organs (i.e., brain, heart, liver). Without full blood flow, the skin is susceptible to burning because the heat, to which it is exposed, cannot be moderated. All attempts should be made to keep a barrier between the heating element and the patient.

There are a variety of heating elements commercially available for veterinary use (Fig. 16.4). See Chapter 10 under temperature monitoring for a complete list and description.

Nasal Oxygen Placement

Indwelling intranasal catheters may need to be placed to provide a means of delivering supplemental oxygen to patients that are extubated. Nasal oxygen lines should be placed before the patient recovers due to the discomfort of placing the catheters. A red rubber or feeding tube can be used. The catheter is passed in the nasal cavity to the level of the medial canthus of the eye. Nasal tubing should not exceed the lateral canthus of the eye. The tubing should be lubricated with water-soluble lubricant to decrease the amount of irritation caused by passing the line. The lines can then be secured in place with sutures, surgical staples, or surgical glue. The lines can then be connected to an oxygen delivery system. The oxygen should be humidified to decrease the irritation of the airways. The oxygen flow rate could vary from 1–3 L/minute depending on the underlying disease process and the size of the patient. Oxygen flow rates higher than 3 L/minute can cause nasopharyngeal irritation.

Bandage Placement

Bandages should be placed on the patient before recovery. Some surgeries performed will require bandage application. Bandages are placed to protect from further damage, prevent wound desiccation, prevent seroma or hematoma formation, immobilize the wound and prevent cellular disruption, minimize surrounding edema, absorb wound exudates, and keep the wound warm, which facilitates wound healing. Bandages must be checked frequently for signs of hemorrhage. They also need to be checked to make sure they are not too tight. Tight bandages can inhibit chest excursions in thoracotomy patients and cut off circulation to distal limbs. Toes should be checked for swelling and warmth several times a day following bandaging. Bandages must also be kept clean and dry. If the bandage becomes wet or soiled, it needs to be changed. Empty fluid bags can be placed over limb bandages for walks outside in the rain or snow. They must be removed immediately once back inside to allow for ventilation of the bandage and limb.

Tracheostomy Patient

Patients undergoing tracheostomy require intensive postoperative care. It is recommended that these patients be recovered in the ICU. A tracheostomy can be temporary or permanent. A temporary tracheostomy usually involves the placement of a single or double lumen tracheostomy tube within a temporary stoma. A permanent tracheostomy is a surgical permanent stoma without the use of a tube. The stoma should be monitored for signs of redness, swelling, discharge, and subsequent occlusion. A temporary tracheostomy requires continual supervision and nursing. The body will produce secretions that require suctioning from the tracheostomy tube. Suctioning should be performed more frequently (every 30 minutes) in the beginning and then less frequently (every 1–3 hours) as the tracheal epithelium adjusts to the dry, cool inspired air. Administer 1 ml of sterile saline before suctioning to break up thick secretions. The site should be closely monitored for blockage and infection. If a blockage occurs in the tracheostomy tube from sections, the tube should be changed. The patient should be monitored to ensure that bedding or other debris cannot occlude the airway.

Urinary Catheter Management in the Recovering Patient

Some patients that undergo anesthetic procedures will receive a urinary catheter. Urinary catheters must be placed using a sterile technique so that microbes are not introduced into the urinary bladder. Female urinary catheters are more difficult to place and take practice. There are many different types of urinary catheter on the market for use in veterinary medicine. The most common long-term indwelling urinary catheters are catheters with or without a pilot balloon. Polypropylene urinary catheters are not recommended for long-term use. Foley catheters contain a pilot balloon on the end that inserts into the urinary bladder; when it is inflated, it holds the catheter in place. Other urinary catheters need to be sutured in place. A Chinese finger trap is recommended to hold the catheter in place. A sterile IV line and sterile fluid bag are connected to the urinary catheter to drain. Sterile technique must always be used when handling and emptying the closed urinary system.

Regurgitation during Recovery

In some cases, patients will regurgitate. It is important to remove this fluid and lavage with saline, because gastric contents are highly acidic and can damage the lining of the esophagus and oral cavity. The patient may also aspirate gastric fluid causing aspiration pneumonia. If the patient regurgitates, ensure that the endotracheal tube pilot balloon is inflated. Using saline or water, rinse and suction out the oral cavity until clean. Ensure that the oral cavity is clean by checking with the laryngoscope to visually ensure that all debris has been cleared.

Analgesia and Tranquilization

It is never certain how animals are going to react recovering from an anesthetic episode. All attempts should be made to aid in a peaceful, pain-free recovery. Reasons for a rough recovery include pain, anxiety, and drug reaction. Analgesia is the freedom from or absence of pain. It is considered humanely necessary to provide sufficient pain control. It is often difficult to distinguish pain from dysphoria. If adequate analgesia was provided in the anesthetic protocol, dysphoria is more likely unless the patient underwent a painful procedure that requires frequent pain assessment and analgesia administration. If a procedure is known to cause pain in a human, it should also be considered to cause pain in animals, and analgesia should be provided.

Patients can become dysphoric and ataxic and may require a form of tranquilization or restraint. Tranquilization relieves anxiety and the patient is relaxed. Patients can also sometimes become fractious during the recovery period. Fractious patients should be safely restrained if possible and/or tranquilized. Tranquilization will aid in the comfort and safety of the animal and the

safety of the person recovering the patient. Chemical restraint should be used if necessary. If needed, benzodiazepines or tranquilizers can be administered intravenously or intramuscularly to sedate the patient. Diazepam, midazolam, and acepromazine can be used for chemical methods of restraint. It is important to remember that the above medications provide no analgesia, and therefore analgesia should be given if there is reason to believe the patient is painful. Medetomidine is an alpha-2 agonist that can be used as a tranquilizer and has analgesic properties as well. The use of medetomidine is controversial in the recovery setting because of the cardiovascular effects and should be considered only for stable patients if other sedatives have not been effective

Feral Cats/Known Fractious Animals

In extreme cases the patient may become too fractious to handle. If obtaining vital signs becomes stressful for the patient it should not be attempted. If the patient is not injuring itself and appears alert, it should be left alone in a quite area.

In some cases a "hands-off" recovery approach is the best option. For many feral cats or known fractious animals, it is better to recover these patients in a small carrier. The patient should be left alone to recover and no vital signs should be attempted. This ensures the safety of the personnel handing the patient and the patient.

Extubation of the Endotracheal Tube

This step of recovery is often considered one of the most important, and if performed too early serious complications can occur. The pilot balloon should be deflated. The only exception to this is when the patient has undergone a procedure where there is excess fluid in the oral cavity. The pilot balloon can be left slightly inflated to prevent fluid from passing down the trachea into the lungs. Once the patient's gag reflex returns, the endotracheal tube can be pulled (Welsh 2003). The patient should be able to swallow and maintain a patent airway before the endotracheal tube is removed. The endotracheal tube should be removed slowly, taking care not to damage the pilot balloon on the teeth. If the patient begins to vomit or regurgitate, the patient's head should be positioned downward to enable fluid to drain by the mouth and not down the airway. The patient should be monitored for signs of dyspnea. Sometimes the patient will have to be reintubated to have supplemental oxygen administered. The patient may need to be reanesthetized and reintubated to maintain a patent airway.

Bedding

There should be padding/bedding to aid in a comfortable recovery for the patient. During the recovery period, patients often urinate and defecate. The patient should be kept clean and dry at all times.

Conclusion

It is important to remember that each recovering patient is different and different problems can arise. Recovery can last a few seconds to hours in some cases. A technician should be aware and prepared to treat problems that could arise in the recovery period. A technician should also be aware of the patient's needs and disease factors that may inhibit a smooth recovery period. Efficient planning inhibits poor performance.

References

Welsh, E. 2003. Anaesthesia for Veterinary Nurses, edited by Welsh, E. Oxford, UK: Blackwell Publishing.

Anesthetic Complications and Emergencies

Samantha McMillan

When we consider that almost all of the anesthetic drugs commonly used cause some degree of reduction in cardiac output, blood pressure, respiratory rate, tidal volume, and body temperature regulation, it is perhaps surprising that anesthetic accidents and emergencies do not occur more commonly. Every anesthetic has the potential to cause harm if not carefully monitored by a proactive anesthetist with a watchful eye for potential complications coupled with the knowledge of how to manage and treat these problems if they occur. Evaluation of patient risk factors, by performing a thorough clinical assessment, will allow the anesthetist to identify any preexisting problems. Where possible, these should be corrected prior to anesthesia. Conditions such as hyperkalemia or hypovolemia should be treated before induction to reduce the patient's anesthetic risk. Conditions and risk factors that cannot be rectified such as breed factors (e.g., brachycephalic obstructive airway syndrome) can be identified and potential complications planned and prepared for. Potentially useful drugs can have their doses and infusion rates calculated and can be prepared for use if required.

Most anesthetic complications and emergencies can be categorized into human error, equipment problems, ventilatory/respiratory problems, cardiovascular problems, and thermoregulatory problems.

Human error is a frequent cause of anesthetic complications and the importance of vigilance by every anesthetist cannot be overemphasized. There are many factors that can contribute to human error, including miscalculation of anesthetic drug doses, an incomplete clinical assessment (i.e., an inadequate history or physical exam), inadequate knowledge of the anesthetic machine or anesthetic drugs being used, and errors in administration of anesthetic drugs (i.e., misidentification of drugs, incorrect route of administration, or incorrect dosage).

It should be noted that most emergencies can be avoided or quickly treated through careful monitoring and early detection because few serious complications and emergencies are truly immediate in onset. Failure to carefully monitor the anesthetic (which may be due to other constraints on the anesthetist's time, complacency, or fatigue) will mean that the anesthetist fails to recognize the early warning signs of a possible complication.

Equipment Complications

True equipment failure is relatively rare, and it is usually human error that causes equipment to fail or malfunction—for example, unrecognized breathing system disconnection or not setting up the anesthetic machine adequately. Probably the most important factor with equipment failure is the inability to deliver an adequate oxygen supply to the patient. This can be due to lack of oxygen in the cylinders, disconnection of piped oxygen supply, a stuck or missing one-way valve in a rebreathing system, leaks in the anesthetic machine/breathing system, or ventilator failure.

A thorough initial check of the anesthetic machine and appropriate breathing system prior to starting the anesthetic, coupled with a good knowledge of the machine, can alleviate many potential equipment problems. Common equipment faults include:

- Exhaustion of carbon dioxide absorber
- Endotracheal (ET) tube complications
- Adjustable pressure limiting (APL, or pop-off) valves
- Vaporizer complications

Although exhausted CO_2 absorbent will change color, if the absorbent is not changed quickly but instead left within the canister, it will gradually return to its original color. This gives the appearance that it is still active, resulting in the patient becoming hypercarbic due to CO_2 not being removed from the breathing system. The patient may show signs of tachycardia and ventricular arrhythmias.

ET tubes may become blocked prior to or during the anesthetic. All ET tubes should be checked thoroughly prior to use and then monitored carefully when in situ. Special care should be taken during procedures around the head and neck area to ensure that the ET tube does not become kinked or twisted. Blood, mucus, saliva, etc. may block the tube while in situ. Regardless of the cause of the blockage it must be quickly rectified. A complete blockage of the patient's ET tube will cause the patient to become dyspneic, hypoxic, and hypercarbic, and possibly progress

to respiratory arrest if not recognized and dealt with rapidly. Reintubation may be required, or the solution may be as simple as repositioning the patient's head or neck to rectify a kink in the tube or suctioning the lumen to remove debris.

Problems with APL valves on the breathing system are created when they are accidentally left in the closed position. This can occur at the start of anesthesia because the anesthetist has not conducted thorough checks or failed to open the valve after pressure checking, or during intermittent positive pressure ventilation (IPPV). The closure of these valves causes the pressure in the breathing system to quickly build up. This pressure causes overinflation of the reservoir bag and consequently the patient's lungs. This causes barotrauma, prevents expiration, may lead to pneumothorax, and reduces venous return impacting on cardiac output and blood pressure. This complication can lead to respiratory arrest and then to fatality in a relatively short period of time. If this is noticed quickly, treatment is generally as simple as opening the valve. Pop-off occlusion valves are available (Smiths Medical) that help prevent this potentially life-threatening complication. By simply pressing a button on the occlusion valve, gas is blocked and accumulates within the system and a positive pressure breath may be given. The button contains a spring that opens the occlusion as soon as the button is released. There is no further adjustment needed. These buttons are highly recommended for use on every anesthesia machine.

Vaporizer complications can also be caused by human error—for example, filling the vaporizer with the wrong anesthetic agent. This may result in the wrong agent being delivered to the patient at an inappropriate concentration. Other vaporizer complications include sticking of the dial (previously associated with the thymol preservative in halothane), underfilling, overfilling, and tilting of the vaporizer. The latter two result in the patient receiving an overdose of inhalant agent, regardless of the percentage on the dial; underfilling causes the patient to not receive any anesthetic agent and potentially wake up. Another complication associated with vaporizers occurs if they are not correctly seated and locked onto the back bar of the anesthetic machine. This may not be immediately obvious, but will cause the patient to become lighter and lighter despite turning the percentage up on the vaporizer dial. The patient will wake up if this error is not recognized and rectified quickly.

Physiologic Complications

Perivascular injection of anesthetic drugs will cause a swelling around the vein and often pain at the injection site. Barbiturate anesthetic agents pose a particular problem when accidental perivascular injection occurs due to their alkalinity. Perivascular administration of these agents can be extremely painful and cause skin and subcutaneous necrosis and sloughing. Prevention simply includes placement of an intravenous catheter prior to induction coupled with careful checking and flushing of the catheter prior to drug administration. Treatment of perivascular injection with barbiturate anesthetics involves dilution by instilling sterile saline (2–10 mL) around the affected vein. Lidocaine can also be administered to neutralize the alkaline pH of the barbiturate and provide local analgesia.

Excitation

Excitation can occur when some drugs (especially benzodiazepines) are used as premedication and induction agents in healthy patients. This can pose a risk of injury to both the patient and the anesthesia team. Appropriate restraint and the administration of further premedication or induction agent are warranted.

Aspiration

Aspiration can occur following vomiting or regurgitation of stomach or esophageal contents or due to aspiration of saliva, blood, or mucus caused as a consequence of either the anesthetic, surgical procedure, or disease process. Vomiting and regurgitation are particularly hazardous during induction and recovery because the patient's airway is not protected. Aspiration,

especially following regurgitation, may be a silent process, and for this reason probably occurs more often than is realized. The initial problem caused by aspiration is airway obstruction with the foreign materials being inhaled into the respiratory tract. This will often result in immediate clinical signs of dyspnea, cyanosis, and bronchospasm. Aspiration pneumonia may develop; signs include dyspnea, tachypnea, cough, pyrexia, and increased lung sounds, and the patient will require treatment. However, this is a more gradual process because it develops usually 1–2 days postanesthesia.

There are some drugs that, through the nature of their action, relax the esophageal sphincter and could predispose the patient to regurgitation. These include volatile agents, anticholinergics, opioids, and barbiturates. There are also some factors that will delay gastric emptying time, causing a possible predisposition to both vomiting and regurgitation. These factors include the use of anticholinergic and opioid drugs, fear, pain, and shock. Other predisposing factors include prolonged anesthesia and increased abdominal pressure, due either to medical or disease factors—pregnancy, pyometritis, obesity, gastrointestinal tract obstruction (particularly pyloric and proximal small intestine), ascites, abdominal effusion—or due to patient positioning (a head-down position during surgery will increase pressure on the stomach).

Treatment will depend on whether the patient is conscious or still anesthetized and whether the airway is protected. If regurgitation/vomiting occurs in the anesthetized patient with a properly inflated cuffed endotracheal tube, the risk is relatively small; the patient should be placed with the head lower than the body and the oral cavity may need to be lavaged and suctioned. Failure to rinse the highly acidic regurgitation from the oral cavity and esophagus can result in esophagitis and even strictures. In the unconscious patient without a protected airway, intubation should be attempted. If this is not possible, the patient should be positioned as before to allow drainage of fluid from the oral cavity and suction should be utilized. The conscious patient that has the ability to swallow should have the ability to protect its own airway, and the anesthetist should ensure that the head and neck are extended with the head lowered.

Apnea

Apnea is commonly seen at induction when drugs such as propofol are given too rapidly. It may also be caused by an overdose of anesthetic drugs, including induction anesthetic agent (e.g., barbiturates, propofol, ketamine), inhalant anesthetics, and the opioid analgesics (e.g., fentanyl). Following induction, breath-holding may also be observed due to an inadequate depth of anesthesia.

Other causes of respiratory arrest include brainstem injury in head trauma patients, hypoxia, severe pulmonary disease, cardiac arrest, iatrogenic hyperventilation of the patient, administration of neuromuscular blocking agents (NMBA), neuromuscular diseases, and equipment failure (i.e., APL valve left closed).

In cases where a drug has been administered too quickly, the apnea is often transient, and spontaneous respiration will return as the initial effect of the drug wears off. SpO_2 and cardiovascular monitoring of the patient through periods of apnea is required to ensure that hemoglobin desaturation and cardiovascular complications do not occur. If the apnea is prolonged and SpO_2 begins to fall, IPPV can be initiated. IPPV must be initiated when apnea is secondary to administration of NMBAs.

Treatment of the underlying cause of the apnea must be established. Anesthetic depth should be evaluated and adjusted accordingly. In the case of respiratory arrest, resuscitation should be commenced (see sections on cardiopulmonary and cerebral resuscitation later in this chapter).

Airway obstruction

Airway obstruction is most likely to occur in the preanesthetic period or during recovery when the patient does not have a protected airway.

Signs of airway obstruction include inspiratory stridor, dyspnea, paradoxical thoracic wall movement (full airway obstruction), increased respiratory effort with prolonged inspiratory time, little or no movement of the reservoir bag (if anesthetized), and cyanotic mucous membranes.

Causes of upper airway obstruction may include soft tissue entrapment—common in brachycephalic patients due to brachycephalic obstructive airway syndrome. The tongue and soft palate are often implicated—laryngeal spasm, laryngeal paralysis, laryngeal edema (often caused by trauma due to intubation), laryngeal or tracheal collapse, foreign material, i.e., blood, mucus, debris, and gastric and esophageal contents (see previous section on aspiration). Upper airway obstruction may also be caused by mechanical obstruction, such as a kinked or blocked ET tube, endobronchial intubation, or a head or neck bandage that is too tight.

Causes of lower airway obstruction may include anaphylactic reaction, bronchospasm, bronchitis, asthma, chronic obstructive pulmonary disease (COPD), tumor, and foreign body.

Treatment for airway obstruction will depend on the underlying cause, but for upper airway obstruction it will generally include extending the head and neck and pulling the tongue forward. This will be especially helpful for patients with soft tissue entrapment. Supplemental oxygen should be provided to any patient in respiratory distress. If vomiting, regurgitation, or obstruction with blood, mucus, or saliva is suspected, the patient should be placed with the head lower than the body to facilitate drainage; suctioning of the airway may be required. Rapid intubation or even emergency tracheostomy may be necessary if the patient is not already intubated. Further treatment, especially for lower airway obstruction, may be required including IPPV and/or drug administration (steroids, antihistamines, or bronchodilators). Planning for the recovery of patients with obstructive airway disease must be thorough and include having essential equipment close at hand, such as a laryngoscope, ET tubes, induction drugs, and tracheostomy tubes. Brachycephalic and other at risk patients should be recovered in sternal recumbency with the head and neck extended and tongue pulled forward.

Laryngospasm

Laryngospasm can occur in cats when the laryngeal tissues are irritated during intubation. This results in airway obstruction due to reflex closure of the laryngeal cartilage. Laryngospasm can be prevented by spraying the larynx with local anesthetic prior to intubation, ensuring adequate anesthetic depth before attempting intubation, and using a gentle intubation technique.

Treatment of laryngospasm involves delaying further attempts at intubation, providing supplemental oxygen, and spraying local anesthetic onto the larynx. This may be enough to encourage the laryngeal cartilage to relax and allow intubation. If this does not work, an NMBA could be considered to paralyze the larynx; however, the patient will need rapid intubation and ventilation due to the paralysis of the intercostal muscles and diaphragm. In severe cases a needle can be placed into the trachea, percutaneously, to provide oxygen, or an emergency tracheostomy may need to be performed. Intubation should never be forced because damage to the larynx can result in edema and may lead to upper airway obstruction when the patient is extubated.

Hypoventilation

Hypoventilation can be defined as reduced minute volume due to a reduction in tidal volume/respiratory rate. This will lead to hypercarbia, which is an increased level of CO_2 in blood (arterial CO_2 tension [$PaCO_2$] will normally read more than 60 mm Hg) and can simultaneously cause hypoxemia. This will normally be recognized by the anesthetist as an increase in end-tidal CO_2. Hypercarbia will cause depression of the central nervous system (CNS) if left untreated. Retention of CO_2 will cause respiratory acidosis and the patient to become acidemic.

Causes of hypoventilation may include:

- Overdose of anesthetic agents, i.e., "too deep"; anesthetic agents depress the respiratory centers in the brain and therefore the normal ventilatory response to hypercarbia, hypoxia, and acidosis.
- Pain such that chest expansion is consciously limited
- Pleural space disease, e.g., pleural effusion
- Pulmonary disease, e.g., pulmonary edema, pneumonia
- Accidental endobronchial intubation
- Abdominal distension increasing pressure on the diaphragm
- Diaphragmatic hernia/rupture
- Severe hypotension leading to reduced cerebral perfusion
- Hypothermia depressing the respiratory centers
- Decrease in functional residual capacity (FRC) during anesthesia, which can lower alveolar ventilation/perfusion ratios and result in ventilation/perfusion mismatch; it can also expand atelectic areas, which can increase intrapulmonary shunting.
- Cervical disease where compression of the spinal cord at the level of the phrenic nerve will compromise respiration
- Paralysis of the muscles of respiration by NMBAs or neuromuscular disease
- Restrictive chest bandages or pain following thoracotomy

Treatment can include reduction in anesthetic depth, reversal of drugs contributing to hypoventilation (e.g., NMBA), IPPV, thoracocentesis, treatment of underlying causes (i.e., abdominal distension, hypotension, hypothermia) and administering analgesia. It is always advisable to check equipment if hypercarbia is suspected (check that sodalime is not exhausted and that one-way valves are moving freely if using a rebreathing circuit). If the patient is in recovery when hypoventilation occurs, administer supplemental oxygen and place in sternal recumbency to minimize the effects of atelectasis, ventilation perfusion inequality, and intrapulmonary shunting. Thoracic bandages should be checked to ensure that they are not the reason for hypoventilation.

Hyperventilation

Hyperventilation can be defined as an increase in minute volume due to an increase in tidal volume/respiratory rate. Common causes are pain, inadequate anesthetic depth (too light), surgical stimulation, overzealous ventilation, hypoxia, hypotension, pyrexia, or hyperthermia. Hyperventilation causes a decrease in $PaCO_2$ and results in a drop in hydrogen ions; this causes respiratory alkalosis and the patient to become alkalemic.

Treatment can include increasing anesthetic depth; administering analgesic agents; reducing IPPV (rate and/or tidal volume); and treatment for hypoxia, hypotension, pyrexia, and hyperthermia if present (see below).

Hypoxemia

Hypoxemia can be defined as low oxygen content in arterial blood. This can be caused by reductions in arterial oxygen tension (PaO_2), decreases in oxygen hemoglobin saturation (SaO_2), and decreases in hemoglobin concentration.

Decreases in PaO_2 are caused by low inspired oxygen levels (FiO_2), hypoventilation, diffusion barrier (i.e., pulmonary edema/pus in alveoli), ventilation/perfusion inequality, and intrapulmonary shunt (causing blood to pass through the lungs without undergoing gaseous exchange).

Decreases in SaO_2 are caused by decreases in PaO_2, and the formation of methemoglobinemia or carboxyhemoglobinemia.

Decreases in hemoglobin concentration are caused by anemia.

Hypoxia

Hypoxia is defined as impaired oxygen delivery to tissues and can be caused by hypoxemia, but can also be caused by decreased cardiac output, decreased perfusion, and increased oxygen extraction by the tissues. Treatment can include oxygen supplementation; IPPV; and, where possible, treatment of an underlying disease, i.e., treatment for hypoventilation, administration of packed red blood cells for anemia, etc.

Cardiovascular

Hypotension

Hypotension is defined as a mean arterial blood pressure of less than 60 mm Hg in small animals. A pressure of greater than this is required to ensure adequate perfusion and oxygen delivery to the brain, heart, and kidneys. Hypotension can lead to signs of shock, ischemia of vital organs resulting in organ dysfunction, and ultimately organ failure.

Causes of hypotension in anesthetized patients include overdose of anesthetic agents (too deep), relative or absolute hypovolemia (hemorrhage, fluid loss, sepsis, systemic inflammatory response syndrome [SIRS]), and drug effects.

There are three main mechanisms that cause hypotension:

- Decreased cardiac output, which can be due to myocardial depression, cardiac arrhythmias, or decreased venous return
- Reduced systemic vascular resistance, which is usually due to vasodilation. Vasodilation is commonly caused by many anesthetic drugs, including barbiturates, phenothiazines, propofol, and all the volatile agents. Vasodilation is also present in patients with SIRS and sepsis.
- Hypovolemia, which can be relative due to vasodilation or can be absolute, caused by factors such as hemorrhage, existing fluid deficits, or third spacing of fluid

Treatment for hypotension will rely on determining the underlying cause, but it will generally include reducing the amount of injectable/inhalational anesthetic agents administered, volume restoration to correct hypovolemia (this may include the use of blood products if the cause is hemorrhage), rectifying oxygenation/ventilation problems to correct hypoxia/hypercarbia, correction of acid-base and electrolyte abnormalities, treatment of arrhythmias, control of hemorrhage, cardiac support if necessary, and vasopressor therapy (refer to Table 17.1).

Hypertension

Causes of hypertension include inadequate depth of anesthesia, pain, hypercarbia, hypoxia, fever, metabolic acidosis, drug effects (catecholamines, ketamine), and systemic hypertension secondary to metabolic disease and secondary to raises in intracranial pressure (Cushing reflex).

Treatment for hypertension will include identifying the underlying cause and correcting this where possible, as in administering analgesia, increasing depth of anesthesia, IPPV treatment of intracranial pressure, etc. Where treatment of the underlying cause is not possible, it may be necessary to administer drug therapy that may include beta blockers or calcium channel blockers.

Arrhythmias

Bradyarrhythmias include sinus bradycardia, atrioventricular (AV) block (1st, 2nd, and 3rd degree), sinus arrest, and atrial standstill. Causes of bradyarrythmias in anesthetized patients include excessive anesthetic depth, drug induction (α_2 agonists, μ opioids, anticholinesterases), increased vagal tone, severe hypoxia, vagal stimulation during surgery, preexisting heart disease, hyperkalemia, intracranial disease causing an increase in intracranial pressure, hypothermia, and severe systemic hypertension.

Many bradyarrhythmias can initially be treated by administration of an anticholinergic (atropine/glycopyrolate). The underlying cause should then be corrected (warm the hypothermic patient, reverse opioids with naloxone, etc). However, anticholinergics are contraindicated if bradycardia is caused by α_2 agonist administration, hyperkalemia, and hypertension (such as with raised intracranial pressure). Where bradycardia is caused by α_2 agonists, reversal can be achieved by the administration of atipamezole if required. Hyperkalemic patients can have their myocardium stabilized with calcium gluconate and the hyperkalemia treated with fluid therapy, dextrose, and insulin administration, or potentially sodium bicarbonate. Patients with increased

intracranial pressure may require treatment with mannitol (Egger 2007).

If the bradycardia is refractory to epinephrine or atropine then isoproterenol can be administered (Egger 2007).

Tachycardia

Tachycardia can be caused by many factors in the anesthetized patient. These include inadequate depth of anesthesia, pain, drug induction (anticholinergics, ketamine, thiobarbiturates, sypathomimetics, pancuronium), hypotension, hyperthermia, hypercarbia, hypoxia, hypokalemia and other electrolyte abnormalities, anemia, hypovolemia, myocardial disease, hyperthyroidism, and pheochromocytoma.

Supraventricular tachydysrhythmias include sinus tachycardia, atrial tachycardia, and atrial fibrillation. Sinus tachycardia can be associated with systemic abnormalities, such as hypotension, hypovolemia, or hypoxia, and can normally be rectified by correcting the underlying problem. It is also associated with patients in chronic heart failure (CHF), but control of the CHF prior to anesthesia should prevent its occurrence.

Supraventricular complexes arise from an ectopic focus above the ventricles. The ventricles will then depolarize in the normal way, resulting in a normal QRS complex. Runs of supraventricular complexes are termed supraventricular tachycardia, and this can greatly reduce cardiac output and consequently tissue perfusion. Where these arrhythmias are severe, diastolic filling is compromised along with myocardial perfusion, and an underlying cause is not obvious, it may be necessary to treat with beta blockers (propanolol, esmolol).

Common ventricular dysrhythmias

The common ventricular dysrhythmias seen in anesthetized patients are ventricular premature complexes (VPCs), ventricular tachycardia, and ventricular fibrillation. These rhythms are associated with primary cardiac disease or a noncardiac cause. Common causes include gastric dilatation and volvulus, trauma, sepsis, acid-base disturbances, hypercarbia, electrolyte imbalances, drugs, hypoxia and myocardial ischemia, splenic, hepatic or atrial hemangiosarcoma, pancreatitis, and traumatic myocarditis.

VPCs arise from an ectopic focus within the ventricles. Depolarization conducts in an abnormal direction across the myocardial cells without using the normal conduction pathways. The complex will appear abnormal, usually wide (due to the prolonged depolarization) and bizarre with the P wave often hidden by the VPC (since the VPC occurs prematurely). Infrequent VPCs will not normally compromise cardiac output, and specific treatment is often unnecessary, but identification of the underlying cause is appropriate to prevent deterioration. VPCs may be caused by pain (a common arrhythmia seen with GDV or splenectomy patients) or hypercarbia. A run of three or more VPCs is termed *ventricular tachycardia* and can cause a significant decrease in cardiac output. Ventricular tachycardia may deteriorate into ventricular fibrillation, which is an arrest rhythm, and its treatment is covered under the section on CPCR. Treatment for ventricular tachycardia includes treatment of the underlying cause and supplemental oxygen, and it may require drug treatment (which would initially be a lidocaine bolus that may be repeated), possibly followed by a continuous rate infusion of lidocaine to prevent the rhythm converting back into ventricular tachycardia. Lidocaine does not work effectively in hypokalemic patients where potassium is <3 mmol/L. Procainamide can be used as a follow-up drug if lidocaine fails to convert the ventricular tachycardia to a normal sinus rhythm (Cooper and Muir 2007).

It should be considered that many dysrhythmias cannot be distinguished without an ECG but that pulse deficits are often indicative of reduced cardiac output due to a cardiac dysrhythmia.

Cardiopulmonary and Cerebral Resuscitation and Crash Protocols

Cardiopulmonary arrest (CPA) can be defined as a sudden cessation of functional ventilation and systemic perfusion. This in turn results in reduced oxygen delivery to tissues with decreased removal of carbon dioxide.

Cardiac arrest and respiratory arrest may occur simultaneously, but often respiratory arrest occurs first; if not quickly treated, cardiac arrest will follow soon afterward. The anesthetist should be able to recognize signs of impending CPA, which may include the following:

- Changes in the patient's respiratory rate, depth, pattern, and effort
- Decreasing end-tidal carbon dioxide
- Hypotension
- Cyanotic, gray, or pale mucous membranes
- Prolonged capillary refill time
- Weak, irregular pulses, irregular heart sounds, tachycardia, ventricular premature complexes
- Bradycardia
- Sudden unexplained increases in anesthetic depth
- Hypothermia despite rewarming efforts

Signs of CPA include

- No detectable heart sounds on auscultation
- Loss of palpable pulses and direct arterial catheter, flat pulse oximeter traces
- Fixed, dilated pupils (occurs within 45 seconds of arrest)
- Absence of ventilation or agonal gasping—this may be masked if the patient is being artificially ventilated.
- Pale, grey, or cyanotic mucous membranes (*Note that mucous membranes and capillary refill time can remain normal for several minutes after arrest*).
- Absence of bleeding at the surgical site; blood may appear dark if the arrest is due to hypoxemia.
- Abnormal ECG tracing; however, with pulseless electrical activity (PEA), the QRS complexes may appear normal on the ECG for several minutes after the arrest, although the myocardium will not be effectively contracting.

- Collapse and loss of consciousness in the awake patient
- Loss of skeletal muscle tone and cranial nerve reflexes

Reasons for Arrest

Reasons for arrest include the following: hypoxemia, hypercarbia, hypotension, hypoglycemia, hypovolemia, electrolyte imbalances (hyperkalemia), vagal stimulation, overdose of anesthetic agent, hypothermia, acid-base abnormalities, preexisting cardiac disease, sensitization of the heart to circulating catecholamines, severe trauma, systemic or metabolic disease, severe underlying cardiac or respiratory disease, CNS (herniation or traumatic brain injury), sepsis, or systemic inflammatory response syndrome (SIRS).

Equipment

It is vitally important to have an adequately stocked crash cart or box comprising essential equipment for both basic and advanced life support techniques. A crash cart allows for more equipment to be stored and is generally used in larger organizations and hospitals. It will normally include space on the top of the cart for an ECG and defibrillator. The box or cart should be kept in a central, easily accessed location and be regularly checked and always immediately restocked after use. This can be encouraged by placing on the crash cart a plastic seal, which is easily broken in an emergency but identifies to personnel that the cart has been used.

The contents of the crash cart or box will vary from hospital to hospital but there are a few essentials that should be included by all:

- Anticholinergic drugs: atropine/glycopyrrolate
- Vasopressor drugs: epinephrine, norepinephrine, vasopressin
- Anti-arrhythmic: lidocaine
- Antagonist drugs: naloxone, flumazenil, atipamazole

- Inotropes: dopamine, dobutamine
- Mannitol
- ET tubes, bandage to secure the tube, laryngoscope and several blades
- Needles and syringes
- I/V catheters, butterfly catheters
- Stylets to aid intubation
- Tracheostomy tubes
- Urinary catheters and connectors to administer oxygen or intratracheal drugs
- Ambubag: not necessary if you always have an anesthetic machine close at hand
- ECG pads: normally preattached to the ECG machine for easy access, but spares should be included in the cart
- Fluids: colloids, crystalloids, and hypertonic saline
- Pressure bags
- Drip sets, including blood filter lines and extension sets
- Surgical kit, including a preloaded scalpel and rib retractors
- Surgical scrub solution, e.g., open chest CPCR
- Defibrillator gel

Attached to the crash cart should be an emergency drug chart that will give the dose in mL per kg for all drugs required in CPCR. This allows quick action by team members when drugs are required in a crash situation.

Emergency drugs should ideally be decanted into multidraw bottles if not already available in this form. This is recommended for drugs that may be needed urgently following CPA, such as epinephrine, atropine, and lidocaine. Glass vials are difficult to negotiate in an emergency situation, especially with larger patients where greater drug volumes are required. These multidraw bottles should be labeled with an expiration date and checked regularly to ensure there is adequate volume remaining. Needles preloaded on assorted labeled syringes are a useful addition kept alongside the appropriate multidraw bottles.

It is useful to think about what is essential to the crash box or cart and what can be obtained from another source if required. The contents should then be prioritized according to emergency use; for example, atropine and epinephrine should be close at hand, whereas drugs that require calculation/dilution/discussion before administration do not have to be so easily accessible. You may decide to include them in your crash box, however, to ensure that there are always some in stock.

Cardiopulmonary and Cerebral Resuscitation (CPCR)

The aim of CPCR is a return to spontaneous ventilation and circulation. During CPCR, we are aiming to restore circulation but also to maximize perfusion to the heart and brain. Cerebral resuscitation is now considered vitally important and has been added to the older resuscitation title "cardiopulmonary resuscitation (CPR)" because studies have shown that there is only a 3-minute window of opportunity in which to restore cerebral perfusion following CPA before irreversible neurological damage will occur (Cooper and Muir 2007).

Speed is therefore of the essence when faced with a patient who has suffered CPA, and all staff should receive training in CPCR techniques and be capable of delivering basic life support techniques. CPCR will be ineffective if performed by only one person, and therefore it is essential that personnel train in CPCR techniques as a team to ensure that they can perform well in a crisis situation.

As soon as a CPA occurs, turn off the anesthetic (if applicable), notify the surgeon and call for help, get someone to hit the alarm button if you have one, and begin initial basic life support procedure:

A—Airway
B—Breathing
C—Circulation

Also consider perioperative drugs that may have precipitated CPA. Reverse opioids using naloxone, benzodiazepines using flumazenil, and medetomidine/ dexmedetomidine with atipamazole.

Airway Management (A)

It is important to quickly establish a patent airway. The most common and effective method is endotracheal intubation. Check existing tubes to ensure that they have not become dislodged or blocked. If the patient is not already intubated, quickly place an endotracheal tube, secure it in place, and inflate the cuff if necessary.

It may be necessary to suction following intubation to remove any mucus or foreign material present within the tube. Remember that suctioning directly from the tube can cause patients to desaturate very quickly. Intermittent oxygen supplementation is recommended between suctioning as well as pulse oximetry.

If the patient cannot be intubated due to respiratory obstruction, oxygen may be provided in a number of ways until an emergency tracheostomy can be performed. An oxygen cannula or urinary catheter may be able to pass the obstruction to allow oxygen administration, or an over the needle catheter can be placed between tracheal rings distal to the obstruction to allow oxygen to be insufflated.

Breathing (B)

Intermittent positive pressure ventilation should be commenced with 100% oxygen using an appropriate anesthetic breathing system. Initially, the patient should be given two breaths 1–2 seconds in duration and then assessed for signs of spontaneous ventilation. If spontaneous ventilation does not occur, ventilation should continue at a rate of 10–12 breaths per minute. Lower ventilation rates have recently been advised following publication of new guidelines for CPCR in humans by the American Heart Association in 2005. Overventilation of CPA patients can cause increased intrathoracic pressure, which will decrease cardiac output and consequently cerebral and coronary perfusion. Overinflation of the lungs can lead to complications such as barotrauma, pneumothorax, inflammation, and hemorrhage and should be avoided. Peak inspiratory pressure should be kept below a maximum of 20 cm H_2O, with tidal volume being approximately 15 mL/kg in patients with normal lungs.

Cats, neonates, and patients with restrictive lung disease (pneumonia and diaphragmatic hernia) will require smaller tidal volumes of 6–10 mL/kg at higher respiratory rates (12–15 breaths per minute) to avoid potential complications.

If the patient is suffering only respiratory arrest, rather than full CPA, use of the Jen Chung (GV26) acupuncture point can be considered (Janssens et al. 1979; Altman 2006). This involves inserting a needle into the bone in the nasal philtrum at the ventral aspect of the nares. This needle is then rotated. This technique is reported to be useful in increasing the respiratory rate in dogs (Janssens et al. 1979; Altman 2006).

Doxapram administration is contraindicated in patients with respiratory arrest because it decreases cerebral perfusion and increases cerebral oxygen consumption and requirement (Plunkett and McMichael 2008).

Circulation (C)

Circulation should be reassessed following intubation and initial commencement of ventilation. If the patient is in cardiac arrest, compressions should be started as soon as possible and not interrupted until return of spontaneous circulation is achieved or a decision is made to cease CPCR attempts.

Closed cardiac compressions: Two mechanisms are employed for closed cardiac compression: the cardiac pump mechanism, which is employed for cats and small, narrow-chested dogs, and the thoracic pump mechanism, which is employed for larger patients.

Cardiac pump mechanism: This method is employed in patients weighing less than 10 kg. The chest is compressed directly over the heart. This action compresses the ventricles to create blood flow. The patient should be positioned in right lateral recumbency with a sandbag placed under the opposing chest wall if required. The heel of one or both hands is used to compress the chest at the fifth intercostal space directly over the heart. In smaller patients, the heart is compressed using the thumb and forefingers on either side of the chest. The chest should be compressed by approximately one-third and excessive pressure should be avoided to prevent intrathoracic trauma (Egger 2007).

Thoracic pump mechanism: This method is suitable for larger patients, over 10 kg, or barrel-chested breeds such as the bulldog. The patient can be placed in either lateral or dorsal recumbency to facilitate this method. If the patient is placed in right lateral recumbency, a sandbag should be placed under the opposing chest wall. The chest wall is compressed by approximately one-third at its widest point. If the patient is in dorsal recumbency, sandbags should be placed to secure the patient in this position and the chest is compressed over the sternum (Egger 2007).

Positive intrathoracic pressure is created by simultaneous ventilation and chest compression. The increase in thoracic pressure causes forward blood flow into the arteries, and back flow into the venous system is prevented by the atrioventricular valves and the collapsing of the great veins due to the pressure. This increased arterial flow will promote cerebral and myocardial perfusion. The relaxation of the chest following compression and the subsequent drop in pressure facilitate venous return.

For both mechanisms the person performing compressions should ideally be situated so that he or she is above the patient's chest.

Interposed abdominal compressions can be performed and may increase venous return.

The chest compression rate in dogs and cats should be approximately 100 compressions per minute, depending on the size of the patient, with a 1:1 ratio of compression to relaxation.

The effectiveness of the chest compressions should be monitored by a person holding a finger on the patient's pulse. Effective compressions should produce a palpable pulse and pink mucous membranes. To monitor pulmonary perfusion a capnograph can be utilized. If there is adequate delivery of blood to the lungs due to effective chest compressions, gaseous exchange will occur due to artificial ventilation resulting in increasing end-tidal CO_2 levels being displayed on the capnograph. An end-tidal CO_2 level above 14 mm Hg is a sign of good CPCR technique (Egger 2007). Assessment of cerebral blood flow can be made using a Doppler ultrasound transducer placed on the cornea.

Open Chest CPCR

The patient may already be having abdominal or thoracic surgery, in which case the decision to opt for open chest CPCR is an easy one. If the patient is not undergoing thoracic or abdominal surgery, a decision must be made by the veterinarian whether open chest CPCR should commence. Indications for open chest CPCR include the following:

- If the chest cavity or abdominal cavity are already exposed, e.g., thoracotomy or laparotomy
- Pneumothorax
- Hemothorax
- Severe chest trauma, including penetrating chest wounds
- Fractured ribs
- Diaphragmatic hernia
- Flail chest
- Pericardial tamponade
- Severe hypovolemia
- Deep-chested dogs and obese patients where closed chest CCPR will not create high intrathoracic pressure
- Coagulopathies
- Septic, anaphylactic, or distributive shock
- Other primary thoracic diseases, e.g., neoplasia, foreign body
- If closed chest CCPR is not effective within 2–5 minutes (Cole 2009; Wingfield 2002) (this last point is controversial and the time at which the chest should be entered following unsuccessful closed CPCR is stated as anywhere from 2 to 10 minutes) (Egger 2007; Cooper and Muir 2007; Wingfield 2002).

Once a decision has been made that open chest CPCR should commence, a strip of hair should be clipped over the fifth intercostal space

and antiseptic solution quickly applied. A lateral thoracotomy is performed at the fifth intercostal space. Once the chest is open, a rib retractor (finnochietos) may be used to increase exposure. An incision is made in the pericardium below the level of the phrenic nerve and the heart is directly compressed. The compression rate remains the same as with closed compressions at approximately 100 per minute (Cole 2009).

Having the chest open allows ventricular filling to be assessed by direct visualization, accurate intracardiac drug administration, direct visualization of the heart rhythm, and occlusion of the aorta if required. The aorta can be cross-clamped if necessary, but increased coronary and cerebral blood flow can be achieved by manual occlusion of the aorta by compressing it against the spine with a thumb (Plunkett and McMichael 2008).

Open chest CPCR will require a surgical team on standby, if the patient is not already in surgery, to repair the thorax postresuscitation. There is also a risk of sepsis because the technique must be performed quickly without much thought to aseptic preparation of the patient or personnel. Further complications associated with excessive force during direct myocardial compression are cardiac trauma, cardiac dysrhythmias, and ventricular fibrillation.

Advanced life support

Advanced life support includes further steps with the aim of establishing and maintaining spontaneous ventilation and circulation via the administration of drugs, appraisal of the electrocardiogram (ECG), and further interventional techniques such as defibrillation.

Drugs (D)

Atropine/glycopyrrolate: These are anticholinergic, parasympatholytic agents that can be used to treat vagally induced bradycardias. They are effective at reducing the effects of parasympathetic stimulation and cholinergic responses and act to increase heart rate, control hypotension, and increase systemic vascular resistence. These drugs are particularly useful in the treatment of vagally induced ventricular asystole. Excessive doses may produce sinus tachycardia and can predispose the myocardium to ventricular dysrhythmias.

Epinephrine: Epinephrine is a mixed adrenergic agonist and a catecholamine. It is generally still the first-choice drug selected for treatment of severe bradycardia that has not responded to anticholinergics, severe hypotension, and cardiac arrest. During CPCR, epinephrine is administered for its α_2 agonist effects, which cause vasoconstriction of the peripheral vasculature, thus increasing coronary and cerebral perfusion. It is believed that epinephrine is less effective in hypoxic, acidotic states. Epinephrine will increase myocardial oxygen demand and can also lead to ventricular dysrhythmias if overdosed.

Vasopressin: Vasopressin is a nonadrenergic pressor that causes vasoconstriction. Unlike epinephrine it is not affected by acidosis and may be effective in cases where epinephrine fails. It works by stimulating receptors in the smooth muscle of vessel walls and appears to cause more vasoconstriction in peripheral tissues than in the coronary and renal vasculature, promoting perfusion of these areas. It is also thought to provide a dilatory effect in the vessels supplying the brain resulting in increased perfusion to this area.

Vasopressin is included in the American Heart Association guidelines for CPCR and could be considered for use with, or instead of, epinephrine in treatment of ventricular tachycardia, ventricular fibrillation, and pulseless electrical activity (PEA) (Cooper and Muir 2007).

Lidocaine: This drug is a class 1b antiarrhythmic (sodium channel blocker). It is indicated for use in cases of atrial fibrillation, some forms of supraventricular tachycardia, ventricular tachycardia, and refractory ventricular fibrillation, which is unresponsive to CPCR techniques including defibrillation and pressor therapy. This drug has been largely superseded by amiodarone in human medicine and this is now the drug of choice for refractory ventricular fibrillation secondary to defibrillation (Table 17.1) (Plunkett and McMichael 2008).

Routes of drug administration during CPCR

The routes of drug administration are listed in order of preference.

Central venous route: A cranial vena cava or jugular catheter is the route of choice for administration of resuscitation drugs as the drugs are deposited in close proximity to the heart.

Peripheral venous route: This route is often the most convenient because most anesthetized patients will already have peripheral intravenous access. It is not ideal because it can take up to 2 minutes for the administered drugs to reach the central circulation during CPCR. A flush of sterile saline intravenously and raising of the extremity will increase the drug's ability to reach the central circulation. If no venous access is present, a surgical cut down may be required to obtain direct access to the vein; however, it may be more appropriate to begin to administer drugs via an alternative route while venous access is obtained.

Chest compressions should be continued for 2 minutes following administration of drugs via a peripheral vein before evaluating the ECG (Plunkett and McMichael 2008).

Intraosseous route: If vascular access is limited, an intraosseous or spinal needle may be placed into the medullary cavity of the wing of the ileum, tibial crest, humerus, or femur. The medullary cavity does not collapse during CPA, uptake is rapid, and large volumes of fluid can be administered via this route if necessary for resuscitation. This is especially useful in small mammals and neonates where vascular access may be difficult.

Intratracheal route: Some drugs may be administered via this route. Remember NAVEL, i.e., naloxone, atropine, vasopressin, epinephrine, and lidocaine. A sterile urinary catheter is passed through the endotracheal tube to administer the drug into the distal trachea. The drug dose for administration via this route should be 2–2.5 times that of the intravenous dose except epinephrine, which should be increased by 3–10 times the I/V dose (Plunkett and McMichael 2008). All drugs should be diluted in sterile water, 5–10 mL, when administered by this

Table 17.1. Drugs commonly used during anesthetic emergencies and following CPA.

Drug	Indications	Dosage
Epinephrine	Severe bradycardia Cardiopulmonary arrest PEA Ventricular fibrillation Ventricular asystole Anaphylaxis	0.01–0.2 mg/kg IV
Atropine sulphate	Sinus bradycardia Atrioventricular block Ventricular asystole	0.01–0.04 mg/kg IV
Glycopyrrolate	Sinus bradycardia Atrioventricular block Ventricular asystole	0.005–0.01 mg/kg IV
Vasopressin	Cardiopulmonary arrest Vasodilatory shock due to sepsis Ventricular fibrillation unresponsive to defibrillation or epinephrine	0.2–0.8 IU/Kg IV
Lidocaine	Atrial fibrillation Some supraventricular tachycardias Ventricular tachycardia Refractory ventricular fibrillation unresponsive to defibrillation or vasopressor therapy	2–4 mg/kg IV
Amiodorone	Atrial fibrillation Some supraventricular tachycardias Ventricular tachycardia Refractory ventricular fibrillation unresponsive to defibrillation or vasopressor therapy	5 mg/kg IV over 10 mins
Dobutamine	Hypotension Myocardial dysfunction	1–10 μg/kg/min IV
Dopamine	Renal failure Low cardiac output Hypotension	2–10 μg/kg/min IV
Naloxone	Reversal of opioid agonists	0.02–0.04 mg/kg IV
Atipamezole	Reversal of α_2 adrenergic agonists	0.1–0.2 mg/kg IV slowly
Flumazenil	Reversal of benzodiazepines	0.02 mg/kg
Furosemide	Cerebral, pulmonary, and laryngeal edema	1–2 mg/kg IV
Calcium gluconate	Hypocalcemia Hyperkalemia Calcium channel blocker overdose	0.5–1 mL/kg of 10% solution IV to effect
Sodium bicarbonate	Metabolic acidosis	0.5 mmol/kg IV over 20–30 minutes

route. This is especially important for epinephrine because it will cause localized vasoconstriction of vessels if given undiluted by this route, and this can delay the absorption of subsequent drugs.

Intralingual: This is a technique that can be considered for use in small mammals and neonates. The base of the tongue has a rich vascular supply and drugs are absorbed readily from this area.

Intracardiac: This is a technique that should be avoided when undertaking closed chest CPCR as potential complications include coronary and pulmonary laceration, myocardial trauma, arrhythmias, and cardiac tamponade. If this route is used during closed chest CPCR, chest compressions must be stopped while the injection is administered to minimize the risk of potential complications.

Intracardiac injections may be indicated to administer drugs when the open chest compression method of CPCR is being performed. This method is normally employed to hasten the delivery of drugs to the coronary arteries and myocardium. The dose for intracardiac administration is generally half that of the intravenous dose (Cooper and Muir 2007).

Electrocardiography (E)

An ECG is essential to monitor the heart rhythm produced immediately following CPA and during CPCR. It allows monitoring of response to treatment and evaluation of the appropriate drug therapy and/or treatment to be delivered according to the rhythm being produced. It should be noted, however, that a normal ECG appearance is not indicative of contractile function of the myocardium or peripheral perfusion.

Do not use alcohol when placing an ECG on a CPA patient because defibrillation may be required during CPCR attempts and the alcohol can cause a fire.

The common arrest rhythms in veterinary patients are asystole, ventricular fibrillation, and pulseless electrical activity (PEA).

Asystole: A flat line will be observed on the ECG, indicating the absence of mechanical and electrical activity. Always check the pulses and ECG connections before you assume that your patient is asystolic! Treatment of ventricular asystole requires rapid basic life support measures—ABC with minimal interruptions. No medications have been shown to be effective in the treatment of asystole (Plunkett and McMichael 2008). However, atropine and epinephrine/vasopressin are still recommended treatments. (Plunkett and McMichael 2008; Matthews 2006; Egger 2007).

Ventricular fibrillation: This is an irregular quivering of the ventricles with no effective cardiac output. The ECG will demonstrate fibrillation waves with no QRS complexes. The patient will have no palpable pulse. All leads should be checked because fine ventricular fibrillation can mimic asystole in some leads.

This rhythm is the least common seen in veterinary patients compared to it being the most common cause of CPA in humans. This is probably fortunate because many smaller clinics do not possess the means to defibrillate.

Direct current cardioversion to defibrillate the heart is the best treatment for this rhythm. Chest compressions should be performed while the defibrillator is being prepared.

Defibrillation

Defibrillation may be attempted externally with paddles, which must be covered with conductive gel to prevent burning the patient. Ideally, each side of the patient's chest should be clipped prior to application of the paddles. The paddles are then placed on either side of the chest, avoiding contact with each other and the table. No personnel should be in contact with the patient, ECG leads, or the table and the operator of the defibrillator should give clear instructions for personnel to "stand clear" before releasing the charge. The initial counter shock is delivered at 2–5 J/kg. Under the 2005 American Heart Association guidelines, one shock should be administered rather than the three successive shocks recommended previously. Chest compressions should immediately be resumed for 2 minutes before reassessing the cardiac rhythm and administration of an additional shock (Plunkett and McMichael 2008).

Open chest defibrillation involves the direct application of specially designed, sterile paddles to the epicardium. Saline-soaked sterile gauze swabs or sponges are placed between the electrodes and the epicardium. One paddle is applied to the base of the heart and the other to the apex. The same precautions should be taken as with external defibrillation. Less energy is required for internal defibrillation, approximately one-tenth of that required for external defibrillation 0.2–0.5 J/Kg (Plunkett and McMichael 2008).

Power settings are selected according to patient size and response to previous attempts. It is useful to have a chart attached to the defibrillator indicating the appropriate settings for different patient body weights for both internal and external cardioversion techniques.

Epinephrine is generally administered every 3–5 minutes if ventricular fibrillation continues after the initial countershock and subsequent 2 minutes of compressions (Plunkett and McMichael 2008). Epinephrine is reported to convert fine ventricular fibrillation to coarse ventricular fibrillation, which is reportedly easier to convert (Egger 2007). Vasopressin can be given as an alternative to epinephrine (Plunkett and McMichael 2008).

Lidocaine cannot convert the heart from ventricular fibrillation to normal sinus rhythm, but it is useful in controlling ventricular dysrhythmias following defibrillation (Cooper and Muir W 2007).

Pulseless electrical activity (PEA): This rhythm was previously referred to as electrical mechanical dissociation. PEA is used to describe patients that have ECG evidence of cardiac rhythm but with an absent or very weak pulse. The waveform can range from having relatively normal QRS complexes to quite wide and bizarre complexes.

Treatment of PEA usually involves treatment of the underlying cause if possible and rapid commencement of basic life support techniques—ABC. Again, no medications have been shown to be effective in the treatment of PEA, and the prognosis is poor for successful resuscitation (Plunkett and McMichael 2008). However, epinephrine/vasopressin and atropine are still administered in PEA cases (Plunkett and McMichael 2008; Matthews 2006; Egger 2007).

Fluid therapy (F)

If CPA is due to hypovolemia, aggressive fluid therapy may be required during CPCR attempts. Shock rate fluids, i.e., 90 mL/kg/hr in dogs and 60 mL/kg/hr in cats, are not normally administered unless the patient was hypovolemic prior to CPA. Fluid resuscitation should be approached cautiously in patients whose volume status was normal prior to arrest, especially those with preexisting lung disease (Cooper and Muir 2007).

Prolonged life support

Once return to spontaneous circulation and ventilation has been achieved through CPCR, there is still intensive treatment to consider to ensure continued support of the patient's cardiovascular and respiratory systems. Postresuscitation patients should be carefully monitored, which will usually involve checking temperature; pulse rate, rhythm, and character; heart rate and rhythm; respiratory rate, depth, and effort; lung sounds; mental status and neurologic function; patient comfort; blood pressure; mucous membrane color; capillary refill time; and urine output at regular intervals. If not already placed, arterial and jugular catheters should be placed to facilitate monitoring of central venous pressure (CVP) and direct arterial blood pressure. The patient will normally be connected to a continuous ECG for at least the first 24 hours post-CPA. Regular blood samples should be taken to monitor the patient's packed cell volume (PCV); total solids (TS); blood glucose concentration; serum lactate concentration; electrolyte, acid-base, and arterial blood gas status.

Oxygen-carrying capacity should be maximized by ensuring that the patient's volume status, blood pressure, and hemoglobin concentration are adequate. Supplemental oxygen should be supplied to these patients initially at

100% immediately post-CPCR and then reduced to less than 60% to avoid oxygen toxicity (Cooper and Muir 2007). Continued ventilation may be required in some patients.

Nutritional support should be considered in these patients and this may require feeding tube placement if enteral feeding is contraindicated.

Common Complications

Common complications following CPA and subsequent CPCR may include cerebral edema, hypoxia, reperfusion injury, acute renal failure, SIRS, abnormal hemostasis, and multiple organs dysfunction syndrome (MODS). These patients are often at risk of further CPAs depending on the underlying cause of the initial CPA.

It should be noted that these patients should not be allowed to become hyperthermic; it is thought that mild hypothermia may improve outcome (Nozari et al. 2004).

Hypothermia can be described as heat loss in excess of heat production and is one of the most common complications seen in the peri- and postanesthetic period. This is mainly due to the fact that all anesthetics impair the patient's thermoregulatory abilities via depression of the central nervous system. Other causes include vasodilation, hypotension, hypovolemia, reduced heat production by skeletal muscles, cold ambient temperature, use of cold intravenous and lavage fluids, cold surgical preparation solutions, overwetting of the patient with surgical preparation solutions and open body cavities. Smaller patients are most at risk of hypothermia due to their large surface area to body mass ratio.

Hypothermia causes depression of the CNS, and as a consequence decreases the requirement for volatile agents (i.e., MAC is decreased in hypothermic patients). Catecholamines are released in hypothermic patients, which will predispose them to cardiac arrhythmias. Hypothermia will also generally cause the patient to shiver on recovery. Shivering increases metabolic rate and oxygen consumption, which can be detrimental in hypoxemic patients.

Hypothermia can cause deficiencies in coagulation interfering with enzymes involved in the clotting cascade and decreasing platelet function.

Prevention of hypothermia will include rectifying the causes outlined above, i.e., warming intravenous and lavage fluids, avoiding overwetting of patients, and maintaining an appropriate ambient temperature. The use of rebreathing anesthetic breathing systems and/or heat and moisture exchange filters will help prevent hypothermia due to respiratory losses. It is important to remember that the main methods of heat loss when considering prevention are evaporation, conduction, convection, and radiation.

Treatment of hypothermia is by actively rewarming the patient. This is most effectively achieved by the use of forced warm air blankets, circulating warm water blankets, and/or the new convective heat blanket units (Hot Dog Warming System). Bladder lavage with warmed fluids is also an effective method of helping to rewarm these patients.

Hyperthermia

Hyperthermia can be defined as heat production in excess of heat loss. This can occur when the ambient temperature is warm and with the use of active external warming devices. There may also be systemic processes responsible for hyperthermia (excessive muscle activity, fever, malignant hyperthermia, or thyroid storm). The organs that are most susceptible to damage caused by hyperthermia are the myocardium, brain, liver, and kidneys. Hyperthermia can also lead to coagulation abnormalities.

Prevention of hyperthermia will generally involve careful monitoring of the patient's temperature. Treatment for hyperthermia may include turning off warming devices; changing the breathing system to a non-rebreathing system to allow heat loss through respiration; cooling the patient with ice packs, cold water and alcohol applications; administering room temperature or slightly cooled fluids and bladder lavage with slightly cooled fluids.

Glucose

Glucose is the major energy source for the central nervous system, and as such a reduction in blood glucose (hypoglycemia) can cause complications associated with CNS depression (unexplained increase in depth of anesthesia, prolonged recovery, tachycardia, hypertension, muscle tremors, and seizures).

Causes of hypoglycemia include sepsis/SIRS, insulinoma, and fasting of patients with diabetes mellitus. Hypoglycemia is also common in small patients and neonatal/pediatric patients.

Prevention of hypoglycemia involves careful monitoring of patients that are predisposed to hypoglycemia.

Treatment generally involves administration of intravenous glucose in the anesthetized patient (bolus and infusions may be required).

Prolonged Recovery from Anesthesia

Prolonged recovery from anesthesia can be caused by many factors, including the following:

- The inability to metabolize the anaesthetic drugs administered (preexisting hepatic and/or renal disease, porto-systemic shunt, breed variation, e.g., sight hounds)
- Hypoventilation, which prevents the expulsion of inhalant agents through adequate respiration
- Hypotension, which reduces tissue perfusion in the hepatic and renal systems and thus slows the metabolism and excretion of anesthetic drugs
- Central nervous system depression, which is caused by systemic factors such as hypoxia, hypercarbia, metabolic acidosis, and hypoglycemia
- Hypothermia

Prevention of these factors should be considered prior to and during the anesthetic period through active attempts to prevent hypothermia, hypotension, etc. Treatment of prolonged recov-

ery will rely heavily on identifying and treating the underlying cause. This may involve reversing anesthetic drugs (opioids, α_2 agonists), administering supplemental oxygen, correction of hypotension, administering glucose, correction of acidosis, etc.

Conclusion

Many of the anesthetic complications and emergencies that have been discussed in this chapter can be either avoided, especially those that are the result of human error, or recognized in their early stages and treated. Prevention of many of these complications involves thorough clinical examination of the patient and patient history, thorough preanesthetic checks of the anesthetic machine and the breathing system, accurate checking of drug dosages, and vigilant monitoring throughout the anesthetic period.

CPA is something that we need to be prepared for as anesthetists. Personnel should be well trained in CPCR techniques and know how to work together as a team when faced with CPA in a patient. A crash cart or box, however small, should be well stocked and kept in an easily accessible and central position. CPCR should not be undertaken lightly and the hard work and monitoring that is required in not only establishing a return to spontaneous circulation and ventilation but also in the immediate postresuscitation treatment and nursing should not be underestimated.

References

Altman, S. 2006. Acupuncture as an emergency treatment. Calif Vet 33:6–8.

Cole, S. 2009. Cardiopulmonary resuscitation. In Small Animal Critical Care Medicine, edited by Silverstein, D, Hopper, K. St. Louis: Saunders Elsevier, p.16.

Cooper, E, Muir, W. 2007. Cardiopulmonary-cerebral resuscitation. In BSAVA Manual of Canine and Feline Emergency and Critical

Care, 2nd ed., edited by King, L, Boag, A. Gloucester: BSAVA, pp.299–306.

Egger, C. 2007. Anaesthetic complications and emergencies. In BSAVA Manual of Canine and Feline Anaesthesia and Analgesia, 2nd ed., edited by Seymour, C, Duke-Novakovski, T. Gloucester: BSAVA, pp.318, 326–330.

Janssens, L, Altman, S, Rogers, PA. 1979. Respiratory and cardiac arrest under anaesthesia: Treatment by acupuncture of the nasal philtrum. Vet Rec 105:273–276.

Matthew, K. 2006. Cardiopulmonary arrest. In Veterinary Emergency and Critical Care Manual, 2nd ed., edited by Matthews, K. Guelph: Lifelearn, pp.135–138.

Nozari, A, Safer, P, Stezoski, SW, et al. 2004. Mild hypothermia during prolonged cardiopulmonary cerebral resuscitation increases conscious survival in dogs. Crit Care Med 32(10):2110–2116.

Plunkett, S, McMichael, M. 2008. Cardiopulmonary resuscitation in small animal medicine: An update. J Vet Intern Med 22:9–25.

Wingfield, W. 2002. Cardiopulmonary arrest. In The Veterinary ICU Book, edited by Wingfield, W, Raffe, M. Teton, WY: NewMedia002, pp.432–433.

Ventilation Techniques in Small Animal Patients

Christine Slowiak

Goals of Ventilation

Manually providing a patient with positive pressure ventilation bagged breaths is an effective and standard practice, but a mechanical ventilator gives the veterinary technician more autonomy to provide sound respiratory support to the animal while allowing other tasks to be performed. A mechanical ventilator is able to give controlled, intermittently timed volume and pressure-sensitive delivery of oxygen and halogenated anesthetic agents.

Goals to be met should always include consideration of the most "normal" and physiologic respiratory function by the patient, attempting to mimic ventilation efficiency when *not* anesthetized. Using a mechanical ventilator allows the anesthetist to potentially ventilate a patient better than it could ventilate itself while under anesthesia. Analgesic agents, stationary positioning, body cavity exposure with temperature loss, and diaphragmatic impairment all can hamper the normal responses of the respiratory system. The job of the veterinary anesthetist is to provide a homeostatic counterpoint to induced and physiologic impairments.

Manual Ventilation versus Mechanical Ventilation

In our hands, the anesthesia machine with a reservoir breathing bag can function much in the same way as a ventilator, but more simplistically. A breath can be given to the patient when the pop-off valve (also known as the APL valve, adjustable pressure-limiting valve) is closed by squeezing the rebreathing bag, delivering a volume of air mixed with anesthetic gas. Differing anesthesia machines may have the option of monitoring total tidal volume delivered via spirometry or a ventilometer. During hand ventilation due to the gross estimation of the reservoir bags, in most cases, the volume delivered to the patient is usually based on peak inspiratory pressures (PIP). Doing this gives a controlled breath via manual ventilation. The biggest concern with this method, along with the labor intensity involved is the fear of forgetting to reopen the pop-off valve once the breath is delivered. Failure to open the pop-off valve while the oxygen flowmeter is still turned on is a potentially life-threatening mistake. Pressure begins to build in the system and in the patient's lungs very quickly (depending on the oxygen flow rate). This mistake can very quickly lead to severe volutrauma (lung damage) and death. Pop-off valve "safety adaptors" that fit most anesthesia machines are available commercially. These fit just behind the actual pop-off valve and involve a spring-loaded "button" that can be depressed during positive pressure ventilation. Once the breath is given and the anesthetist releases the button, it springs open, releasing pressure buildup. These are inexpensive and highly recommended for placement on every anesthesia machine in the practice.

Mechanical ventilation is the act of placing the patient on a machine that will provide timed delivery of a volume of oxygen and anesthetic gases to the patient. Mechanical ventilators are also used in the critical care department where microprocessor controlled ventilators, as opposed to bellows-driven units, are usually found. Advanced functions are available on ICU microprocessor-controlled units, which may not be of direct applicability in the anesthesia or surgical theater setting.

Common Ventilation Terms

Understanding common terminology is essential in setting and effectively utilizing ventilation techniques in your patients. Many of these terms will be reflected either in abbreviations on the faceplate of the ventilator or in the user manual.

Intermittent positive pressure ventilation (IPPV) refers to artificial inspirations applied to the airway. They may be applied manually or mechanically with the use of a mechanical ventilator. IPPV airway pressure during inspiration is higher than that of ambient pressures. During exhalation, pressures fall to ambient pressures, which allows for passive exhalation (Hartsfield 2007).

The *respiratory rate* (RR) is a set number of breath cycles to be administered to the patient over 1 minute. IPPV is more efficient than spontaneous breathing; therefore, lower respiratory rates are warranted. Because of this efficiency, ventilated patients also need to be closely monitored for anesthetic depth. Patients given regular, controlled ventilation will maintain a steadier plane of anesthesia because the delivery of inhaled anesthetics remains constant. Usually, once the patient is "captured" by the ventilator completely, inhalant concentrations can be reduced. Generally, a respiratory rate of 8 to 14 breaths per minute is considered within normal limits for a small animal patient on a ventilator.

Tidal volume is the volume of air that moves in and out of the patient during a full respiratory cycle. Common values for small animal patients are between 7–15 mL/kg.

Minute volume is the product of multiplying respiratory rate and tidal volume. The minute volume reflects the total gas exchanged to the patient over 1 minute. Reference ranges have been reported between 150–250 mL/kg/min in the small animal patient (Johnson 2007).

Hypocapnia is a decreased amount of carbon dioxide in the blood. Patients who are painful or hyperventilating can cause themselves to blow off too much carbon dioxide. $ETCO_2$ of <35 mm Hg indicates hypocapnia. Attention should be paid to a patient that is hyperventilated for a long period of time, because an ensuing respiratory alkalosis will occur. *Hypercapnia* is an increased retention of carbon dioxide. $ETCO_2$ of >60 mm Hg indicates hypercapnia. Hypercapnia will lead to respiratory acidosis in patients who do not have this corrected. Evaluation of hypo- or hypercapnia can be done with a capnograph or via arterial blood gas analysis (Hall et al. 2001).

Hyperventilation is an increased respiratory rate causing hypocapnia. Hyperventilation can also be referred to as a technique in ventilating a patient, by increasing the rate and depth of ventilations to assist in decreasing carbon dioxide that is being retained. Spontaneous breaths are frequently shallow and sharp in hyperventilation. *Hypoventilation* is a decrease in the rate or depth of ventilations. Hypoventilation eventually leads to hypercapnia and thereby should be corrected early. Changes in ventilation rate can be due to alkalosis, narcotics, or too low a set ventilation rate and/or tidal volume. Hypothermia is also a contributor to physiologic hypoventilation.

Hypoxemia is reduced blood oxygen content caused by inadequate ventilation or inadequate gas exchange. Numerically, it can reflect a partial arterial oxygen content of 60 mm Hg or less. There are five clinical listings of possible hypoxemia in animals: shunting, V/Q mismatch, hypoventilation, diffusion impairment, and low inspired oxygen concentration. Hypoxia is defined as impaired oxygen delivery due to systemic delivery issues. A patient may have appropriate blood oxygen content, but still be hypoxemic due to low cardiac output and, therefore, decreased delivery of oxygen to tissues (Robertson 2002).

V/Q mismatch is the abbreviated term for ventilation-perfusion inequality. V/Q mismatch occurs when there is ventilation to the alveoli but the alveoli are not perfused (blood flow is somehow restricted or shunted) (Papadakos and Lachmann 2008).

Resistance can be simply defined as anything that causes an increase in work to attain adequate ventilation. Resistance can be in either the upper or lower airways. A good example of resistance is ventilating the pneumonia patient, where difficulty in providing ventilation to the patient is caused by congestion due to inspissated fluids in the terminal alveoli. An iatrogenic equipment-induced resistance can be anatomical patient neck positioning, causing a reduction in air to flow to and from the lungs, for example, via the torqued endotracheal tube or an overinflated endotracheal tube cuff, which crushes the inner lumen of the tube. An anatomic resistance may be a geriatric patient with calcified chostochondral junctions, making thoracic expansion difficult. In feline patients, commonly the accumulation of salivary secretions in the endotracheal tube can eventually occlude the lumen, creating resistance in breathing.

Compliance is the evaluation of distensibility and allowance of tidal filling to the lungs and lower airways. Another way to consider compliance is the "flexibility" or allowance of filling in the pulmonary space. Disease processes and airway obstructions are examples where a patient may have a decrease in compliance. Asthmatic patients may have inflamed airways; while chronic obstructive pulmonary disease (COPD) patients have dense, thickened pulmonary tissue.

Atelectasis refers to a diminished volume or lack of air in part or all of a lung lobe. Causes of atelectasis are many, including improperly placed endotracheal tubes, inflammation in asthmatic patients, aspiration of a foreign body causing obstruction of the airway, mucous plugs, or bronchial and pulmonary tumors. Atelectic lung tissue is neither able to fill appropriately or empty appropriately due to alveolar impairment. During anesthesia, the diaphragm relaxes, which causes it to be less able to maintain differential pressures between the abdomen and thoracic cavity. Intercostal muscles may be blocked with a local anesthetic, impaired from injury or recumbent due to position and body weight (Papadakos and Lachmann 2008). These reasons will cause compression of the lung tissue rendering it less able to fill and empty, thereby decreasing effective gas exchange. Some amount of atelectasis is normal and tolerated; however, hypoxemia is a primary complication and should be monitored and treated accordingly, frequently with ventilation support for extended periods of time.

Functional residual capacity (FRC) is the amount of air left in the lungs after normal expiration. The FRC is important to the veterinary anesthetist because during apnea it is the reservoir to supply oxygen to the blood (Ward 1992).

Equipment definitions

Controlled ventilation occurs when respiratory rate and volume are completely controlled, either mechanically or manually. This is the method used when spontaneous ventilations are not active due to level of anesthesia (deep), use of neuromuscular blockers, or during intrathoracic surgery.

Peak Inspiratory Pressure (PIP) is the numeric pressure value of gas delivery to the patient at the peak of inspiration. PIP can be monitored by watching the pressure manometer on the anesthesia machine during peak inspiration. The pressure manometer should be monitored whenever positive pressure ventilations are given to the patient. In general, in healthy small animal patients, PIP should not exceed 20 cm H_2O so as to avoid trauma to the lung tissues. There are, however, some instances in which higher pressures are needed to deliver adequate tidal volumes (obese patients in dorsal recumbency; patients with large, space-occupying lesions in the abdomen that are pushing on the diaphragm). A PIP of 12–15 cm H_2O in the closed thorax patient is sufficient to accomplish adequate respiratory function provided that respiratory rate is acceptable (Robertson 2002). Feline patients may require less pressure to adequately ventilate, usually 10–15 cm H_2O. An open thorax may require an increased PIP for expansion of the lung fields, which would normally be assisted by the negative pressure system of a closed thorax. When starting a case and transitioning through the stages, attention needs to be paid to trending these patients with capnography and arterial blood gas samples. Ventilation should be evaluated based on capnography and arterial blood gas sampling (Stoelting and Dierdorf 1983).

In cases where long-term atelectasis is suspected, only conservative pressure should be provided during IPPV, because if the alveoli were to be forced into immediate expansion, a condition called *reexpansion pulmonary edema (RPE)* is possible. As stated, pulmonary edema is formed from the "blowing open" at high pressures and the alveoli rupture and weep, causing fluid to leak out into the bronchioles. Usually, healthy inflated lung portions will incur trauma before long-term atectalectic lung can be reexpanded. Almost always, RPE patients will need extended oxygen and possibly ventilatory support, diuretic therapy, and possibly the addition of steroids to their treatment protocol (Benumof and Alfery 1994). Preventing RPE by responsible and thorough decision making during administration of ventilatory support is a big step in successful recovery.

The driving gas is usually atmospheric air piped into the bellows chamber that, when pressurized, compresses the bellows and delivers the preset tidal volume to the patient. The bellows is filled with oxygen and inhalant gas. For the ventilator to deliver a breath the area surrounding the bellows becomes pressurized, the electronic control of the ventilator fires, and the driving gas exerts pressure on the bellows, compressing the preset volume or pressure into the anesthesia breathing circuit to the patient (Clutton 1999).

Positive End Expiratory Pressure (PEEP) refers to maintaining a degree of pressure in the lungs at the end of exhalation. PEEP valves, which can be directly applied to the anesthesia machine, are commercially available (Hallowell EMC) in various cm H_2O pressures. Be aware that although PEEP can be very useful, it can affect cardiac output by maintaining constant positive pressure in the thoracic cavity, which can affect venous return to the heart (Hines and Marschall 2008). Blood pressure measurements should be monitored. Use of PEEP in thoracotomy/open chest patients can be very helpful. Using PEEP allows the anesthetist to prevent alveolar collapse and keeps terminal airways partially inflated. The evaluation of SpO_2 during the use of PEEP can help determine its effectiveness. It may not be necessary to employ PEEP during the entire thoracotomy (or other) procedure. The *Inspiratory to Expiratory Ratio (I:E ratio)* is used to determine the time of inspiration versus the time allowed for expiration by the patient (Fig. 18.1). The I:E ratio should be 1:2 for all mechanically ventilated animals (Hartsfield 2007).

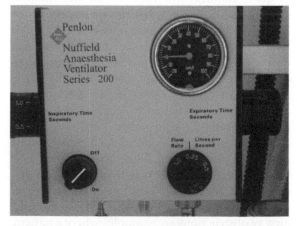

Figure 18.1. The Nuffield Anaesthesia Ventilator 200 (Penlon) faceplate close-up with I:E parameters and in line with the anesthesia circuit. Of note on this unit is the inline pressure manometer. (Photo courtesy of Heather Deering-McPherson.)

Setting too short an I:E ratio could potentially cause circulatory issues, because the thoracic pressure is not allowed to sufficiently drop to allow for refilling of the vascular and cardiac structures. This would cause a decrease in cardiac output overall. Different ventilators have variable flexibility. Some designs may have an adjustable I:E ratio, with 1:2 through 1:4 being the most common available. On simpler models, a preset ratio of 1:2 is a standard acceptable setting.

Types of Ventilators

Pressure limited or pressure cycled: These ventilators deliver a tidal volume based on a preset pressure. Once the preset pressure is reached, inspiration ceases. These ventilators are considered safe because regardless of the size of the patient being ventilated, inspiratory pressure (PIP) will remain constant and, therefore, overly large tidal volumes can be avoided. There is no adjustment that needs to be made between patients as long as a reasonable PIP was selected originally. The tidal volume is in a sense determined by the pressure limit set by the anesthetist. To increase tidal volume, choose a higher pressure setting and vice versa. Usually an alarm will sound if the pressure selected is exceeded (as when a patient spontaneously breathes during IPPV) or if the set pressure is not reached. This is usually the case in a disconnect situation. These ventilators are sensitive to patients with preexisting disease and varying degrees of lung compliance that may cause resistance, so monitoring of CO_2 and blood gases can ensure that adequate tidal volumes are being delivered.

Volume cycled: These ventilators have the ability to deliver a tidal volume independent of the pressure achieved in the airways. Most are equipped with safety valves that allow the release of excess pressure in the system. Usually, these are set at 60 cm H_2O. These ventilators may have an ascending or descending bellows (Fig. 18.2). Ascending bellows are more helpful in signaling leaks in the system because if there is a leak or

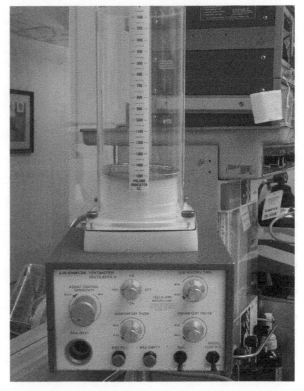

Figure 18.2. Air-Shields Ventimeter Ventilator II with ascending bellows. (Photos courtesy of Heather Deering-McPherson.)

disconnect, the bellows will not reach the top of the housing.

Time cycled means that the breaths are given at fixed intervals (chosen as rate), independent of the patient's respiratory efforts (Davey and Diba 2005). Minute volume is chosen by adjustment of the inspiratory flow control and the rate control. The Hallowell EMC models 2000 and 2002 also have a maximum working pressure limit (MWPL) control. This works somewhat like the pressure limited ventilator in that it allows for a certain maximum airway pressure to be chosen. When this pressure is reached, inspiration is terminated.

Many ventilators in veterinary medicine are a combination of one or more types of ventilatory control, giving greater manipulation of values to the anesthetist. Most commonly a pressure limited/time cycled design has been the basis for veterinary ventilator designs (Fig. 18.3).

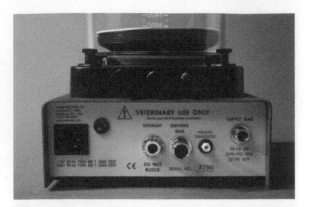

Figure 18.3.   The reverse of the Hallowell EMC 2000. The rear faceplate is labeled (from R to L). A threaded oxygen port, pressure transducer port (and a provided line and adaptor, which connects to the patient circuit, frequently placed at the site of the reservoir bag or in the expiratory limbs), and driving gas, which correlates the baseplate to the upper bellows housing port (unlabeled but on the R side). The two additional connections on the bellows housing are to the breathing circuit (L) and exhaust system (M). (Photo courtesy of Max S. Hallowell.)

Setup of the Ventilator

Each ventilator will vary to some degree on its functionality in the veterinary patient because many units have been extrapolated from human medicine. In choosing a unit for your practice, the preference is to choose a ventilator that works well in the hands of the veterinary technician, with minimal complication and ease in maintenance, and with the availability of repair parts. Always refer to the manufacturer's guidance in the proper setup and directions on the use of your particular model.

Power to the ventilator should be connected and the breathing circuit functional. Affix oxygen supply connections to the appropriate connections on both the anesthesia machine and the patient ventilator. Often this requires the use of an oxygen wye. Double-check the connections on your ventilator, which usually are standard to include the breathing system inlet, the exhaust port to a scavenging system, and a driving gas port that may be an independent source from your base unit. Choose a bellows for use in your patient based on approximate tidal volume to be delivered. If you are on the cusp of a smaller- to

larger-sized bellow, choose the larger of the two. Although it is not always convenient to read the graduations on the larger bellows housing, it is advantageous to have the larger tidal volume able to be delivered if, for some reason, the patient is dynamic and higher PIP and T_v need to be produced. Before installing, check the bellows for tears, dirt, or hair (Dorsch and Dorsch 1999). The corrugated tubing from the ventilator's breathing hose terminal should be connected to the anesthesia machine where the rebreathing bag goes.

Depending on your model, decide whether the pop-off valve needs to be closed or a control arm needs to be switched over to change to mechanical ventilations from your anesthesia machine. Most ventilator units will have a low-pressure alarm, a high-pressure alarm, and an oxygen-flow alarm, which alerts the operator to deficiencies in oxygen line pressure. Getting to know your unit the first time you place a patient on the system could be disastrous; therefore, it is advised to do a test run of this setup prior to any patient application until the operator is familiar and proficient with operation. Prior to placing the patient on the ventilator system, a pressure test should be performed, duplicating many of the steps mentioned above in regard to machine connections.

Pressure testing the ventilator and presetting

Just as important as pressure checking the anesthesia machine prior to use, the ventilator should also be pressure tested prior to use each time, especially when the bellows are changed out or the circuit is disconnected. Pressure testing verifies the correct system configuration, monitors the ventilator for consistent cycling, and checks for leaks. It ensures patient safety. To perform a pressure check:

1. Install the appropriate bellows assembly.
2. Using your chosen bellows, connect a reservoir bag (use as a "test lung") to the patient end of the wye and close the pop-off valve or move the control arm attached to the anesthesia machine.

3. Fill the breathing system with the oxygen flow meter turned up adequately until the bellows reaches the top of the bellows housing.

4. Turn the volume control to the minimum setting, set the rate as desired and turn on the ventilator.

5. Increase the volume controls until the peak pressure of each breath is approximately 30 cm H_2O.

6. If your model of ventilator is equipped, depress the inspiratory hold button long enough to verify that the breathing system is not leaking. The pressure should remain constant. Observe that the ventilator is continuing to cycle, and that over a few minutes the bellows continues to hold pressure and is not losing significant volume.

Following this pressure check, turn the inspiratory flow rate back to the anticipated volume range for your patient so that large tidal volumes are not delivered when the patient is connected. Set the rate where it should be and do a trial run before the patient is induced.

When preparing a case for surgery that is going to be anesthetized and then moved to an OR for the procedure, it may be helpful to consider using two ventilators if possible. The first ventilator unit can be set up in the OR ahead of time.

Prime this unit and choose a reservoir breathing bag (to represent the patient's lungs—based on tidal volume) to be placed at the patient end of the anesthesia circuit. Choose an appropriate bellows, using your patient's calculated tidal volume with an additional 20% volume added. This should encompass any physiologic anomalies (for example, large-breed, deep-chested dogs with lean body mass that have a higher tidal volume than a moderate dog of equal body weight with higher body mass index but smaller thoracic cavity). Calculate the proposed oxygen flow to the patient, close the pop-off valve and start oxygen flowing to the bellows chamber to verify for circuit patency and leak testing. Allow for the bellows to fill completely with oxygen and power on your unit. Set the proposed respiratory rate and peak inspiratory pressure and gradually dial

up the volume to be delivered until the bellows reflects the appropriate proposed tidal volume. After this is confirmed, you may turn off the OR ventilator unit, leaving all settings the same.

Be prepared to make changes to these settings, using only values that you have set as a baseline. A patient lung is much more dynamic than a rubber breathing bag. This setup is to ready the machine, streamline the transfer of the patient from prep to OR, and acclimate the patient early in the anesthesia period without having to disconnect and reconnect all parts of a ventilator setup, thereby hopefully reducing total anesthesia time to the patient. Continue to anesthetize your patient outside the operating room, setting up exactly as the prepared unit in the OR but affixing the patient to the circuit instead of the reservoir breathing bag. Beginning to acclimate your patient to the ventilator during the preparation stage helps with a smoother transfer to the operating room. Evaluating compliance, resistance, and tidal volume issues prior to the surgery theater is helpful, allowing for the veterinary technician to be able to prepare mentally for changes in the patient and surgical needs that may arise in the early stages of ventilation care.

"Bucking" the ventilator is an expression that means the animal is trying to breathe against the set respiratory rhythm and volume being delivered by the mechanical ventilator. Bucking is a normal step in progression during introduction to the ventilator (unless the patient was apneic) and during the weaning phase of discontinuing ventilation. If the patient is bucking the ventilator during the procedure, investigation is warranted. Check patient depth; perhaps the patient is too light under anesthesia. If this is the case, ask the surgeon to stop any stimulation to the patient, increase the inhalant percentage (make sure the vaporizer is full), and turn up the oxygen flow rate. To change inhalant anesthetic concentration in the system quickly, the flow rate must be increased. The respiratory rate may be increased briefly as well in an effort to recapture the patient. It is imperative to monitor for changes in anesthetic plane during this time. Changes can happen rapidly. Once the patient stops bucking and is once again under control, be sure to readjust the respiratory rate and flow rate. Consider altering your plan of anesthesia and analgesic support so as not to peak and trough your patient during the remainder of the procedure.

If anesthetic depth is not deemed the cause of the patient bucking the ventilator, immediate investigation as to the cause is necessary. Assess the patient. Be sure that the patient is not experiencing agonal breaths. Check all ventilator and anesthetic machine functions and search for a disconnect at the patient wye interface. Blood gas analysis may be warranted to ensure that the patient is being ventilated adequately.

Discontinuing ventilation support

When the procedure is nearing conclusion and ventilatory support is no longer necessary, the process of transferring primary work responsibility from the ventilator back to the patient begins. This process is referred to as "weaning" from the ventilator. Most anesthesia patients will make the transition back to spontaneous ventilations with little trouble. The baroreceptor center in the brain signals to the body that a breath is necessary when carbon dioxide is higher than physiologically desired. By starting to decrease the set respiratory rate and tidal volume to be delivered by the ventilator, greater opportunity for carbon dioxide to build in the patient's bloodstream will signal the brain to respond by the patient taking a voluntary breath. Special attention should be paid to capnography at this point to ensure acceptable levels. Patients that are on neuromuscular blocking agents, in deep planes of anesthesia, or on higher constant rate infusions of opiates will take considerably more time to efficiently and safely be weaned from mechanical ventilation. Discontinuing mechanical ventilation warrants judicious monitoring. Patients should be able to maintain normal $ETCO_2$ before being taken away from oxygen.

Evaluation of Ventilation Efficiency

All patients that are receiving mechanical ventilation should be placed on a capnograph, at minimum, to verify efficiency in gas exchange and adequate ventilation. Blood gas analysis can also be a useful tool when using IPPV.

References

Benumof, J. and Alfery, D. 1994. Anesthesia for thoracic surgery. In Anesthesia, 4th ed., edited by Miller, R. New York: Churchill Livingstone.

Clutton, RE. 1999. Anaesthetic equipment. In BSVMA Manual of Small Animal Anaethesia and Analgesia, edited by Seymour, C., Gleed, R. Mid Glamorgan, UK: British Small Animal Veterinary Association.

Davey, AJ, Diba, A. 2005. Ward's Aneaesthetic Equipment, 5th ed. China: Elsevier Limited.

Dorsch, JA, Dorsch, SE. 1999. Understanding Anesthesia Equipment, 4th ed. Baltimore: Williams & Wilkins.

Hall, LW, Clarke, KW, Trim, CM. 2001. Veterinary Anaesthesia, 10th ed. England: Harcourt Publishers Limited.

Hartsfield, S. 2007. Equipment and monitoring. In Lumb & Jones' Veterinary Anesthesia and Analgesia, 4th ed., edited by Tranquilli, WJ, Thurmon, JC, Grimm, KA. Ames, IA: Blackwell Publishing, pp.514, 516.

Hines, RL, Marschall, KE. 2008. Stoelting's Anesthesia and Co-Existing Disease, 5th ed. Philadelphia: Churchill Livingstone.

Johnson, LR. 2007. Respiratory Physiology, Diagnostics, and Disease, Veterinary Clinics of North America, Vol 37, Number 5. Philadelphia: Elsevier Inc.

Papadakos, PJ, Lachmann, B. 2008. Mechanical Ventilation: Clinical Applications and Pathophysiology. Philadelphia: Saunders Elsevier.

Robertson, S. 2002. Oxygenation and ventilation. In Veterinary Anesthesia and Pain Management Secrets, edited by Greene, SA. Philadelphia: Hanley & Belfus, Inc., pp.15.

Stoelting, RK, Dierdorf, SF. 1983. Anesthesia and Co-Existing Disease. New York: Churchill Livingstone.

Ward, S. 1992. Respiratory physiology. In Principles and practice of Nurse Anesthesia, 2nd ed., edited by Waugaman, W.R., Foster, S.D., Rigor, B.M. Norwalk: Appleton & Lange.

19
Anesthesia for Ophthalmology Patients

Kim Lockhead

General Considerations

Unlike humans, veterinary patients that undergo ocular procedures require the use of general anesthesia. Even in healthy patients, there is always some risk of anesthetic complications or even death. This risk can be minimized by carefully considering the health status of each patient and developing an anesthetic plan tailored to the patient's individual needs. Patients requiring anesthesia for ocular procedures may have unique anesthetic needs. Other than emergency patients, the majority of ophthalmic patients are either pediatric or geriatric. The needs of these age groups should be considered in addition to the specific needs of the ophthalmic patient undergoing anesthesia. General anesthetic concerns revolve around maintaining an appropriate level of anesthesia while maintaining normal cardiopulmonary function. A few additional factors should be taken into account when dealing with ophthalmic patients. The main goals when anesthetizing the ophthalmic patient are:

1. To provide analgesia where appropriate
2. To maintain or lower intraocular pressure (IOP)
3. To prevent activation of the oculocardiac reflex (OCR)
4. To provide a level of anesthesia that allows surgical manipulation of the eye and surrounding structures while maintaining normal cardiovascular function

Determinants of Intraocular Pressure (IOP)

Normally, intraocular pressure in the dog ranges from 10–26 mm Hg. In the cat it ranges from 12–32 mm Hg. An IOP exceeding these values is considered abnormal (Thurmon et al. 1996). There are many factors that will cause changes in IOP. Struggling and excitement in a poorly sedated pet; pressure on the jugular vein from neck leads, restraint, or blood draws; and certain anesthetic drugs can all increase IOP. Vomiting, gagging, and coughing increase IOP as well. Even a smooth tracheal intubation without coughing or gagging can cause IOP to increase. It is important to prevent increases in pressure since it may result in permanent loss of vision and/or globe rupture. Table 19.1 shows some factors that affect intraocular pressure.

Table 19.1. Factors affecting intraocular pressure

Struggling, restraint	Increase
Coughing, gagging, vomiting	Increase
Tight neck leads	Increase
Jugular compression	Increase
Ketamine	Increase
Succinylcholine	Increase
Pressure on eye	Increase
Sudden ↑ in BP	Increase
Hypercapnia	Increase
ET intubation	Increase
↓ BP	Decrease
Hypocapnia, hyperventilation	Decrease
Pentothal	Decrease
Propofol	Decrease
Alpha-2 agonists	Decrease
Benzodiazepines	Decrease
Acepromazine	Decrease
Opioids	Decrease

The Oculocardiac Reflex (OCR)

The oculocardiac reflex is a spontaneous drop in heart rate associated with traction or pressure on the eye or surrounding structures. Pressure on the trigeminal and vagus nerves of the parasympathetic nervous system is responsible for this sudden, and sometimes life-threatening bradycardia. Arrhythmias can also be seen and include atrioventricular (AV) block, bigeminy, ectopic beats, and occasionally cardiopulmonary arrest (CPA). The OCR is most likely to occur during ophthalmic procedures in patients that are very young and patients that are brachycephalic, such as the Pug and Shih Tzu. Pediatric and brachycephalic patients generally have higher vagal tone than adults of other breeds, which predisposes these patients to the bradycardia and arrhythmias seen after activation of the OCR.

Although gentle manipulation of the eye and surrounding structures is the best prevention, administration of an anticholinergic drug as part of the premedication is helpful in preventing bradycardia. Glycopyrrolate is the anticholinergic of choice with ocular procedures and can be given at a dose of 0.01 mg/kg intramuscularly (IM) or intravenously (IV). Atropine can be given but is much more likely to cause tachycardia and cardiac arrhythmias. Also, atropine will cross the blood-brain barrier and cause dilation of the pupil (mydriasis). This may be problematic, depending on the patient's condition and the procedure being performed. If atropine is chosen as an anticholinergic, it can be given at a dose of 0.02 mg/kg IM or SQ. Intravenous administration of atropine is not recommended for routine preemptive use because of its pronounced cardiac effects.

If the OCR is activated during the procedure, pressure or traction on the eye or surrounding structures should immediately be discontinued. This, in itself, may resolve the bradycardia. If it does not, an anticholinergic should be administered. Glycopyrrolate (0.01 mg/kg) or atropine (0.02 mg/kg) should be given as a rapid intravenous bolus. Atropine has a more rapid onset than glycopyrrolate and is a better choice if the bradycardia is severe or if CPA has occurred (emergency situation). A second dose may be given if the heart rate does not respond initially. If a response is not seen after a repeat dose and the bradycardia is thought to be life threatening, a retrobulbar block with lidocaine may be performed. This block has been shown to be effective in treating an episode of OCR because infusion of lidocaine into the retrobulbar space will inhibit vagal stimuli to the central nervous system (Thurmon et al. 1996).

Premedication

When choosing a premedication for most ocular procedures, minimizing stress is extremely important. If a patient is struggling or is tightly restrained, it causes an increase in IOP that could potentially worsen ophthalmic problems. Increases in IOP can cause pain, proptosis of the eye, damage to the optic nerve, or rupture of the globe. Acepromazine is a good choice as a sedative in most patients. However, some geriatric or pediatric patients may not be able to tolerate the hypotension that is sometimes associated with this drug. With these patients, it may be better to choose a very low dose of acepromazine (0.01 mg/kg) or a different type of sedative. A benzodiazepine, such as midazolam (0.1–0.2 mg/kg), is an alternative choice.

These sedative drugs can be combined with an opioid as part of the premedication. The combination of an opioid and a sedative (neuroleptanalgesia) will provide analgesia for the procedure and sedation to allow placement of an intravenous catheter without a struggle. The choice of opioid (and whether to include an opioid as part of the premedication) will depend on the procedure. One problem with opioid administration is the likelihood of causing vomiting and a subsequent increase in IOP. There are several things that can be done to minimize the risk of vomiting. One possibility is to choose a partial agonist, such as buprenorphine, or an agonist/antagonist, such as butorphanol, as part of the premedication. Very rarely is vomiting associated with these two drugs. The drawback, however, is that they may not provide enough analgesia for the procedure if the patient is especially painful. Also, if it is decided later that a pure agonist opioid is needed, the other drugs administered may interfere with its action somewhat. A second possibility is to wait until after induction and placement of an ET tube to administer an opioid. Once the patient is under general anesthesia, the likelihood of vomiting is greatly reduced. A third possibility is to administer a pure agonist opioid in the premedication but combine it with acepromazine because this drug has antiemetic properties. That being said, a patient that is already painful is less likely to vomit after administration of an appropriate dose of an opioid analgesic.

The level of pain from the ophthalmic condition and the surgery that is being performed will determine what analgesic is appropriate. The cornea is a highly enervated region so any procedure or condition that affects the cornea is generally very painful. Corneal ulcers and desmetoceles are conditions seen that can be quite painful. Pure agonist opioids such as hydromorphone or oxymorphone are the best choices for these types of conditions. It is best that morphine be avoided, despite its excellent analgesic qualities, because it is very likely to cause vomiting after administration.

Induction and Maintenance of Anesthesia

For intraocular procedures or procedures where an increase in IOP is of concern, ketamine should be avoided as an induction agent. Patients with extraocular problems can be induced with ketamine/midazolam (or diazepam). This induction protocol may be beneficial because ketamine can provide supplementary analgesia and generally helps to support heart rate and blood pressure. Other induction options include propofol, thiopental, or etomidate. These three drugs will decrease IOP, but each one has pros and cons. Etomidate may not be the best choice for patients with increased IOP because it commonly causes excitement, gagging, and retching at induction, especially without adequate premedication. This drug should be reserved for patients with severe cardiac disease and those that are heavily sedated from premedication. Thiopental and propofol are both good choices but thiopental should be avoided in very old patients or those with liver dysfunction. Mask and box inductions should generally be avoided since excitement and struggling may cause in increase in IOP.

Most volatile inhalant anesthetics are appropriate for maintenance of anesthesia in ophthalmic patients. Nitrous oxide, however, is uncommonly used for intraocular procedures. This drug is contraindicated in ocular procedures where air may be injected into a chamber of the closed eye because nitrous oxide will diffuse into the bubble and increase IOP (Thurmon et al. 1996).

Local Blocks for Ophthalmic Procedures

Local infiltration of anesthetic

A simple line block can be performed for some ocular procedures, including enucleation and surgeries involving the eyelid. This type of block is helpful when the eyelid is cut during enucleation surgery. A line block involves injecting local anesthetic into the tissue of the eyelid. Local anesthetic can also be injected around the globe in the subconjunctival tissues before removal of the globe (Giuliano 2007). Lidocaine can be used to provide local analgesia for 1–2 hours. If bupivicaine is used, it can provide analgesia for up to 6 hours. The two drugs can also be mixed together to provide a rapid onset of analgesia with a prolonged effect. When using these drugs it is important to calculate appropriate doses to prevent inadvertent overdose.

Retrobulbar block

A retrobulbar block is another type of local block that can be performed for ocular procedures. This block is done much more commonly in large animals than small due to the degree of technical difficulty and the risk of complications. The risks are numerous and include retrobulbar hemorrhage, perforation of the globe, damage to the optic nerve, and injection of local anesthetic into the subarachnoid space (Giuliano 2007). This final complication is potentially the most serious since infiltration of local anesthetic into the subarachnoid space can cause respiratory or cardiac arrest. The advantages to performing the retrobulbar block include a reduction in other anesthetic drug needs, complete analgesia/anesthesia of the eye, and elimination of the need for peripheral muscle relaxants (neuromuscular blocking drugs) for ocular muscle relaxation. The anesthetist performing the retrobulbar block should have an excellent understanding of the anatomy in the area and should be fully aware of potential complications.

Neuromuscular Blockade

One of the difficulties with ocular and intraocular procedures is the requirement of a central eye position. Normally, a deep level of anesthesia is necessary to achieve this eye position. One way to avoid this possibly dangerous level of anesthesia is the use of neuromuscular blocking drugs. Neuromuscular blockers (NMBs) are used in ophthalmic surgeries to prevent movement of the eye during the procedure and to maintain the eye in a central position. NMBs are also known as peripheral muscle relaxants or "paralytic" drugs. They do not provide analgesia or sedation and therefore should never be used without provision of concurrent anesthetic and analgesic drugs. Patients that wake during neuromuscular blockade can experience extreme anxiety and pain. This has been described by human patients because paralytic drugs are used much more commonly with humans than with veterinary patients. Signs of insufficient anesthesia in the patient under neuromuscular blockade include an increase in heart rate and blood pressure.

Use of NMBs for ophthalmic procedures

Neuromuscular blocking drugs are helpful in ophthalmic procedures that require the eye to be in a central position. Cataract removal surgery (phacoemulsification), conjunctival flap surgery, and removal of iridial masses will all require the eye to be in this position. Without the aid of NMB drugs the only way to maintain the desired eye position and an adequate level of anesthesia would be to keep the patient at a very deep anesthetic plane. This is not recommended or desirable. As the level of anesthesia deepens, the cardiovascular effect of anesthetics becomes more profound. This means that heart rate decreases, cardiac contractility decreases, and vasodilation increases, often resulting in severe hypotension and reduced cardiac output. These cardiovascular effects are not well tolerated by most patients, especially the geriatric and pediatric patients that commonly present with ophthalmic conditions. Excessively deep levels of anesthesia also result in hypoventilation or apnea. Hypoventilation causes arterial carbon dioxide levels to increase, sometimes to dangerous levels. This can result in hypoxemia and acidemia, which leads to cardiac arrhythmias, cardiovascular collapse, and death. Neuromuscular blocking drugs allow the concentration of anesthetic to be reduced to a safer level while maintaining a central eye position and allowing surgical manipulation of the eye.

Before using NMB drugs it is important to understand the anatomy of the neuromuscular junction and how these drugs work to prevent skeletal muscle movement.

The neuromuscular junction

The neuromuscular junction is where a motor neuron synapses with skeletal muscle fibers. In order for the neuron to communicate with the skeletal muscle fiber it releases a neurotransmitter, acetylcholine, into the synaptic cleft. Acetylcholine will then bind to receptors on the postsynaptic muscle cell in order to activate an action potential, which is then converted into muscle contraction. The acetylcholine will immediately be broken down by an enzyme, acetylcholinesterase, to discontinue activation of the muscle fiber and allow the membrane to repolarize.

Types of NMBs

Depolarizing NMBs

Depolarizing NMBs cause depolarization of the neuromuscular junction. Nondepolarizing NMBs work by blocking transmission of the nerve impulse at the level of the postsynaptic muscle fiber. Depolarizing NMBs are used infrequently in veterinary medicine. One that may be of clinical significance is succinylcholine. Succinylcholine works by first stimulating the postsynaptic muscle fiber, causing depolarization and then muscle contraction manifesting as muscle fasciculations. Muscle fasciculation is characteristic of depolarizing NMBs. After this initial phase, skeletal muscle paralysis will occur from pro-

longed depolarization of the motor endplate (Muir et al. 2000). Neuromuscular blockade ceases when the drug is metabolized by another enzyme, pseudocholinesterase. Depolarizing NMBs cannot be antagonized (reversed) by anticholinesterase drugs. These drugs are not often used for ocular procedures because they can potentially cause an increase in IOP.

Nondepolarizing NMBs

Nondepolarizing NMBs are much more commonly used in veterinary medicine. Muscle fasciculation does not occur because there is no depolarization of the muscle fiber. Nondepolarizing NMB drugs will recognize the acetylcholine receptor on the muscle fiber and bind to it, but they do not trigger an action potential. By doing so, they occupy the receptors and prevent acetylcholine from binding to those sites. The enzyme acetylcholinesterase is unable to break down the NMB drug so it will continue to block transmission of the nerve impulse until the drug is metabolized or until its concentration is so low that acetylcholine can once again compete for binding sites (Karas and McCobb 2005).

Specific neuromuscular blocking drugs

Atracurium is a commonly used nondepolarizing NMB. This drug has very few cardiovascular effects and does not depend on hepatic metabolism or renal excretion for elimination. This makes it a good agent for patients that have renal or hepatic insufficiency. Atracurium is eliminated from the body through a process called *Hoffman elimination*. This process is pH- and temperature-dependent, so elimination may be prolonged in hypothermic or acidotic patients. Generally the first dose of atracurium is given at 0.25 mg/kg IV. If additional doses are needed throughout surgery, half of the first dose (about 0.1 mg/kg) may be given. Atracurium has a short half life and generally lasts only 15–30 minutes. The level of neuromuscular blockade may be evaluated using a nerve stimulator. Also, the surgeon can alert the anesthetist if the eye has moved out of position and additional drug may be administered. Wait 3–7 minutes to assess the level of blockade before administering additional drug.

Ventilation

Once the patient is under anesthesia and prepped it should be placed into position for surgery. Anesthetic monitors should be placed, including ECG, SpO_2, BP, and $ETCO_2$. The patient should be at a medium anesthetic plane. Before paralytic drugs are administered, it is important to make sure that manual or mechanical ventilation is available. If a mechanical ventilator is to be used, proper function should be verified prior to induction and approximate settings dialed in. Once the patient is attached to the mechanical ventilator, proper ventilator settings should be set and appropriate ventilation should be confirmed. Only after it is determined that the ventilator is functioning normally and the patient is able to be normally ventilated should the NMB be administered. Ventilator function must be confirmed as a safety precaution because the patient will not be able to ventilate on its own once the drug is administered. A normal breathing system and bag should be readily available should there be mechanical failure of the ventilator during the procedure. If manual ventilation is to be provided, it is important to pressure-check the anesthetic machine and visually inspect the bag and circuit for holes, obstruction, or foreign objects. It is recommended that, with manual ventilation, a pop-off occlusion valve be used as opposed to the normal screw-down pop-off valve. This makes it significantly easier to give regular breaths and makes it less likely that the APL valve will be accidentally left closed.

Monitoring neuromuscular blockade

In addition to the usual anesthetic monitoring devices, the level of neuromuscular blockade should be monitored as well. It is important to monitor the level of blockade to provide the correct amount of muscle relaxation for surgery but to prevent drug overdose. Monitoring will also help to determine when neuromuscular blockade has ceased or can be reversed. This can be accomplished using a device called a *nerve stimulator*. This device will electrically stimulate a peripheral nerve to cause a muscle contraction. The degree of muscle contraction from before and after neuromuscular blockade is then compared to determine the degree of muscle relaxation. Commonly used nerves for this purpose include the ulnar, peroneal, tibial, and facial nerves. The peroneal nerve is the most easily utilized in small animal patients undergoing ocular surgery. Figure 19.1 shows a nerve stimulator device in place over the peroneal nerve of a dog. The electrodes are placed on either side of the stifle joint and when the device is activated, a twitch of the leg should be observed.

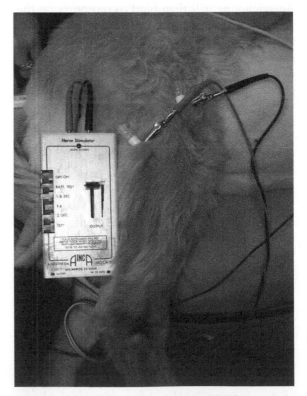

Figure 19.1. Nerve stimulator in place, peroneal nerve of the dog.

There are various patterns of nerve stimulation that may be used. A single twitch is the simplest. When activated, the device will show one twitch of the selected muscle group. Once the NMB has been administered, the muscle twitch should diminish or be completely abolished. A more common nerve stimulation pattern is called the "Train of Four" (TOF). This pattern is more useful than a single twitch because it gives the anesthetist some qualitative information about the level of the block. Four electrical stimuli are given over two seconds, and four corresponding muscle twitches should be observed. As the degree of muscle relaxation increases, the muscle twitches will be abolished, starting with the fourth. If all four muscle twitches are abolished, it means that at least 95% of the acetylcholine receptors have been blocked (Karas and McCobb 2005). Once the neuromuscular blockade begins to wear off, the twitches should start to reappear, starting with the first. The level of muscle relaxation can be determined by comparing the height of the fourth to the first twitch.

Reversal of neuromuscular blockade

Nondepolarizing NMBs, such as atracurium, are reversible by anticholinesterase drugs. These reversal agents work by inhibiting acetylcholinesterase. This allows acetylcholine to build up in the neuromuscular junction for restoration of muscle movement. Before giving an anticholinesterase drug, it is important to wait for signs of recovery from neuromuscular blockade. Because of this, monitoring with a nerve stimulator is very helpful. At least two twitches from a TOF nerve stimulation pattern should be present before the reversal agent is given. This is important because adequate reversal may not occur if signs of recovery are not seen first. Commonly used reversal agents include neostigmine (0.02 mg/kg) and edrophonium (0.5–1 mg/kg). An anticholinesterase drug should be preceded by an anticholinergic to prevent side effects, bradycardia in particular. Glycopyrrolate (0.01 mg/kg IV) should be given about 5 minutes before reversal. After the anticholinergic drug has taken

effect, the reversal agent may be given slowly over 5–10 minutes while watching for bradycardia. If an anticholinergic is contraindicated (severe heart disease), the reversal agent may be administered slowly and, if excessive bradycardia is observed, the anticholinergic may then be given. Recovery from neuromuscular blockade has occurred when the TOF has returned to pre-blockade levels and the patient is able to maintain an adequate tidal volume. A respirometer or capnograph can be used to establish whether ventilation is adequate. Only after reversal has occurred should anesthesia be discontinued. If the patient were to wake up before adequate reversal of the block, extreme anxiety could result.

Anesthesia for Electroretinogram (ERG)

For ERG, generally only light anesthesia or deep tranquilization is necessary. Propofol may be a good choice for this procedure because it can easily be titrated to effect. It is helpful that a light plane of anesthesia be maintained so that the patient will remain still but the eye may stay in an adequate position for examination. Some clinicians may want the eyes covered with a towel or drape for about 10 minutes once the patient is sedated or asleep so that the eyes have time to adjust to the dark.

Anesthesia for Extraocular Procedures

Generally, for extraocular procedures, no special considerations are needed. Analgesia should be provided as needed and a combination of opioids and NSAID pain relievers may be helpful. Even with extraocular procedures, premedication with an anticholinergic should be considered because pressure on the muscles surrounding the globe can occasionally activate the OCR. This is particularly important in pediatric and brachycephalic patients.

Anesthesia for Ocular and Intraocular Procedures

Enucleation

Enucleation is generally considered a very painful procedure. It may be difficult to maintain an adequate level of anesthesia. The increase in blood pressure caused by insufficient analgesia may also cause excessive bleeding during surgery. A pure agonist opioid, such as hydromorphone, should be included in the preanesthetic protocol. A sedative and an anticholinergic should be included as well. Normal anesthetic induction and maintenance regimes may be used. Additional analgesia may be provided in the form of a constant rate infusion (CRI) during the procedure. Fentanyl, lidocaine/ketamine, or morphine/lidocaine/ketamine (MLK) are some possible choices. The addition of an NSAID can help potentiate the analgesia provided by these drugs. Local anesthetic infusion into the eyelid before it is cut and anesthetic splashed into the orbit before closure can be helpful. The retrobulbar block is also a possible choice, though it is associated with more complications and may be difficult to perform in smaller patients. Applying an ice pack to the surgical site before the patient is awake is also helpful in reducing pain from inflammation. These techniques together can help maintain a smoother anesthesia and provide a quiet recovery with a reduced risk of bleeding and self-injury.

Conjunctival flap

The main anesthetic concerns for this procedure are reducing pain, maintaining proper eye position for surgery, maintaining or reducing intraocular pressure, and providing a smooth recovery. This procedure is performed as treatment for corneal ulceration, which is generally quite painful. The drugs chosen should provide analgesia and sedation to prevent struggling in the preanesthetic period. Drugs that increase IOP should be avoided. Ketamine and succinylcholine are the anesthetic drugs most commonly associated with increases in IOP. Neuromuscular blockade is usually necessary to maintain the eye in a central position, so ventilation support must be provided and proper monitoring of neuromuscular blockade should be available. Additional sedation in the recovery period may be necessary to prevent self-injury.

Cataract removal

Patients that present with cataracts frequently have systemic disease that may increase their anesthetic risk. Often, these patients are geriatric or diabetic and additional precautions may need to be taken. Diabetic patients should have their blood glucose (BG) checked frequently in the perianesthetic period. Generally, a BG should be taken at the beginning of surgery and then every hour during the procedure. These patients should be given drugs that will not prolong recovery so that they will be awake and able to get back on their usual eating schedule. Insulin and dextrose can be given as needed. Geriatric patients may have heart or renal disease, and the anesthetic protocol will have to be adapted to whatever condition is present. Patients presenting for cataract removal also will require the use of NMB drugs to maintain the eye in a central position, so ventilation and proper monitoring must be provided. In addition, intraocular procedures, such as cataract removal, require dilation of the pupil. Opioid pure agonists cause miosis (constriction of the pupil) in dogs and may be contraindicated preoperatively. It is important to discuss with the surgeon his or her preference about the preoperative administration of opioids.

Positioning

Many ocular and intraocular procedures require positioning in dorsal recumbency for surgery. This can be a problem because, while the patient is on its back, the head and nose must be positioned toward the chest so that the surgeon has access to the eye. Figure 19.2 shows a

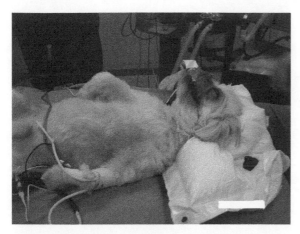

Figure 19.2. Patient in position for conjunctival flap surgery. Note the position of the head and the potential for kinking of an unguarded endotracheal tube.

patient in position for a conjunctival flap. This head position can cause normal endotracheal tubes to become kinked and cause an occlusion of the airway. Signs of airway occlusion include increased respiratory effort or apnea, difficulty in providing positive pressure ventilation, lack of chest wall motion, lack of breath sounds, and decreased or absent end-tidal carbon dioxide values. The incidence of this positional complication can be greatly reduced by using a wire-reinforced (guarded or armored) endotracheal tube. These tubes have a wire coil embedded in the wall, which helps to prevent the tube from kinking and occluding. It is highly recommended that a wire-reinforced ET tube be used for ophthalmic procedures that require the neck to be pulled forward into this position.

Recovery

Keeping the patient sedated and comfortable in the recovery period is essential to a successful outcome when dealing with ophthalmic procedures. Pain and/or anxiety cause an increase in blood pressure that can cause an increase in IOP, which can jeopardize the repair or damage the animal's vision. An increase in blood pressure can also lead to hemorrhage in procedures where this is a potential complication, such as enucleation. There is also the potential that the patient will cause self-trauma by scratching or rubbing the affected eye. A sedative, such as acepromazine, may be needed in the recovery period. Additional narcotic analgesics should be provided preemptively if possible. An e-collar is a wonderful tool in preventing self-trauma in postoperative ophthalmic patients. The e-collar should be in place very soon after extubation. It is helpful to make sure that the recovery area is dark and quiet to prevent excess stimulation postop. It is important to remember that patients that have received opioids are often light- and noise-sensitive and may have a strong reaction to a stimulating environment.

Any patient that has received NMB's as part of their anesthetic protocol should be monitored closely during the recovery period. Though uncommon, reparalyzation is a possible complication. Hypoventilation from incomplete recovery from the effects of NMB's is also a concern. The patient's respiratory rate, respiratory effort, and mucous membrane color should be monitored for several hours postop.

References

Giuliano, EA. 2007. NAVC Proceedings. Local Blocks in Ophthalmic Surgery. North American Veterinary Conference, IVIS, Ithaca, NY.

Karas, A, McCobb, E. 2005. Clinical Use and Monitoring of Neuromuscular Blocking Agents. Technician and Student Guide, Tufts Cummings School of Veterinary Medicine.

Muir, WW, et al. 2000. Handbook of Veterinary Anesthesia, 3rd ed. St. Louis: Mosby, Inc.

Thurmon, JC, et al. 1996. Lumb & Jones' Veterinary Anesthesia, 3rd ed. Baltimore: Lippincott, Williams & Wilkins.

Figure 13-2.

Anesthesia for Patients with Cardiac Disease

20

Wendy Curtis-Uhle and Katy W. Waddell

Small animal patients with cardiac disease may require anesthesia for a number of reasons. Such patients may present for diagnostic, interventional, or surgical treatment of their congenital or acquired cardiac abnormalities, or they may need to be anesthetized for unrelated procedures. In any case, an understanding of the physiology of the particular cardiac disease, the effects of anesthetic agents on the cardiovascular system, and appropriate measures to support these compromised patients is a step toward providing them with quality care.

General Measures to Optimize Outcome

There are a variety of concerns with different types of heart disease, but there are general measures that can be taken to optimize patient outcome.

Reduce stress

Because stress activates the sympathetic nervous system and increases cardiac work, techniques should be employed to reduce/avoid stress in the cardiac-compromised patient. Each patient must be individually assessed to determine whether a particular procedure will create more stress than the benefit afforded.

Premedications

The beneficial aspects of providing preoperative tranquilizers and/or analgesics are significant. A reduction of fear/anxiety coupled with a preemptive analgesic state will potentially decrease the need for a full dose of induction agents and provide a MAC-sparing effect for inhalant agents. A fearful, struggling patient during induction will have an increased heart rate, blood pressure, and myocardial oxygen demand. Catecholamine release can potentiate ventricular arrhythmias. Conversely, withholding sedation is appropriate in patients who cannot endure any respiratory or cardiovascular depression.

Balanced anesthesia

A balanced anesthetic protocol utilizing multiple agents serves to decrease doses of each agent, thereby reducing detrimental side effects. It also serves to provide multimodal analgesia. Anesthetic agents should be selected based on cardiac dysfunction to cause the least amount of disturbance to normal function. Suggested agents will be discussed later in the chapter as dictated by each disease. Regional and local blocks should be employed whenever possible.

Preoxygenation

Preoxygenation before anesthesia induction can increase the alveolar oxygen concentration. This enhances the amount of oxygen to be transported by the hemoglobin after administration of induction agents until an endotracheal tube is placed and oxygen delivered through it. One hundred percent oxygen delivered via a tight-fitting mask is most advantageous but is often objectionable to the patient (Pascoe and Bennett 1999). Although not as effective, holding the breathing hoses close to the mouth or nares is usually tolerated and will provide some benefit.

Ventilatory support

Oxygen delivery and carbon dioxide removal should be monitored using a capnograph, a pulse oximeter, inspiratory pressure, a respirometer, and observation of chest excursions. If required (i.e., low tidal volume, high end-tidal carbon dioxide partial pressure), manual or mechanically assisted ventilation should be applied. However, positive pressure ventilation can impede venous return and decrease cardiac output. Tidal volume should be adjusted accordingly to minimize this effect (Muir et al. 2000).

IV fluid support

Crystalloids and/or colloids should be given to maintain normovolemia, hydration, and blood pressure, and if necessary to correct electrolyte imbalances. However, because pulmonary edema due to fluid overload is of particular concern in patients with left-sided heart failure, fluid restrictions may be required. Fluid overload in right-

sided failure will increase ascites and hepatic hypertension and may ultimately lead to pulmonary edema as well. However, because many heart patients have been on diuretics, hydration may be needed. A balance must be achieved in providing needed fluid therapy, while avoiding overload and edema. Currently, the most effective way to monitor this balance is by measuring central venous pressure, which approximates the pressure of the blood entering the right atrium (Johnson 1999). The volume of any other agents, such as injectable anesthetics, IV catheter flushes, and any infusions for blood pressure support, should be considered as part of the fluid volume calculation.

Perioperative blood work evaluation

Serum electrolytes and acid-base status may need repeated monitoring. Calcium, potassium, and magnesium serve critical roles in cardiac muscle cell conduction. Imbalances should ideally be corrected before undertaking any anesthetic procedure. Blood pH can influence drug interactions and protein-binding, thereby increasing the chance of toxicity of some drugs or decreasing the effectiveness of others (Cornell 2007). Most patients with congenital defects that are undergoing repair are pediatric and should have serial blood glucose monitoring and supplementation as needed. Any anemia should be managed to ensure a PCV of 22–35% in feline and 25–45% in canine patients in order to optimize oxygen-carrying capacity (Thurmon et al. 1999).

Classification of Patients with Cardiac Disease

Decisions regarding anesthesia for patients with heart disease should be based on degree of disease and type of disease. The American Society of Anesthesiologists' classification for patients with regard to anesthetic risk is described in a previous chapter. Classification of patients with heart disease has also been devised in order to determine risk to anesthesia and treatment guide-

Table 20.1. ASA classification of patients with heart disease.

Class I	Disease confirmed by radiographs, echocardiography No clinical signs of failure, may be receiving medications	**ASA category II** Those not receiving drugs **ASA category III** Those receiving cardiac medications Safe to sedate or anesthetize without stabilization
Class II	Mild to moderate signs of failure at rest/ mild exertion	**ASA category IV** Should be stabilized with cardiac medication and be free of signs of heart failure for several days prior to receiving sedation or anesthesia Drug therapy to continue during anesthesia and recovery phase Higher risk of debilitation/death during perianesthetic period
Class III	Signs of fulminate heart failure, may present in shock	**ASA category V** Aggressive therapy to stabilize before anesthesia is considered Once stable, ASA category IV–V because patient may decompensate and death may occur during perianesthetic period

Source: This table is adapted from guidelines provided by the International Small Animal Cardiac Health Council, 1994.

lines (Table 20.1). As described, patients with mild cardiovascular changes may require little change in protocol. On the other hand, patients with congestive heart failure present the need for additional monitoring, blood pressure support, and careful anesthetic administration.

Heart Failure

Heart failure is defined as the inability of the heart to move blood forward effectively enough to meet metabolic needs. This may be caused by valvular insufficiencies or stenoses, cardiomyopathies, heartworm disease, arrhythmias, or other conditions causing poor cardiac output.

Whatever the cause, there are several physiological compensatory mechanisms in order to maintain blood pressure. During a hypotensive event, feedback from baroreceptors in the aortic arch and the carotid body cause an increase in heart rate. Neurotransmitters activate the sympathetic nervous system and depress parasympathetic responses. Consequently, the heart rate increases, and blood vessels constrict in order to increase venous return and cardiac output. Decreased intravascular pressure causes fluid to shift from the tissues to the intravascular space. The kidney secretes renin, which indirectly causes an increase in Angiotensin II, a potent vasoconstrictor. Angiotensin II stimulates thirst and the secretion of aldosterone from the adrenal glands. Aldosterone causes retention of sodium and water by the kidneys. Antidiuretic hormone (ADH; also called *vasopressin*), secreted by the pituitary gland, decreases urinary output and produces vasoconstriction. In addition, low levels of atrial natriuretic peptide (a hormone secreted from atrial myocytes in response to high pressure) causes retention of sodium and water.

These compensatory mechanisms are physiologically beneficial in the short term; however, over time, the enhanced intravascular volume and vasoconstriction result in volume overload, increased peripheral resistance, and increased myocardial work. An increase in cardiac muscle mass or chamber size will occur.

In left-sided failure, increased volume and pressure will impede forward flow from the pulmonary system. Resulting increased hydrostatic pressure in the lungs causes fluid to leak out of the vessels inciting pulmonary edema (Tranquilli et al. 2007). In right-sided failure, back pressure will result in ascites and increased hepatic pressure.

At the same time, ischemia (due to inadequate oxygen supply to the heart muscle in the face of increased workload) and changes in myocardial structure (increased muscle mass or chamber size) can lead to conduction disturbances. Eventually, if left untreated, heart failure will

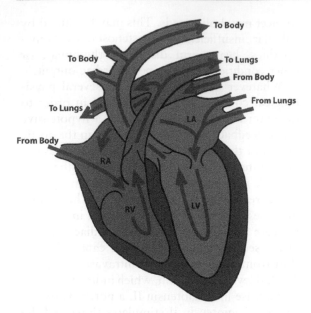

Figure 20.1.   Normal blood flow through the heart.

result in life-threatening pulmonary edema, inadequate tissue perfusion, and/or detrimental arrhythmias.

Medications used in the treatment of heart disease are aimed at reducing compensatory mechanisms in order to break the cycle and slow progression of the disease. The effects of drugs prescribed for cardiac disease may be exacerbated by anesthetic agents. For example, vasodilatory effects of medications will be compounded by inhalants and other anesthetics, and dehydration from chronic diuretic administration will increase the need for support of hydration and blood pressure. (Fig. 20.1 illustrates normal blood flow through the heart.)

Cardiac Diseases

Dilated cardiomyopathy

Dilated cardiomyopathy is most commonly seen in certain large-breed dogs (Oyama 2008). This condition is characterized by stretching and weakening of the heart muscle so that chamber size is increased while contractility is compro-

mised. Stroke volume is reduced resulting in decreased blood pressure. Compensatory mechanisms for hypotension ensue.

Chamber enlargement may alter the shape and function of the mitral valve, leading to valvular insufficiency. In addition, changes in myocardial architecture effect cell communication and disrupt organized depolarization. Atrial fibrillation, premature ventricular contractions, and ventricular tachycardia may develop. These patients are at grave risk of developing pulmonary edema/congestive heart failure.

When anesthetizing a patient with dilated cardiomyopathy, the goal is to maintain preload, contractility, and a normal heart rate. Bradycardia, tachycardia, and vasoconstriction should be avoided (Pascoe 2005).

The following doses are those generally used by the Section of Anesthesia at the Ryan Hospital of the University of Pennsylvania. Premedication may consist of glycopyrrolate at 0.01 mg/kg dependent on the patient's heart rate, with hydromorphone or oxymorphone. Should patients be of a brachycephalic breed where respiratory difficulties may be present, butorphanol can be used in place of hydromorphone. Low doses of acepromazine (5 mcg/kg) might be considered in case of excessive vasoconstriction or to add to sedative effects of opioids.

Following preoxygenation, induction may be achieved with diazepam at 0.2 mg/kg given IV followed by etomidate at 1–2 mg/kg given IV to effect. Hydromorphone or oxymorphone (0.1 mg/kg) may also be included. A ketamine top-up calculated at 1–4 mg/kg IV might follow to provide a deeper plane of anesthesia and facilitate intubation. It may also help stabilize heart rate due to an increase in sympathetic tone. However, ketamine may not be advisable in patients that are tachycardic or have had arrhythmias.

Anesthetic maintenance may include isoflurane or sevoflurane if tolerated with regard to blood pressure. A constant rate infusion of fentanyl (0.1–0.8 mcg/kg/minute) and midazolam (3–8 mcg/kg/minute) may be used in order to decrease inhalant agent administration. Ventilatory support may be required with the administration of this CRI due to the potent respiratory depression caused by fentanyl. Toward the end of the procedure the CRI should be discontinued or reduced in order to avoid reversal, which may compromise postoperative analgesia (although fentanyl's duration of action is short).

Hypotension may be corrected with the use of positive inotropes or beta agonists such as dobutamine. These drugs focus on improving contractility without increasing afterload. Dobutamine should be diluted and administered as a constant rate infusion, beginning at 2 micrograms (mcg) per kilogram per minute, and increased as needed (up to 20 mcg/kg/min). Dopamine as a CRI may also be used to support blood pressure and is calculated to be delivered at a starting rate of 2 mcg/kg/minute. High doses of dopamine cause vasoconstriction and should be avoided. Ventricular arrhythmias may be exacerbated with the use of beta agonists (e.g., dobutamine), so close monitoring of the EKG is necessary (Cole and Drobatz 2008).

Fluids must be administered conservatively to avoid overload and pulmonary edema. Assessment of hydration status should be accompanied by CVP monitoring in order to determine appropriate fluid administration.

Contraindicated anesthetic agents are ketamine (when arrhythmias or tachycardia are present), any alpha-2 agonist, and halothane. Caution should be taken with propofol and thiopental administration, because they are negative inotropes (Pascoe 2005).

Hypertrophic cardiomyopathy

Although hypertrophic cardiomyopathy (HCM) is not commonly seen in dogs, it is the most common heart disease in cats (Kienle 2008). Feline HCM is a common sequela of hyperthyroidism. but generally its etiology is not known. HCM is considered a disease of diastole and is characterized by thickening of the left ventricular wall and decreased chamber size. Reduction of space within the chamber and the inability of the heart to relax during diastole leads to diminished filling volume and consequently inadequate stroke volume.

This makes cardiac output particularly rate-dependent so bradycardia must be avoided. On the other hand, tachycardia will impede relaxation and perfusion of the myocardium, increase myocardial oxygen demands, and reduce filling time.

When handling patients with HCM, particularly cats with hyperthyroidism, avoidance of stress is vital because they are prone to tachyarrhythmias. Because most drugs do not produce reliable sedation in cats, the benefits of acepromazine may outweigh the risk of the vasodilation it causes, especially in fractious cats. Along with a sedative, butorphanol may be well tolerated in order to facilitate IV catheter placement. Mu agonists such as hydromorphone are needed to provide analgesia and allow reduction of inhalant but will be less likely to cause excitement if given after sedation has been achieved. Ketamine should be avoided. However, in the intractable cat a small dose of ketamine with acepromazine, in addition to butorphanol or hydromorphone, may be better than the degree of stress that can accompany an induction without adequate sedation.

Induction of anesthesia may be achieved with diazepam at 0.2 mg/kg IV followed by etomidate at 0.52 mg/kg IV titrated to effect. Hydromorphone or oxymorphone at 0.05–0.1 may also be included (Ryan Hospital).

Maintenance may include isoflurane or sevoflurane if the patient can tolerate the subsequent vasodilation. Opioids and benzodiazepines may be used intraoperatively to decrease inhalant needs. Bradycardia subsequent to opioids may necessitate treatment with .005–.02 mg/kg of atropine or glycopyrrolate. Adequate IV crystalloid therapy should be administered in order to prevent hypovolemia and decreased filling volumes. A balanced electrolyte solution may be administered at a rate of 5 mL/kg/hour. Alpha agonists such as phenylephrine are useful for their vasoconstrictive properties if blood pressure support is needed. An increase in contractility or heart rate is undesirable, so beta agonists are not recommended.

Alpha-2 agonists are generally contraindicated. Recently, it has been suggested that the decreased heart rate and vasoconstriction produced by alpha-2 agonists may be beneficial in cats with left ventricular outflow obstruction. Studies are being currently developed to test this hypothesis.

Mitral valve insufficiency

One of the most common cardiac disorders in dogs is mitral valve insufficiency (Abbott 2008). A normal mitral valve will close during ventricular contraction, thereby ensuring that all blood moves forward to systemic circulation. A defective valve will allow some blood to be pumped back into the left atrium (Fig. 20.2). This reduces cardiac output and systemic blood pressure. Compensatory mechanisms in response to lowered blood pressure will increase the total fluid volume in circulation and cause vasoconstriction. Increased peripheral vascular resistance causes the left side of the heart to enlarge. Increased pulmonary pressure will follow and lead to pulmonary edema.

When anesthetizing a patient with mitral valve disease, the goals are similar to that of dilated cardiomyopathy: maintaining heart rate, preload, and contractility, while avoiding increased afterload (Pascoe 2005). Opioids, benzodiazepines, and etomidate are considered good choices in an anesthesia protocol. Ketamine is often avoided because it increases myocardial oxygen needs. Propofol should be avoided or used with extreme care due to its vasodilating and hypotensive effects, and thiopental due to its depressant effect on myocardial function.

Judicious use of anticholinergics is warranted in order to avoid either tachycardia or bradycardia. Tachycardia will increase the oxygen needs of the heart, so the prophylactic use of an anticholinergic as a premedicant is usually not recommended. However, low doses can be used if indicated by bradycardia that is causing hypotension.

Untreated mitral valve disease may benefit from the vasodilating effects of anesthetics. However, patients who have been on ACE inhibitors or hydralazine may not tolerate the compounded effect, and drugs such as acepromazine, propofol, and isoflurane are best minimized. In

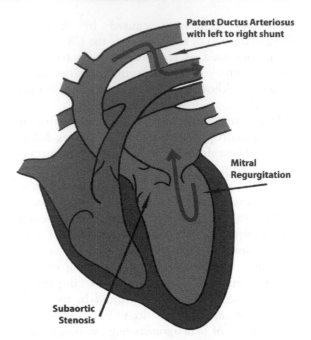

Figure 20.2.   Locations of mitral regurgitation, patent ductus arteriosus, and subaortic stenosis.

the event of hypotension, beta agonists such as dobutamine may be used to improve contractility. Pure alpha agonists such as phenylephrine may exacerbate systemic resistance and are not recommended (Pascoe 2005).

Fluids must be delivered with caution to avoid overload. Evaluation of hydration status should be coupled with CVP monitoring in the determination of fluid rate. A rate of 2.5–5 mL/kg/hour may be a reasonable starting rate, and adjustments should be made according to estimated fluid losses, arterial blood pressure, and central venous pressure.

Patients with mitral insufficiency are also prone to infection of the heart valve, so antibiotics should be administered during any situations in which bacteria may enter the bloodstream (dental procedures, wounds, skin infections).

Patent ductus arteriosus (PDA)

The ductus arteriosus is a vascular connection between the pulmonary artery and the aorta in the fetus. While in the womb, much of the blood leaving the right ventricle travels from the pulmonary artery through the ductus to the aorta and then to systemic circulation, thus bypassing the lungs. Because the fetus is supplied with oxygenated blood through the placenta, it is not necessary for all blood to travel through the lungs before entering systemic circulation. At this time the alveoli are not expanded with air, and vascular resistance is higher in pulmonary than systemic circulation, thus encouraging shunting through the ductus from the pulmonary artery to the aorta.

Within hours to days after birth the ductus normally closes, thereby ensuring that all blood leaving the right ventricle goes through the lungs to receive oxygen before entering systemic circulation.

In animals with patent ductus arteriosus the ductus fails to close. Because the left ventricle pushes with greater force than the right, the blood is shunted from the aorta, through the ductus, back to pulmonary circulation. This is called a "left to right shunt." When this occurs, blood that has already gone through the lungs and received oxygen will travel through the lungs again and into the left atrium (see Figure 20.2). Left heart enlargement occurs due to volume overload, and congestive heart failure may ensue.

In some cases if the shunt is large, pulmonary vascular injury or pulmonary hypertension may occur. Increased pulmonary resistance may reverse the direction of the shunt, thereby sending deoxygenated blood to systemic circulation. Patients with a right to left shunt will suffer from hypoxemia, resultant polycythemia, and the condition will continually deteriorate.

A patient with a PDA will have a characteristic ("machinery") murmur that is easily detectable and therefore often diagnosed at an early age. Correction of a PDA with left to right shunting can be accomplished by surgical ligation of the ductus or by using occlusion devices with the use of cardiac catheterization.

When anesthetizing a patient with a PDA, agents that cause vasodilation and decrease systemic vascular resistance should be avoided because this will potentiate right to left shunting. If pulse oximetry indicates oxygen desaturation or the patient shows moderate to severe hypotension, an alpha agonist such as phenylephrine may be used (Harvey and Ettinger 2007).

During ligation or occlusion of the ductus, a reflex bradycardia may be seen due to sudden increase in blood pressure. If hypotension results from the bradycardia, an anticholinergic can be administered (Harvey and Ettinger 2007).

Irritation of the heart may occur from surgical manipulation or cardiac catheterization, so antiarrhythmics such as lidocaine should be available.

Pulmonic stenosis

Pulmonic stenosis (valvular, supravalvular or subvalvular) is a congenital defect characterized by the narrowing of the outflow tract of the right ventricle. This limits the ability of the right ventricle to move blood out through the pulmonary artery to the lungs. The systolic pressure rises in the right ventricle and hypertrophy occurs over time. Relaxation of the hypertrophic muscle is subnormal and diastolic blood pressure increases. Cardiac output is maintained by an increase in heart rate as stroke volume is compromised. With the increase in cardiac work and decrease in output across the stenotic valve, these patients may experience exercise intolerance or syncopal episodes (Tranquilli et al. 2007). Interventional catheterization and balloon valvuloplasty can be performed on many of these patients. For this procedure, a specialized catheter with an inflatable balloon is strategically placed in the stenotic area with the use of fluoroscopy. The balloon is inflated for short periods of time in order to stretch the fibrotic area.

If the disease progresses, however, tricuspid regurgitation and right atrial enlargement will develop, resulting in right-sided heart failure.

In providing anesthesia for a patient with pulmonic stenosis, the goals are to maintain as close as possible a normal resting heart rate and support right ventricular preload with adequate balanced crystalloid administration (rate based on hydration status, blood pressure, and central venous pressure). Should it be necessary to support contractility, a positive inotropic agent such as dobutamine or dopamine may be added to the anesthetic protocol.

Premedication to be considered would be an opioid with or without a benzodiazepine for stress reduction and IV catheter placement.

Induction may be accomplished with either hydromorphone or oxymorphone at 0.1 mg/kg or 0.05 mg/kg IV followed by a benzodiazepine. This may be followed with etomidate calculated at 0.5–1.5 mg/kg and titrated to effect to obtain the airway.

Anesthesia maintenance should be provided by either isoflurane or sevoflurane. The addition of a fentanyl/midazolam CRI is beneficial in decreasing MAC requirements. As with any ventricular hypertrophy patient, there is an increased likelihood for developing arrhythmias. Preoxygenation would help prevent hypoxia during the intubation. These patients may already be on beta blocker medication that will impede the results of positive inotropes. Multiple agents may be needed to provide blood pressure support.

Aortic stenosis

Aortic stenosis is usually a congenital abnormality. The stenosis may be subvalvular, valvular, or supravalvular and is caused by the development of extra fibrous tissue sometime during the first few months in life (see Fig. 20.2). The result is a partial left ventricular outflow obstruction, which causes increased left intraventricular pressure and subsequent thickening of the left ventricular walls. Other sequelae include cardiac ischemia, arrhythmias, aortic or mitral regurgitation, and left-sided congestive failure.

Diagnosis is usually made at an early age due to a murmur caused by the increased turbulence of blood flow in the affected area. Mildly affected dogs may lead fairly long lives, whereas severely affected animals develop CHF or may die suddenly of ventricular arrhythmias (Tilley and Smith 2000).

Surgical correction requiring open heart surgery and cardiac bypass is usually not an option and carries a poor prognosis. Dilation of the stenotic area can be accomplished with varying degrees of success via cardiac catheterization and balloon valvuloplasty.

Medical management of patients with aortic stenosis most often begins with the administration of beta blockers in order to limit myocardial oxygen consumption and prevent tachycardia and ventricular arrhythmias. However, as heart failure ensues, increased heart rate is necessary for maintaining cardiac output and beta blockers become counterproductive.

As the heart walls thicken and the muscle becomes less compliant, cardiac output is dependent on adequate filling pressure. Thus, diuretics and venodilators must be used with caution. ACE inhibitors, calcium channel blockers, or other arteriolar dilators may also negatively affect the ability of the heart to produce adequate cardiac output due to a decrease in preload. Positive inotropes may exacerbate outflow obstruction and ventricular arrhythmias (Tilley and Smith 2000).

In a patient with aortic stenosis an increase in heart rate should be avoided. Opioids and benzodiazepines are appropriate choices for a premedication and induction. Etomidate can be titrated to effect once sedation has been achieved, and isoflurane or sevoflurane may follow. Using a fentanyl/midazolam CRI is wise to diminish inhalant levels. Lidocaine should be readily available and a lidocaine CRI calculated (50 mcg/kg/min) because VPCs would not be unexpected. If bradycardia warrants it, a low dose of an anticholinergic may be necessary. Both ketamine and acepromazine are not recommended.

As previously stated, pediatric patients should have blood glucose checked sequentially and be supplemented as needed.

Heartworm disease

Heartworm disease, dirofilariasis, may be evidenced by the presence of circulating microfilaria in the bloodstream. In occult infections there are only adult heartworms present. Depending on the stage of the disease, heartworm infection does not always result in or produce changes seen radiographically, on ECG or echocardiogram, or produce clinical signs. The adult heartworms can be found primarily in the right pulmonary artery but may also inhabit the right ventricle, right atrium or vena cava. Depending on worm burden, adult heartworms may cause mechanical interference with the outflow of blood from the right ventricle to the lungs (right outflow tract obstruction). Common ECG findings with an adult worm burden would be seen as an increase in the T wave of a lead II ECG due to right ventricular hypertrophy found in those patients with advanced disease. In those heartworm-positive patients requiring anesthesia, it would be best to consider protocols consistent with a right-sided heart-compromised patient.

Premedication for patients with heartworm disease may or may not include an anticholinergic, depending on the patient's heart rate, and dose of opioid. Maintaining a normal resting heart rate is ideal. An opioid such as oxymorphone or hydromorphone may be used, or butorphanol may be considered if the patient is brachycephalic.

Intravenous induction agents may include an opioid of choice, followed by a benzodiazepine. Propofol may be slowly titrated to effect if needed. Ketamine should be avoided because it increases sympathetic tone and causes an increase in heart rate. Alpha-2 agonists should also be avoided. (See Tables 20.2 and 20.3 for a summary of cardiac diseases and the effects of anesthetic agents.)

Perianesthetic arrhythmias

Encountering arrhythmias in those patients with existing cardiac disease should not be unexpected, depending on the nature of the disease. Those patients with conditions causing atrial enlargement are predisposed to the development of supraventricular arrhythmias (SVT), atrial premature contractions (APCs), atrial fibrillation, or atrial flutter. Those with ventricular enlargement may be predisposed to ventricular premature contractions (VPCs), ventricular tachyarrhythmia, or ventricular fibrillation. Indeed, the act of providing anesthesia may predispose patients with normal myocardial function to show arrhythmias.

Supraventricular rhythms are rapid rhythms arising from the atria or the atrioventricular junction. SVTs may be broken by the use of a vagal maneuver. Applying pressure to the eyes or carotid massage may increase vagal tone, thereby resulting in the slowing of the sinoatrial node discharge and the atrioventricular nodal conduction time. Failing response to a vagal maneuver, procainamide at 20 mg/kg may be administered over a 20-minute period or to effect. If the tachyarrhythmia persists, diltiazam at 0.125–0.35 mg/kg may be given slowly IV. Diltiazam is a calcium channel blocker and should not be considered if the patient is hypotensive or has sick sinus syndrome. Adverse side effects may be seen as bradycardia, hypotension, or heart block. Esmolol, an ultra–short-acting beta blocker, may also be used should rhythm conversion fail with previous treatments. This requires a loading dose of 200–500 mcg/kg IV to be given over a 60-second period, followed by a CRI of 25–200 mcg/kg/minute. If esmolol administration precedes diltiazem therapy, a 30-minute wait is recommended. Transient hypotension and bradycardia may be seen with esmolol administration. These doses and those in the remainder of the chapter are those used at Texas A&M, Section of Cardiology.

Ventricular premature contractions (VPCs) may be the result of poorly managed pain, electrolyte abnormalities, hypoxemia, hypercarbia, and underlying organic dysfunction. The key is to recognize the arrhythmia, try to determine the cause, and provide an intervention for correction. Those patients exhibiting the occasional VPC, unifocal VPCs less than three in a row, should not require intervention unless they are hemodynamically unstable. If the VPCs occur more often than approximately 10 per minute, occur as a "run" of more than three in a row, are multifocal, or cause a decrease in systemic blood pressure, therapy should be instituted. A 2 mg/kg bolus of lidocaine given IV should be the first line of treatment. Lidocaine is a Class IB antiarrhythmic agent and works by inhibiting sodium channels. If the arrhythmia persists, up to four boluses, for a total dose of 8 mg/kg, may be delivered over a 15-minute time frame. If the bolus is given too rapidly, a fall in blood pressure

Table 20.2. Cardiac diseases.

Heart Disease	Description	Sequalae and Concerns	Considerations	Cardiovascular Support
Dilated cardiomyopathy	Increased ventricular chamber size Decreased contractility	Poor cardiac output Valvular insufficiency Conduction disturbances	Maintain contractility. Maintain normal heart rate. Avoid vasoconstriction. Conservative fluid therapy; CVP monitor	Dobutamine Dopamine (low dose only)
Hypertrophic cardiomyopathy ± hyperthyroidism	Thickened ventricular walls Decreased chamber size Compromised diastolic function	Decreased chamber filling Decreases cardiac output Tachyarrhythmias Left ventricular outflow obstruction	Optimize diastolic relaxation and filling. Minimize stress. Avoid increased contractility or heart rate. Avoid ketamine if possible.	Phenylephrine
Mitral valve insufficiency	Backflow into left atrium Reduced forward flow	Enlarged left atrium Increased pulmonary pressure Valvular endocarditis	Maintain normal heart rate. Avoid vasoconstriction. Conservative fluid therapy; CVP monitor. Give prophylactic antibiotics.	Dobutamine Dopamine (low dose)
Patent ductus arteriosus	Open vessel from aorta to pulmonary artery Left to right shunt, usually Right to left shunt may occur.	Left heart enlargement Pulmonary hypertension Arrhythmias during correction procedure Hypoxemia, polycythemia if right to left shunt occurs	Avoid decreasing systemic vascular resistance. Conservative fluid therapy; CVP monitor Lidocaine for ventricular arrhythmias during PDA correction	Phenylephrine
Pulmonic stenosis	Congenital narrowing of right ventricular outflow tract	Compromised flow to pulmonary circulation Right ventricular hypertrophy Increased diastolic pressure Exercise intolerance/ syncope Ventricular arrhythmias	Maintain normal heart rate. Support right ventricular preload. Conservative fluid therapy; CVP monitor	Dobutamine Dopamine
Aortic stenosis	Congenital narrowing of left ventricular outflow tract	Compromised flow to systemic circulation Left ventricular hypertrophy Ventricular arrhythmias	Maintain normal heart rate and contractility. Avoid decrease in systemic vascular resistance.	Dopamine (low dose) Phenylephrine
Heartworm disease	Adult heartworms inhabiting the pulmonary artery, right ventricle, right atrium, or vena cava	Mechanical interference with the outflow of blood from the right ventricle to the lungs Right ventricular hypertrophy	Maintain normal heart rate.	Dopamine

Note: This table serves as a general review. Some suggested drugs may be inappropriate for particular cases, as elaborated in the body of the chapter.

Table 20.3. Anesthetic agents and their cardiovascular effects.

Drug	Cardiovascular Effects
Anticholinergics	Counteract bradycardia from drugs and other events May cause tachycardia
Opioids	Bradycardia (responsive to anticholinergics) Minimal myocardial depression
Benzodiazepines	Minimal cardiovascular effects
Phenothiazines	Vasodilation, antiarrhythmic
Alpha-2 agonists	Bradycardia Vasoconstriction; transient hypertension Decreased cardiac output; hypotension
Dissociogenics	Increase heart rate and blood pressure Increase cardiac workload Increase arrhythmogenicity
Thiobarbiturates	Myocardial depressant Increase parasympathetic and sympathetic tone; may potentiate atrial or ventricular arrhythmias
Propofol	Myocardial depression Vasodilation
Etomidate	Relatively minimal change in cardiac output, rate, blood pressure Does not sensitize heart to catecholamine-induced arrhythmias
Lidocaine	Retards cell depolarization; treatment for ventricular tachyarrhythmias
Halothane	Myocardial depression Vasodilation; hypotension Sensitizes heart to catecholamines; may potentiate arrhythmias
Isoflurane	Relatively minimal cardiac depression; cardiac output maintained Vasodilation; hypotension Does not sensitize heart to catecholamine-induced arrhythmias
Sevoflurane	Similar to isoflurane

may be seen. The onset of action is two minutes; duration is 10–20 minutes. If the arrhythmia converts to a normal sinus rhythm, a CRI may be initiated. The usual starting rate for arrhythmia control is calculated at 50 mcg/kg/minute and may be up-titrated to 100 mcg/kg/minute. If a CRI is being administered, this may be considered as an adjunctive analgesic agent. It will have a MAC-sparing effect, thus allowing the anesthetist to decrease the vaporizer setting accordingly. Procainamide, a Class IA antiarrhythmic agent, works by slowing conduction velocity and is used for the treatment of VPCs that are not controlled by lidocaine administration. Typically,

a dose calculated at 20 mg/kg is given IV over a 20-minute period or until the rhythm converts. If conversion is successful, a CRI may be delivered for further control. Long-term treatment is usually achieved by using a beta blocking agent, if indicated, once the patient has recovered from anesthesia. Blood pressure monitoring is mandatory when administering Class I antiarrhythmic drugs because they may cause a precipitous drop in systemic pressure.

Ventricular arrhythmias may also occur as escape beats, and it is critical to distinguish these from premature ventricular contractions. Although they may look identical in configuration, the distinguishing feature is heart rate. An escape rhythm is slow rather than rapid; an escape beat is preceded by a long pause during which the atria fail to depolarize. When the ventricular pacemaker takes over because cells earlier in the pathway fail to fire, these beats are physiologically life saving. Slowing conduction with lidocaine is therefore contraindicated. Instead, an anticholinergic should be administered to enhance conductivity.

Bradyarrhythmias

Bradycardia is commonly seen with the anesthetized patient. Large-breed dogs are usually considered bradycardic with rates less than 60 beats per minute and small-breed dogs with rates less than 80 bpm. A feline patient may be considered bradycardic if the heart rate is less than 100–120 bpm. Decreased heart rate may negatively impact cardiac output (stroke volume × beats per minute), thereby having a negative effect on blood pressure.

In the awake patient, bradycardias arise from electrical disruption or dysfunction, increased vagal tone due to gastrointestinal, respiratory, or neurological disease. Hyperthyroid and hypothyroid conditions, hyperkalemia, and hypothermia may be incriminated as causes of bradycardia as well. It is advisable to determine the underlying cause of the bradycardia and correct it if possible prior to administering anesthesia. If anesthesia is necessary to perform diagnostics or surgery, a rescue dose of an anticholinergic should be drawn up and available at all times.

During anesthesia, commonly the cause of bradycardia is dose-related to the anesthetic and/or analgesic agents used. If the heart rate is low with a normal sinus rhythm and it is supporting blood pressure, the anesthetist should be aware and prepared to treat, but tolerant of a slow rate. If hypotension is noted in addition to a slow rate, an anticholinergic may be indicated to increase cardiac output; this is particularly true with pediatric and juvenile patients whose blood pressure can be dependent on heart rate. The plane of anesthesia should be assessed to decide whether the inhalant setting may be lower in order to assist rate. Patient body temperature should be supported, because the body is less able to respond to anticholinergic administration if hypothermic.

Other causes of bradycardia include increased vagal tone during intubation, administration of alpha-2 agonists or opioids, and manipulation of the eyes or viscera. In addition, hypothermia and profound hypoxia may cause bradycardia.

1st degree AV block

In 1st degree atrioventricular block, there is a P wave associated with every QRS complex; however, there is a prolongation between the P and the QRS complex. Typically, no treatment is warranted.

2nd degree AV block

In 2nd degree AV block, one or more P waves are unaccompanied by QRS complexes. The atrial rate is faster than the ventricular rate. In the anesthetized patient, this may be caused by increased vagal stimulation on the part of the surgeon when manipulating the airway or viscera.

There are two types of 2nd degree block. Mobitz type I shows a progressive lapse between the P wave and QRS complex. Mobitz type II is seen as a regular P wave rate with the QRS complex periodically dropping out. Either type may respond to anticholinergic agents; however, a worsening of the block may also be seen.

Advanced 2nd degree block is diagnosed when the heart rate is greater than 40 beats per minute, but there is no relationship between the P wave and the QRS complex.

3rd degree AV block

In 3rd degree AV block, there is no association between the P waves and the QRS complexes. Frequently, this ventricular rate is based solely on escape or fusion beats and is lower than 40 beats per minute. Often, these patients present with episodes of syncope and are nonresponsive to an atropine challenge. These patients should be referred to a cardiology service for pacemaker

Table 20.4 Cardiac arrhythmias.

Type of Arryhythmia	Definition of the Arrhythmia	Possible Treatments
Supraventricular tachyarrhythmias	Rapid rhythms arising from the atria or atrioventricular junction	Vagal maneuver Procainamide Diltiazam Esmolol
Ventricular tachycardia or premature ventricular contractions	Rapid rhythm arising from the ventricles	Lidocaine Procainamide
Ventricular escape rhythm or escape beats	Rhythm arising from the ventricles after a prolonged pause	Anticholinergic
Bradyarrhythmias		
1st degree AV block	Prolongation between the P wave and the QRS complex	No treatment warranted
2nd degree AV block	One or more P waves without a QRS	Anticholinergic
3rd degree AV block	No association between the P wave and the QRS complex	Pacemaker implantation

implantation because they are at a high risk for sudden death. The ventricular escape beats should never be treated with antiarrhythmic agents because this is the only driving ventricular beat.

In sick sinus syndrome, arrhythmias seen will include sinus bradycardia, sinus arrest, alternating brady-tachycardia, and escape beats. These patients should receive a temporary or permanent pacemaker should anesthesia be indicated for diagnostics or a surgical procedure (Cornell 2007).

Atrial standstill

Atrial standstill produces no P waves, and little or no contractility of the atria is seen with echocardiography. This is nonresponsive to anticholinergic agents or exercise. (Table 20.4 summarizes cardiac arrythmias and their possible treatments.)

Conclusion

The goal of maintaining oxygen delivery to the tissues in the face of diminished cardiac function is a challenge indeed. Because there are no agents without some degree of cardiovascular impedance, understanding the disease process and pharmacology of anesthetic agents will help in choosing those that are least deleterious in a particular circumstance. Intensive monitoring is necessary in order to titrate drugs and intravenous fluids with accuracy. Attention to details such as patient temperature, hematologic values, and ventilation is essential in these critical patients.

Acknowledgment

The authors would like to thank M. Paula Larenza DVM, DECVAA, for reviewing and providing constructive criticism to improve this chapter.

References

Abbott, J. 2008. Acquired valvular disease. In Tilley, et al., Manual of Canine and Feline Cardiology, 4th ed. St. Louis: WB Saunders Company, pp.110–115.

Cole, S, Drobatz, K. 2008. Emergency management and critical care. In Manual of Canine and Feline Cardiology, 4th ed., Tilley, et al. St. Louis: WB Saunders Company, p.345.

Cornell, C. 2007. Cardiovascular emergencies. In Small Animal Emergency and Critical Care for Veterinary Technicians, edited by Battaglia, A. St. Louis: WB Saunders Company, pp.243–253.

Harvey, RC, Ettinger, SH. 2007. Cardiovascular disease. In Lumb and Jones' Veterinary Anesthesia and Analgesia, 4th ed., edited by Tranquilli, WJ, Thurmon, JC, Grimm, KA. Ames, IA: Blackwell Publishing Company.

Johnson, C. 1999. Patient monitoring. In BSAVA Manual of Small Animal Anesthesia and Analgesia, Seymour, C, Gleed, R. United Kingdom: British Small Animal Veterinary Association, pp.52–53.

Kienle, R. 2008. Feline cardiomyopathy. In Manual of Canine and Feline Cardiology, 4th ed., Tilley et al. St. Louis: WB Saunders Company, pp.151–160.

Muir, H, Skarda, JAE, Bednarski, RM. 2000. Handbook of Veterinary Anesthesia, 3rd ed. St. Louis: Mosby, pp.235–236.

Oyama, M. 2008. Canine cardiomyopathy. In Manual of Canine and Feline Cardiology, 4th ed., Tilley et al. St. Louis: WB Saunders Company, pp.139–142.

Pascoe, PJ. 2005. Anesthesia for Patients with Cardiovascular Disease. Proceedings of the Spring Meeting of the Association of Veterinary Anaesthetists. Rimini, Italy, April, 3005.

Pascoe, P, Bennett, R. 1999. Thoracic surgery. In BSAVA Manual of Small Animal Anesthesia and Analgesia, Seymour, C, Gleed, R. United Kingdom: British Small Animal Veterinary Association, pp.184–191.

Thurmon, JC, Tranquilli, WJ, Benson, GJ. 1999. Essentials of Small Animal Anesthesia and Analgesia. Baltimore: Lippincott, Williams and Wilkins.

Tilley, L, Smith, F. 2000. The 5-Minute Veterinary Consult Canine and Feline, 2nd ed. Baltimore: Lippincott, Williams and Wilkins, pp.448–449.

Tranquilli, WJ, Thurmon, JC, Grimm, KA. 2007. Blackwell's Five Minute Veterinary Consult: Canine and Feline, 4th ed., edited by Tilley, L, Smith, F. Ames, IA: Blackwell Publishing, pp.286,1156.

21

Anesthesia for Small Animal Patients with Head Trauma or Increased Intracranial Pressure

Ellen LoMastro

The incidence of veterinary patients requiring general anesthesia for cranial surgical procedures and diagnostics such as computed tomography (CT) and magnetic resonance imaging (MRI) is relatively common. When a patient presents with head trauma or suspected brain abnormalities it is important for the anesthetist to recognize the signs, understand the physiology, and proceed cautiously with an appropriate anesthetic plan (Fig. 21.1). The cranial injury may be obvious on initial physical exam, as is sometimes the case with animals that are hit by a car or have sustained bite wounds to the skull.

In some instances cranial injury or abnormality is not apparent until a thorough neurologic exam is performed.

Patients with intracranial disease may present with one or more of a variety of signs that may indicate the presence of a brain lesion (Fig. 21.2).

Signs include a history of seizures, circling, head tilt, abnormal gait, facial paralysis, head pressing, disorientation, changes in behavior or temperament, uneven pupil size, full or partial blindness, loss of hearing or sense of smell, and change in appetite. A patient who has sustained head injuries or is suspected of having a brain lesion is at risk of increased intracranial pressure as a result of hemorrhage, cerebral edema or a space-occupying lesion. Patients who exhibit more severe signs, such as a profound depression of mental status, are at greater risk for cerebral ischemia, brain herniation, and death. Understanding the autoregulation of cerebral blood flow and the changes that anesthetics produce can dramatically improve the patient's outcome.

Autoregulation, Cerebral Blood Flow, and Intracranial Pressure

The brain is contained within the skull, which is effective for protection but leaves little space for any increase in intracranial mass or intracranial pressure (ICP). Cerebral blood flow must be maintained to ensure a constant delivery of oxygen and glucose to the brain tissue. Autoregulation is a compensatory mechanism that causes cerebral blood vessels to dilate or constrict in order to maintain a relatively constant blood flow to brain tissue. Autoregulation of cerebral blood flow and intracranial pressure occurs in the normal brain when the partial pressure of carbon dioxide is maintained between 30 and 40 mm Hg, when the partial pressure of

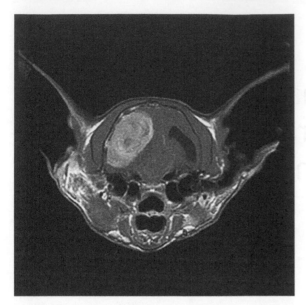

Figure 21.1. Magnetic resonance image of a canine brain with a lesion in the thalamic region of the left hemisphere.

arterial oxygen is above 50 mm Hg, and when mean arterial pressure is between 50 and 150 mm Hg (Wilson 1992). The protective action that autoregulation provides may fail in patients who develop intracranial disorders, such as an

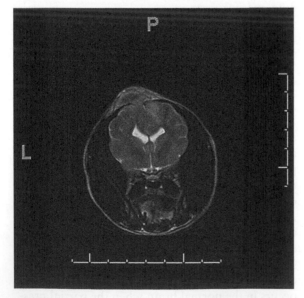

Figure 21.2. Magnetic resonance image of a bite wound on the top of the skull of a Pomeranian. Brain matter protrudes into the wound.

increase in tissue mass from a tumor, swelling, edema, hemorrhage, or obstruction of outflow and also in patients that experience hypercapnia, hypoxia, severe hypertension, or hypotension.

If the brain becomes enlarged, initially some blood and cerebrospinal fluid (CSF) escape to avoid the concurrent rise in intracranial pressure. CSF production may decrease as well, in order to maintain a normal ICP. If the pathological process continues to cause increasing pressure within the cranial vault, eventually this compensatory response will reach its limit. Cerebral swelling may lead to herniation of the brain. If cerebral perfusion pressure (CPP) falls to a point where there is no cerebral blood flow, death occurs.

CPP is defined as the difference between mean arterial pressure (MAP) and intracranial pressure (ICP):

$$CCP = MAP - ICP$$

To perfuse the brain, the mean arterial blood pressure must be greater than the intracranial pressure. As previously stated, constant cerebral blood flow is maintained when mean arterial pressure is between 50 mm Hg and 150 mm Hg. Cerebral blood flow may become blood pressure dependent in a patient with abnormal brain pathology or in a patient receiving vasodilator agents such as the inhaled halogenated agents. As arterial pressure rises, cerebral blood flow will rise, causing an increase in cerebral volume. As arterial pressure falls, cerebral blood flow will decrease, along with intracranial pressure; but this may lead to inadequate perfusion to the brain. Therefore, it is critical to maintain normal blood pressure during the anesthetic period. The use of fluid therapy and drugs that support blood pressure may be indicated.

The Cushing Reflex

Cerebral perfusion pressure declines as intracranial pressure increases. When arterial pressure is less than intracranial pressure, a reflex called the CNS ischemic response is initiated by the hypothalamus in the brain. The sympathetic nervous system causes peripheral vasoconstriction and increased cardiac output. These two effects increase arterial blood pressure, thus restoring blood flow to the brain. The increased arterial blood pressure stimulates baroreceptors in the carotid bodies, slowing the heart rate, often to the point of bradycardia. The presence of hypertension and bradycardia associated with increased intracranial pressure is referred to as the *Cushing reflex*. As the condition becomes more life threatening, decreased perfusion to the brainstem may cause respiratory abnormalities. If irregular respiration accompanies the hypertension and bradycardia, the term *Cushing's triad* applies (Bledsoe 2007).

Effects of CO_2 and O_2 on Cerebral Blood Flow

Carbon dioxide causes cerebral vasodilation. When a patient experiences hypercapnea ($PaCO_2 > 60\,mmHg$), cerebral blood flow increases along with intracranial pressure. Therefore, controlled ventilation is necessary to maintain a normal $PaCO_2$ in anesthetized patients. $PaCO_2$ can be measured through serial arterial blood gases. Additionally, the measurement of end-tidal CO_2 through capnography is extremely useful. Patients exhibiting severe signs of increased ICP should be hyperventilated to an end-tidal CO_2 of 25–$30\,mmHg$ (Wilson 1992). Controlled hyperventilation also counteracts the effects of inhalation anesthetics (at lower concentrations) on ICP and is useful for reducing brain size during neurosurgery. Excessive hyperventilation ($PaCO_2 < 25\,mmHg$) leading to low cerebral perfusion pressure can be detrimental to patient survival. In addition, positive pressure ventilation should be carefully adjusted to minimize the side effects (increased intrathoracic pressure leading to decreased cardiac output) that may lead to a low mean arterial pressure.

Low arterial oxygen tension also has a profound effect on cerebral blood flow. Hypoxia ($PaO_2 < 50\,mmHg$) increases cerebral blood flow, which in turn can cause an increase in ICP.

Other things to consider

Several other factors can cause an increase in intracranial pressure that may be detrimental to the patient. Neck leashes, application of pressure on the jugular veins, and placement of jugular catheters should be avoided (Harvey et al. 2007). Excitement, struggling, straining, or coughing may also increase intracranial pressure. Patient position is also important to consider, because the head-down position or excessive flexion and rotation will increase ICP or occlude jugular venous drainage. Patients should be placed at a slight incline (10–$20°$) with the head level slightly above the level of the heart. Excessive fluid therapy, positive pressure ventilation, and pain can also increase intracranial pressure. Seizures should be controlled because epileptic activity causes an increase in cerebral metabolism, which in turn increases blood flow, and cerebral swelling.

Effects of Anesthetic Agents on Intracranial Pressure

The anesthetic agents used in veterinary medicine today have different effects on cerebral metabolic rate, cerebral blood flow and intracranial pressure. Most injectable anesthetics cause a reduction in these parameters, with ketamine being an exception. Inhalant anesthetics increase cerebral blood flow and intracranial pressure.

Injectable Anesthetics

The direct effects of opioids on cerebral blood flow and intracranial pressure are minimal, however, respiratory depression caused by the use of opioids indirectly increase CBF and ICP by raising $PaCO_2$. In patients whose mental status or respiration is not depressed, opioids are used as a preanesthetic, alone or in combination with other drugs, for sedation, if necessary. Opioids are used for induction in combination with hypnotics and benzodiazepines. Constant rate infusions of opioids such as fentanyl and remifentanil are commonly used in neuroanesthesia. Rapid recovery and the ability to reverse these agents augment their usefulness. Pain can cause physiological changes that may lead to increased intracranial pressure. The judicious use of opioids may be indicated for neuropathological patients who are experiencing pain. In all situations it is important to avoid hypercapnia by choosing opioids that cause the least respiratory depression or by titrating doses to provide maximum pain control with minimum respiratory depression.

Barbiturates reduce cerebral blood flow by both direct cerebral vasoconstriction and indirectly by a reduction in metabolism. Thiopental potently decreases intracranial pressure and is often used in general anesthesia as an induction agent either alone or in conjunction with other agents. Large doses or prolonged use of thiopental should be used with caution in patients with increased intracranial pressure because it may lead to hypotension and prolonged recovery (Walters 1998a). Thiopental can also be used to treat seizures.

Propofol reduces cerebral blood flow, cerebral blood volume, intracranial pressure, and cerebral metabolism. Propofol is frequently used as an induction agent either alone or in conjunction with other agents. Propofol is suitable for continuous infusion and is often used, either alone or with an opioid CRI, to maintain total intravenous anesthesia and to avoid the use of inhalation agents. Propofol CRIs have been used to treat status epilepticus.

Etomidate reduces cerebral blood flow, intracranial pressure and cerebral metabolism (Bramwell et al. 2006). The benefits of using etomidate on patients with cardiovascular disease would make it an appropriate induction agent for patients with both cardiac and neurological pathologies.

Benzodiazepine tranquilizers such as diazepam and midazolam decrease cerebral blood flow and intracranial pressure (Harvey et al. 2007). Benzodiazepines, especially midazolam, are used as premeds and as induction agents. Diazepam has long been the first choice for treatment of seizures.

Phenothiazine and butyrophenone tranquilizers (e.g., acepromazine and droperidol, respectively) demonstrate no effect or decrease intracranial pressure (Greene 2002). The controversy over whether or not these agents potentiate seizure activity still compels many clinicians to avoid their use in the epileptic patient.

Studies have indicated that the alpha-2 agonists medetomidine and dexmedetomidine lower cerebral blood flow and intracranial pressure in mechanically ventilated dogs anesthetized with isoflurane (Sinclair 2003; Harvey et al. 2007). The effects that may be caused by alpha-2 agonists such as hypoventilation, bradycardia, hypertension ± hypotension, seizures, vomiting, and hyperglycemia make them a risky choice for patients with head trauma or neurological disease. They are still used for sedation and as a preanesthetic by some clinicians however. Appropriate patient selection is always indicated when using alpha-2 agonists.

Ketamine increases cerebral metabolic rate, cerebral blood flow, and intracranial pressure. It is commonly suggested that the use of ketamine, as well as other phencyclidine derivatives, be avoided in patients with head trauma or neurological disease. If there is a compelling reason to use ketamine as part of an anesthetic protocol, hyperventilation and the inclusion of thiopental or propofol and benzodiazepines should be considered prior to the use of ketamine to reduce the effects on CMR, CBF, and ICP.

Lidocaine decreases cerebral metabolism and reduces cerebral blood flow and cerebral blood volume. Endotracheal intubation can cause a rise in intracranial pressure. An intravenous bolus of lidocaine has often been given before intubation and at extubation to reduce the urge to cough (Wilson 1992).

A more recent study in dogs anesthetized with propofol concluded that the use of 1 mg/kg of lidocaine administered intravenously before intubation to attenuate cough was not supported (Jolliffe et al. 2007).

Neuromuscular blocking drugs are occasionally included in anesthetic protocols for patients with neurologic disease. Most neuromuscular blocking agents have no effect on intracranial pressure. Vecuronium and cisatracurium are preferred because they provide cardiovascular stability. Pancuronium may cause histamine release, which may lead to cerebral vasodilation. Succinylcholine has been reported to cause a direct increase in intracranial pressure; therefore, its use is generally not recommended.

Inhalant Anesthetics

Halothane reduces autoregulation, increases cerebral blood flow, and increases intracranial pressure. As the concentration of halothane increases, cerebral autoregulation is abolished. Among the inhaled anesthetics used today, halothane severely increases ICP, therefore, other choices are recommended.

Isoflurane causes a reduction in cerebral metabolic rate. Cerebral blood flow and cerebral blood volume, in the normal brain, are not affected by concentrations of less than 1.1 MAC isoflurane, and there is less impairment of autoregulation when compared to halothane. Higher concentrations of isoflurane will increase cerebral blood flow and increase intracranial pressure. In the damaged or pathological brain, small concentrations of isoflurane may result in some cerebral vasodilation and increases in intracranial pressure. Despite these side effects, isoflurane has become a useful drug for neuroanesthesia because of its ability to reduce cerebral metabolic rate and to cause less vasodilation than other inhalants (Walters 1998b).

Sevoflurane and desflurane have similar properties to isoflurane on the brain, cerebral blood flow, cerebral blood volume, and intracranial pressure. Rapid recovery may be a compelling reason to use either of these inhalation agents; however, the expense may be prohibitive.

Nitrous oxide causes the most dramatic increase in cerebral blood flow and intracranial pressure of all the inhaled anesthetics. The combined use of nitrous oxide and a volatile anesthetic gas can produce even greater increases in CBF and ICP. Additionally, the risk of expansion of air emboli and pneumocephalus in craniotomies indicates that nitrous oxide is contraindicated for intracranial surgery and for patients

with increased intracranial pressure (Harvey et al. 2007).

The use of inhalant anesthetics in patients with head trauma or brain pathologies remains controversial; however, low concentrations of inhalant anesthetics (less than 1 MAC), combined with controlled ventilation, are used by many clinicians.

Anesthetic Management

The patient should be assessed as to cardiovascular, respiratory, and neurologic status, and laboratory results reviewed. Correct the patient's fluid, electrolyte, and acid-base imbalances before anesthetizing. Intravenous fluids such as isotonic crystalloids, colloids, hypertonic saline, and blood products may be used to achieve normovolemia. Once fluid deficits are replaced, the patient should receive a maintenance rate of an isotonic crystalloid. Measure urine output and other ongoing losses, such as blood loss, and replace with the appropriate intravenous fluid. Glucose-containing crystalloid solutions are contraindicated because studies suggest that cerebral ischemia may worsen with hyperglycemia (Cornick 1992). Diuretic administration can be useful before, during, or after the procedure if increased intracranial pressure is suspected. Furosemide lowers intracranial pressure when used alone or with mannitol. Mannitol is effective in reducing brain edema and intracranial pressure. Do not use diuretic therapy on hypovolemic patients or on patients in shock. The administration of glucocorticoids, such as dexamethasone and methylprednisolone, in patients with brain pathology is common, yet remains controversial.

Anesthetic protocol selection is dependent on the patient's physiological status. While there is no ideal anesthetic agent or protocol for patients with intracranial trauma or disease, choose the most appropriate agents tailored to the patient's specific needs. Preoxygenate the patient before induction.

The following are examples of balanced anesthetic protocols:

Induction:

Fentanyl (5 µg/kg) IV **or** hydromorphone (0.1 to 0.2 mg/kg) IV **or** oxymorphone (0.1 to 0.2 mg/kg) IV

AND

Midazolam (0.2 mg/kg) IV **or** diazepam (0.2 mg/kg) IV

AND

Thiopental (2 to 6 mg/kg) IV **or** propofol (1 to 2 mg/kg) IV **or** etomidate (1 to 2 mg/kg) IV. In addition, you may decide to administer lidocaine (1 mg/kg for cats and 2 mg/kg for dogs) at induction. A rapid, stress-free induction and smooth intubation followed by immediate hyperventilation with 100% oxygen should reduce the risk of increased intracranial pressure caused directly or indirectly by the anesthetics.

Maintenance:

(You may use one or more of the following as the situation or procedure indicates.)

Fentanyl CRI (0.7 to 1 µg/kg/min) **or**

Remifentanil CRI (0.3 to 0.7 µg/kg/min)

AND/OR

Propofol CRI (0.1 to 0.2 mg/kg/min)

AND/OR

Isoflurane (<1 MAC) **or** sevoflurane (<1 MAC)

Anticholinergics such as atropine and gylcopyrrolate may be used as needed.

Monitoring patients with neurological disease ideally includes all of the following:

- ECG
- Blood pressure measurement
- End-tidal CO_2 measurement
- Agent monitoring
- Pulse oximetry
- Temperature monitoring

An arterial line should be placed to measure arterial blood gases. The first arterial blood gas should be measured 20 to 30 minutes after hyperventilation begins and then every 30 minutes thereafter to most accurately assess patient's ventilatory status. Intraoperative laboratory analysis of sodium, potassium, chloride, and glucose is recommended. Correct electrolyte imbalances and treat hypoglycemia as necessary.

Avoid extremes in patient's body temperature by providing support to maintain normothermia. Proper positioning is critical for any kind of procedure performed on patients with neuropathology. The head should be slightly elevated above the heart level, and compression of the jugular veins should be avoided as to not impair venous return.

Mean arterial blood pressure of 80 to 100 mm Hg is desirable during anesthetic maintenance. Hypotension may result from hypovolemia, vasodilation, decreased myocardial contractility or bradycardia. Depending on the cause, hypotension may be treated with a modest fluid bolus (6 to 8 mL/kg), by decreasing anesthetic depth, by administering vasopressors, inotropic agents or anticholinergics.

Recovery from Anesthesia

Recovery from anesthesia is a critical time that should be carefully executed. After the anesthetic agents have been discontinued, gradually decrease ventilation by reducing the rate or tidal volume to allow CO_2 to increase to encourage spontaneous ventilation. If opioids were used in the anesthetic protocol, naloxone may be given in small boluses to reverse the respiratory effects. Avoid coughing and excitement during extubation. A well-controlled emergence and recovery in the postanesthetic period is optimal.

References

Bledsoe, BE. 2007. Understanding the Cushing Reflex. Street Medicine Society, pp.1–2.

Bramwell, KJ, Haizlip, J, Pribble, C, VanDerHaden, TC, Witt, M. 2006. The effect of etomidate on intracranial pressure and systemic blood pressure in pediatric patients with severe traumatic brain injury. Pediatric Emergency Care, p.1.

Cornick, JL. 1992. Anesthetic management of patients with neurologic abnormalities. Compendium 14, No.2, pp.163–168.

Greene, SA. 2002. Anesthesia for the patient with neurologic disease. In Veterinary Anesthesia and Pain Management Secrets, edited by Seymour C, Gleed, R. Philadelphia: Hanley & Belfus, Inc.

Harvey, RC, Greene, SA, Thomas, WB. 2007. Neurological disease. In Lumb & Jones' Veterinary Anesthesia and Analgesia, edited by Tranquilli, W, Thurmon, JC, Grimm, KA. Ames, IA: Blackwell Publishing.

Jolliffe, CT, Leece, EA, Adams, V, Marlin, DJ. 2007. Effect of intravenous lidocaine on heart rate, systolic arterial blood pressure and cough responses to endotracheal intubation in propofol-anaesthetized dogs. Vet Anesth Analg 34(5):322–30.

Sinclair, MD. 2003. A review of the physiological effects of α2-agonists related to the clinical use of medetomidine in small animal practice. Canadian Veterinary Journal, p.1.

Walters, FJM. 1998a. Intracranial Pressure and Cerebral Blood Flow, Update in Anaesthesia, Issue 8, pp.1–4.

Walters, FJM. 1998b. Neuropharmacology—Intracranial Pressure and Cerebral Blood Flow, Update in Anaesthesia, Issue 9, pp.1–5.

Wilson, D. 1992. Anesthesia for patients with head trauma. In The Veterinary Clinics Of North America Small Animal Practice, edited by Haskins S, Klide, A. Philadelphia: WB Saunders Company.

Anesthesia for Thoracotomies and Respiratory-Challenged Patients

22

Susan Bryant

Patients with respiratory compromise include those with a reduced ability to ventilate adequately due to upper airway disease, patients admitted with trauma that affects their ability to ventilate effectively, and those presented with primary lung diseases that have difficulty oxygenating adequately. Some patients may be battling more than one of these problems. Patients unable to ventilate and oxygenate themselves adequately represent one of the most challenging anesthetic patients because oxygen is so vital to survival and because most anesthetics affect ventilation in some way. Some may relax the muscles used for ventilating and others can alter the body's sensitivity of the respiratory center to the effects of CO_2 (Paddleford and Greene 2007). Proper preparation and a plan for dealing with potential complications are important factors in a successful anesthetic event involving a patient with respiratory compromise.

As always, any patient requiring anesthesia should have a workup by the anesthetist prior to induction. Every effort should be made to get the patient as stable as possible before anesthetic agents are administered. Ideally, a complete physical exam including auscultation of the upper airway and lungs is indicated. The absence of lung sounds on one side or area of the thorax

can give some indication of how well the pulmonary system is working. Chest excursions and respiratory effort should be noted. Patient history, blood work (complete blood count, chemistry profile) and other indicated laboratory testing (coagulation profile?) should be completed prior to induction when possible. Chest radiographs are obviously indicated for patients with lower airway symptoms to help determine the cause of the compromise and to rule out metastasis when masses or tumors are suspected. Unfortunately, with cases of acute respiratory/airway compromise, this is not always possible. Simply restraining the patient for radiographs and changing its recumbency can be catastrophic. Patients that cannot ventilate adequately are usually extremely anxious and are working very hard to attempt to ventilate themselves. Oxygen consumption in these patients rises with the anxiety level so that pets have difficulty keeping up with their oxygen demands. These patients are often overheated and frequently near exhaustion, depending on the severity of the disease or trauma. In these patients, often the best thing to do is to induce anesthesia and capture the airway as soon as possible, or, if an upper airway obstruction is suspected, have the veterinarian perform an emergency tracheostomy. In an extreme, acute obstruction, a large-bore catheter or needle can be used to quickly puncture the trachea below the obstruction, and 100% oxygen can be provided through it while further stabilization takes place. This may be a lifesaving tactic. Further workup can follow once the patient has a patent airway, is intubated, and is stabilized. In all cases, supplemental oxygen should be supplied in some way.

Preoxygenation of any patient is never a bad idea as long as it is tolerated and doesn't add to preexisting stress levels. Some patients are extremely agitated by mask application. For these patients, the "flow by" method, using either a mask with the diaphragm removed or just the wye, can be placed near the nose/mouth to provide supplemental oxygen with minimal stress. Preoxygenation is a technique that can buy time before the onset of hypoxemia. In cases where intubation may be difficult or prolonged or if the patient may be become apneic due to induction drugs, preoxygenating increases the oxygen content within the functional residual capacity (FRC, see chapter 1) of the lungs. It takes only 90 seconds for a patient that has not been preoxygenated to become hypoxemic in the event of an airway obstruction, as compared to 3–4 minutes in a preoxygenated patient (Robertson 2002). It's a simple technique that is highly recommended.

Premedication

As mentioned previously, most anesthetic agents cause respiratory depression to some degree. The anesthetist must consider the side effects of any potential premedication drug before it is given in order to anticipate potential worsening of hypoventilation and hypoxemia. The procedure that is to be performed must also be considered. Patients in need of thoracic surgery will obviously require potent analgesics. Patients in need of further diagnostic testing, such as radiographs or ultrasound, may need only mild sedation. In all situations a balanced anesthesia approach in which several different anesthetic and analgesic drugs are used is ideal for reducing dose require-

ments and therefore the negative side effects of all drugs used.

The pure agonist opioids (oxymorphone, hydromorphone, morphine, and fentanyl) are potent analgesics but also potent respiratory depressants. Although the effects are dose-dependent, in the most critical cases where patients are having difficulty ventilating adequately, they might not be the best option for administration prior to induction. In nonpainful patients, opioids can cause vomiting. For the respiratory-challenged patient where aspiration is a big concern, this should be a consideration prior to administration. The opioid agonist-antagonist butorphanol causes minimal respiratory depression and good sedation, but it will not provide adequate analgesia for thoracic surgery. If it is used as part of a premedication protocol, larger doses of an agonist opioid analgesic may be needed intraoperatively to override the butorphanol's antagonist effects. In emergency cases, if IV catheterization is possible without causing undo stress and anxiety, it may be possible, and necessary, to administer analgesics after induction and intubation. The opioid drugs however, particularly fentanyl, are ideal for use as low-dose constant-rate infusions intraoperatively to provide analgesia (following a loading dose) and to help reduce inhalant requirements during surgery.

If the patient is critical but stable and ventilating adequately, a neuroleptanalgesic technique can be used for premedication. Usually, this entails using a benzodiazepine such as diazepam or midazolam, along with an opioid. This combination can be given IM or, if the patient has an IV catheter already in place, the two drugs can be titrated separately, IV, to effect. Benzodiazepines have minimal effects on the respiratory system at therapeutic doses and so are considered good choices for use in respiratory-compromised patients. When used alone in otherwise healthy dogs, excitement can be seen. For that reason, in the healthy dogs, it is best to titrate in a bit of the opioid dose first, flush it in, and then administer the benzodiazepine. Some anesthetists feel that titrating in the opioid dose to effect rather than giving the full dose IV makes dogs more prone to vomiting after administration. Although this has not been proven, the anesthetist must follow hospital protocol. In general, patients that are already painful are less likely to vomit after opioid administration. In critical patients and those exhausted from the work of trying to maintain ventilation, titrating to effect makes sense because much lower doses of each drug may be needed to reach the desired effect. Many of the critical patients can be intubated with a neuroleptanalgesic technique, eliminating the need for an induction agent. Usually for this to occur, a quiet, darkened room is necessary. In case quick intubation is not possible with the neurolept technique, a dose of induction agent should be drawn up and available for rapid rescue. Any leftover opioid drug may be taken into the OR for "top-ups" as needed. Be sure to note how much of the drawn-up drug was used preoperatively so that anesthesia records are accurately filled out.

Acepromazine is the most commonly used phenothiazine tranquilizer used in veterinary medicine. It has minimal effects on ventilation, although higher doses can have depressant effects. Acepromazine can lower the respiratory rate in some patients, but minute volume usually remains unchanged because tidal volume increases (Paddleford and Greene 2007). Low doses (0.02–0.04 mg/kg) can be useful in patients that are anxious and distressed over acute respiratory dysfunction. The side effects of acepromazine include vasodilation, which can exacerbate hypotension. Acepromazine also decreases the hematocrit by 20–30% (Lemke 2007). Because of this, along with the fact that its effects are not reversible and are generally long lasting (several hours in some cases, depending on dose), it may not be the drug of choice in patients that will undergo general anesthesia and surgery right away. It can be ideal, however, in patients that are anxious about being hospitalized or those whose distress from the effort of maintaining ventilation worsens their upper airway obstruction. It can also be an ideal drug to use for postoperative anxiety in these patients. Acepromazine's peak onset of action is approximately 30 minutes.

The α_2-adrenergic agonists (xylazine, dexmedetomidine) have variable effects on the respiratory system, depending on the dose and the patient (Paddleford and Greene 2007). Some patients will have only slight respiratory depression while others show a marked effect. These drugs cause vasoconstriction and therefore can cause mucous membranes to blanch or appear bluish in color. This can be mistaken for cyanosis when in fact arterial partial pressure of oxygen is normal or near normal (Paddleford and Greene 2007). α_2-adrenergic agonists also cause a degree of hypotension and cardiovascular depression. Although the effects of these drugs can be reversed with atipamazole, they are not recommended for use in the critical patient.

The anticholinergic drugs atropine and glycopyrrolate work by blocking stimulation of the vagus nerve, reversing parasympathetic effects. These effects include bradycardia and reduced cardiac output (McKelvey and Hollingshead 2003). In patients with high existing vagal tone, such as the brachycephalic breeds, anticholinergic use as part of the premedication protocol is recommended. These drugs also decrease salivary and bronchial secretions, which can be beneficial in some patients as well. In the critical or highly stressed animal, administration of anticholinergics is contraindicated. Usually, these patients are already tachycardic or cardiovascularly compromised, and the increase in myocardial work and subsequent increase in oxygen consumption caused by anticholinergics can be detrimental.

Regardless of the premedication chosen, respiratory-compromised patients should not be left unsupervised once the drugs have been given. Premedication can cause muscle relaxation of the upper airway muscles, which can lead to worsening obstruction, or the compensatory mechanisms employed by patients with airway compromise may be obtunded requiring immediate induction and intubation. In most cases, the benefits of premedication outweigh the risks as long as careful supervision and monitoring take place.

Induction

Any induction agent that allows for rapid intubation should be used in a respiratory-

Table 22.1.   The morphine/lidocaine/ketamine (MLK) recipe used at Tufts Cummings School of Veterinary Medicine.

The MLK recipe below is for use on dogs *during anesthesia*. Infuse at 10 mL/kg/hr. DO NOT BOLUS. Use a separate catheter and bag of fluids for bolusing.

MLK	Conc mg/mL	Add to 250 mL Bag	Add to 500 mL Bag	Add to 1 L Bag	Dose Rate to Animal
Morphine	15	0.4 mL (6 mg)	0.8 mL (12 mg)	1.6 mL (24 mg)	0.24 mg/kg/hour
Lidocaine	20	3.75 mL (75 mg)	7.5 mL (150 mg)	15 mL (300 mg)	50 μg/kg/hour
Ketamine	100	0.15 mL (15 mg)	0.3 mL (30 mg)	0.6 mL (60 mg)	0.6 mg/kg/hour

Note: Dosages used at Tufts Cummings School of Veterinary Medicine (Anesthesia Section).

compromised patient. As always, the side effects of each drug need to be considered, especially in patients that are surgical candidates. Propofol induces anesthesia quickly but can cause transient apnea and hypotension following induction. If there is any indication that intubation may be difficult or prolonged it may be best to look at another induction agent. Pentothal also induces patients quickly, but may cause a brief excitement phase, and its side effects need to be considered especially in fragile patients. Ketamine/midazolam (or diazepam) may be a good choice because the ketamine can indirectly support the cardiovascular system and provide some analgesia and the midazolam provides good muscle relaxation. Etomidate may not be a good choice when quick airway control is the goal because it can also cause transient respiratory depression and apnea. Unless the patient is well sedated, or the drug is combined with a benzodiapine for induction, excitement is sometimes seen. Etomidate may be the drug of choice, however, in a fragile patient with cardiovascular compromise.

Mask or chamber inductions are very risky and poor choices for the respiratory-compromised patient.

To decrease doses of inhalant anesthetic necessary for maintenance and the hypotension associated with higher inhalant doses, a concurrent opioid CRI is recommended during surgery.

Fentanyl, remifentanil, or hydromorphone may be used. Alternatively, the MLK (morphine, lidocaine, ketamine developed by Dr. William Muir at Ohio State University) infusion may be used in dogs, although more control of opioid dosing may be desired in painful thoracotomy surgeries (Table 22.1). If that is the case, a separate opioid CRI in a syringe pump with small bolus capabilities may be a better choice.

The "LK" portion of the MLK drip may be given without the morphine. A ketamine CRI is also a good option, especially for cats, at CRI of 0.1–0.6 mg/kg/hr. Ketamine CRIs should be used as part of a multimodal analgesic approach (Table 22.2).

Ventilation

During intrathoracic surgery the negative pressure that normally exists in the thoracic cavity and is necessary for lung expansion is disrupted by surgery. Therefore, these patients need to be provided with positive pressure ventilation. This can be done manually, which can be very labor intensive for the anesthetist, or by the use of a mechanical ventilator, which is recommended. Usually normal tidal volumes of 10–15 mL/kg are acceptable unless there is significant pathology in the lung parenchema that renders it friable

Table 22.2.   Various CRI dosages.

CONSTANT RATE INFUSIONS (CRIs)				
Drug	Conc mg/mL	Units	Dose Range	Rate
Fentanyl	50	**microg**/mL	0.3–0.9	**microg**/kg/min
Hydromorphone	2	mg/mL	0.025	mg/kg/hour
Ketamine	100	mg/mL	0.1–0.6	mg/kg/hour
Lidocaine	20	mg/mL	40–80	**microg**/kg/min
Oxymorphone	1.5	mg/mL	0.3	mg/kg/hour

Note: Dosages used at Tufts Cummings School of Veterinary Medicine (Anesthesia Section).

and easily damaged. Peak inspiratory pressure (PIP) is normally limited to 15–20 cm H_2O (Muir et al. 2000). In some cases where there is significant pressure on the diaphragm from enlarged abdominal organs or in the case of a diaphragmatic hernia, higher pressures may be needed to deliver adequate tidal volumes. Respiratory rates of 8–12 breaths per minute are usually adequate. It is important to maintain adequate tidal volumes to help prevent atelectasis. The use of capnography to monitor the adequacy of ventilation is ideal. $ETCO_2$ levels should be maintained at 35–45 mm Hg.

Special Considerations

Brachycephalic breeds

The brachycephalic breeds typically have anatomical abnormalities that cause some degree of upper airway obstruction. These include hypoplastic tracheas, stenotic nares, elongated soft palates, laryngeal saccule eversion, laryngeal collapse, and very large, thick tongues (Fig. 22.1).

These abnormalities are often the reason these pets are presented to the veterinarian. They can cause snoring, respiratory stridor, exercise intol-

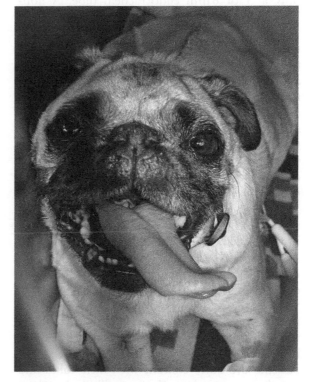

Figure 22.1.   The very large tongue of a brachycephalic dog can act as an obstruction, especially when the dog is sedated.

erance, cyanosis, and collapse (Cuvelliez and Rondenay 2002). Obesity often exacerbates these abnormalities. Surgical intervention can improve some of these conditions (soft palate reduction, everted saccules), but even after surgery these patients can be difficult and challenging anesthetic candidates (Fig. 22.2). The brachycephalic breeds have, for the most part, learned to live with their functional limitations and have found ways to compensate for their respiratory insufficiencies. They learn to maintain their own airways. Sedating these patients removes these protective mechanisms and mannerisms and so the anesthetist must take over and become the keeper of the airway. These patients should never be left alone once they are sedated. They may need assistance in positioning their heads in a way that maintains a patent airway. Bulldogs in particular have extremely small tracheas in proportion to their body size. For instance, a 35 kg bulldog may be able to take only a 5 or 6 mm endotracheal tube. A non-brachycephalic breed dog of that body weight would require twice that size. When preparing to anesthetize a brachycephalic patient, it is wise to have many different-sized endotracheal tubes available. In general, only mild sedatives are needed and should be chosen for premedication of these patients. They tend to be somewhat sensitive to the sedative effects of most drugs. Often these patients are exuberant and excitable when they are feeling well, so choosing larger doses seems necessary. Overall, it is better to dose too low and add more if needed than to overdose. Low doses of acepromazine (0.01–0.02 mg/kg) work very well in taking the edge off of healthy brachycephalics presented for routine surgery. Ace can also help ease anxiety (and therefore upper airway obstruction) without respiratory depression in postop airway surgery patients. Some of these patients may need ongoing oxygen therapy postoperatively. The brachycephalic breeds are famous for being unwilling to be extubated at the end of a procedure. Very often these patients are quite content with their tubes and may be very much awake, yet still intubated.

In general, it's best not to rush extubation. Be prepared to reintubate in recovery if an upper airway obstruction occurs after extubation. These patients should be monitored long after extubation because reobstruction can occur. The oral cavity should be cleared of blood and debris after airway surgery and prior to extubation to

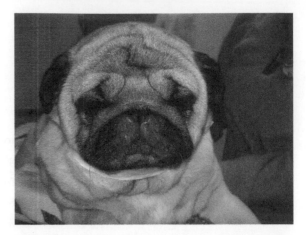

Figure 22.2. Severely brachycephalic pug puppy. Breeders charge more for puppies with more wrinkles. The owners chose not to pursue any corrective procedures because of this fact.

eliminate the possibility of aspiration. If opioids are indicated postoperatively, doses should be titrated to effect and lower dose ranges used. For airway surgeries, the partial agonist, buprenorphine often provides adequate analgesia with minimal respiratory depression.

Intrathoracic Surgery (Thoracotomy)

Depending on the lesion or reason for the thoracotomy, these cases can be especially challenging. Some of the potential reasons for a thoracotomy include diaphragmatic hernia, cardiac surgery (heart-based tumor, pericardial window), space-occupying lesions in the thorax, impalement, lung lobe torsion, spontaneous pneumothorax, chylothorax, or any condition that restricts chest wall excursions. These lesions are referred to as "extrapulmonary lesions" because they affect lung expansion. Other lesions involving the pulmonary system, such as pneumonia, pulmonary edema, atelectasis, and interstitial disease affect perfusion and diffusion at the site of oxygen and CO_2 transfer in the lungs. These are called "intrapulmonary lesions," and most are not the primary reason for surgery (Paddleford and Greene 2007). These intrapulmonary conditions should be stabilized prior to surgery when possible. In any case, thoracotomy patients are considered critical patients, and the presurgical prep should include placement of at least two large-bore IV catheters for the administration of maintenance fluids, rapid fluid administration in cases with moderate to severe blood loss, constant rate infusions, drug administration, and possible transfusions if indicated. Depending on the nature of the surgery (cardiac surgery, mass removal, impalement), it may be wise to make sure the patient is blood-typed prior to surgery and that blood/plasma is available. Ideally, these patients will have an arterial catheter placed during prep to allow for blood gas and direct blood pressure monitoring. Pulse oximetry monitoring is instrumental in these patients for quick detection of desaturation. Monitoring of the electrocardiogram for potential arrhythmias is also highly recommended. Manipulation of the heart during thoracotomy surgery usually results in at least a few ventricular premature contractions (VPCs). Aggressive manipulation of the heart during surgery may cause runs of VPCs or worse. The negative effects of the manipulation and/or arrhythmia on cardiovascular stability (including effects on blood pressure) should be communicated to the surgeon. Usually, simply stopping the manipulation treats the arrhythmia and allows hypotension to resolve. Occasional "breaks" are needed between manipulations to allow the patient to stabilize if possible. Sometimes the surgeon requires that one set of the lungs be "packed off" to prevent inflation and improve visibility and access to certain parts of the heart or thorax. This is usually accomplished by gently stuffing damp lap sponges over the lung lobes so that they can't expand. Careful monitoring of ventilator pressures, $ETCO_2$, and pulse oximetry during this time is mandatory. Blood gas analysis is ideal. Normally, patients do fine with one lung ventilation. The advantage of having the chest open is that either the anesthetist or the surgeon can see how well the other lung is inflating and whether adequate pressures are being used. Atelectasis can be visible and an indicator that higher tidal volumes are needed. When it becomes time to release the packed-off lung, be aware that

increasing peak inspiratory pressures in an attempt to "blow open" the deflated lung usually backfires. In most instances, applying excessive pressure (by increasing tidal volume) results in volutrauma (damage) to the functioning lung lobes long before atelectasis in the packed-off lung is reversed. The healthy packed-off lung will reinflate with time. It is best not to force it.

Desaturation

Assume that the patient will desaturate at some point during the procedure, so a plan for dealing with it should exist. Desaturation can occur at any time with a respiratory-compromised patient. It often seems to occur just after induction during the surgical prep. If it is a case of pneumo/chylo/hemothorax, a thoracocentesis or aspiration of existing chest tubes usually helps saturation return to acceptable levels. If possible, the affected side of the chest should be put down. This is not always practical, though, especially in the case of a lateral thoracotomy. Ideally, respiratory-compromised patients should be placed in sternal recumbency, but this is also not practical for surgery. Very often, especially in severe cases of diaphragmatic hernia (DH), turning a patient onto its back for surgical prep can have catastrophic results. In the case of a DH, some of the abdominal organs can push into the thoracic cavity, leaving no room at all for lung expansion. Patients can actually arrest when they are flipped into dorsal recumbency. If at all possible, prep these patients "side to side" and build an incline on the surgery table so that the head remains higher than the tail; in cases of severe DH it is advantageous to attempt to gently "shake" the abdominal organs out of the chest cavity. This is done, either before or immediately after induction and intubation, by setting the patient on its haunches and literally shaking the upper body in an effort to have gravity help remove the abdominal organs from the chest cavity. This obviously needs to be done gently, depending more on gravity than motion, because organs can be injured as they move through the vent in the diaphragm.

Flushing the thoracic cavity with saline prior to closing or while searching for a spontaneous pneumothorax will cause the patient to desaturate. Fluid in the chest cavity, whether it is supplied by the surgeon or the patient (as in pneumonia, hemothorax), disrupts perfusion and oxygen delivery. Usually, suctioning the cavity quickly restores saturation. Communication with the surgeon about the status of the patient throughout surgery is imperative to a positive outcome.

The use of positive end expiratory pressure (PEEP) can be extremely helpful in treating desaturation during surgery. PEEP can be applied manually or with PEEP valves, which are commercially available in various sizes. To apply PEEP manually the patient must be removed from the ventilator and hand-bagged. At the end of expiration, the bag remains squeezed so that 5–10 cm H_2O pressure is shown on the pressure manometer and remains in the airways as the next breath is initiated. This can help reopen small airways and prevent atelectasis. Flow rates may need to be adjusted and some gas released through the APL valve periodically so that pressures do not continue to rise in the system. Some amount of PEEP can be applied by using very high oxygen flow rates as well. High oxygen flow rates will exacerbate hypothermia and dry out airways. PEEP, although useful, adds pressure to the thoracic cavity, which can impede venous return to the heart, especially in hypovolemic patients. Judicious cardiovascular monitoring is warranted during the use of PEEP.

Recovery and Postop Analgesia

Often, recovery is the most difficult period to manage in thoracic surgery patients. During anesthesia the patient is intubated, ventilated, and provided with 100% oxygen. All body systems are being supported under anesthesia. Attempting to wean the patient off of the ventilator and eventually off of 100% oxygen can be tricky. As the surgeon is closing, ventilator and inhalant settings can be reduced in an effort to raise CO_2 levels and stimulate the respiratory center. At this time, it may be wise to discontinue any opioid CRIs as well. A plan for postoperative analgesia should be in place. Thoracotomies are considered highly painful surgeries and analgesics are essential to promote adequate ventilation and chest excursions in the postoperative period. Patients with inadequate pain relief are at risk of hypoventilation due to small tidal volumes (breathing hurts). Respiratory depression from opioid administration is always a concern, but they should not be withheld and the drugs can be titrated to effect and antagonized if necessary. Use of opioids as a constant rate infusion postoperatively often eliminates the peaks and valleys of intermittent dosing and the side effects that go along with spiking and diminishing blood levels. The partial agonist opioid buprenorphine may cause less respiratory depression but is likely not a potent enough analgesic for immediate postop relief of thoracotomy patients. The patient may be "stepped down" to buprenorphine several days postop. For these patients, a multimodal approach to pain relief is often the best option. Patients may benefit from an epidural of preservative-free morphine (Duramorph at 0.1 mg/kg) at the lumbosacral space prior to surgery. This provides good pain relief with fewer systemic side effects. Local analgesia techniques are a great adjunct to systemic analgesics in this patient group. Local and regional analgesia allow for lower doses of the systemic analgesics to be used and therefore also decrease the side effects. Intercostal blocks can be performed prior to surgery. Patients with a chest tube should have local anesthetic infused into the tube prior to recovery and at regular intervals thereafter. Human beings report chest tubes to be extremely painful. A very effective local anesthesia technique involves the use of a wound soaker or diffusion catheter placed into the wound/incision. These catheters have a closed end with several perforations around the catheter that allow seepage of local anesthetic to diffuse into the wound bed. Use of these catheters can significantly reduce the dose of systemic analgesics needed to control pain in postop thoracotomy patients (Fig. 22.3, Table 22.3).

After weaning from the ventilator and discontinuing anesthesia, the patient will need to be

Table 22.3. Wound Soaker Protocol. Protocol Design by anesthesiologists at Tufts Cummings School of Veterinary Medicine.

SOAKER CATHETERS

What is a soaker catheter?

A soaker catheter, also called a *diffusion catheter*, works just like a soaker garden hose. The catheter is polypropylene with a sealed distal tip and many tiny perforations along the catheter length down to the distal tip that allows drug diffusion into a tissue bed. A black mark indicates the start of the perforations.

The catheters are produced with different diffusion lengths to suit different sizes of wound, e.g., 9 inch, 7.5 inch, 6 inch, and 4 inch. The proximal (exterior) end has a butterfly connection to fit a syringe or IV administration set.

What are the indications for use?

Amputations are the most common indication.

Large wounds, e.g., mass removal

Median sternotomy incisions

What about cats?

Soaker catheters are OK to use in cats but you need to be more careful with dosing. Cats metabolize the drugs more slowly and are more sensitive than dogs to the cardiotoxic and neurotoxic effects of local anesthetics. Therefore we use only the intermittent injection technique and not a constant rate infusion. A problem we've noted is that cats are more prone to pulling the catheter out, just because they are cats.

How is the catheter placed?

- We sometimes prime the catheters first with local anesthetic before inserting into the wound but this is not essential with the commercially available catheters (vol ~0.4 mL). It is *essential* to prime if using red rubber catheters to confirm that the distal end is sealed. Without a firm seal the drug will exit from the tip and not diffuse throughout the wound bed.
- Insert the catheter with the distal tip in the deepest layer of the closure and then suture in place so it can't be accidentally pulled out. It is essential that all perforations are below the skin. Place a purse string suture and Chinese finger trap to secure the catheter. After this placement do two friction sutures deeply to catch fascia plus skin. For the friction sutures place suture through skin and deep fascia and tie two throws. On the next throw create a surgeon's knot around the catheter with slight crimping and finish with three more throws. Placement of the friction sutures will keep the catheter from pulling out.
- Suture the butterfly connector to the skin. Cover with tegaderm and seal the catheter end with an injection cap. Add a clear label to the soaker catheter site to avoid confusion with an IV injection cap.
- For aggressive dogs add an extension line and secure this to the rump or other convenient place.
- If making a soaker catheter from a red rubber one allow about 10–15 minutes for completion before it is to be sutured in place.

How are the drugs calculated and administered?

Use either of two methods, periodic injection (dog or cat) or constant rate infusion (dog only).

Injection:

- Fill the catheter with local anesthetic at the end of surgery and repeat the injection every 6 hours.
  - A lidocaine/bupivacaine mixture is ideal for the first injection. Lidocaine works immediately, and bupivacaine is slower in onset but has longer duration. Subsequent injections need only be bupivacaine.
  - The maximum dose of **bupivacaine** to use is 1.5 mg/kg. For a large dog such as a German shepherd (45 kg, 100 lb) the volume would be 13.5 mL. For a medium dog such as a Border Collie (20 kg, 44 lb) the volume would be 6 mL.
  - The maximum dose to use for **lidocaine** is 2 mg/kg. For a German shepherd the volume would be 4.5 mL and for the border collie the volume would be 2 mL.
  - The bottom line is that **6–12 mL** is the ideal *total* volume to use depending on dog size. The initial injection of mixed drugs makes up half the total volume with each drug. In the case of the border collie use 2 mL lidocaine + 4 mL bupivacaine.
  - Most of our soaker catheter use is in large breeds but occasionally a really small dog may need a soaker catheter. For example, a dachshund (7 kg, 15 lb), would require volumes of 2 mL bupivacaine and 0.7 mL lidocaine. This may not be sufficient to reach the entire tissue bed so you can dilute the final mix to reach a total volume of about 4–5 mL. One percent lidocaine seems to be as effective as 2%. The limiting factor in smaller dogs is the length of catheter with perforations.
  - Use only bupivacaine for injections after the initial one because of its longer duration.
  - For cats use the same protocol as for dachshunds and limit the volume to 4 mL.
  - Always inject slowly to allow more even distribution.

Table 22.3.   *Continued*

Constant rate infusion (not for cats)
- Fill the catheter with local anesthetic and start a slow infusion for the next 24–48 hours.
    - Lidocaine is sufficient for this because of the constant infusion.
    - For infusion the *dose rate* should be **2 mg/kg/hour**, and the *flow rate* should be approximately **5 mL/hour**. This could be reduced for small dogs that have a smaller catheter in place. The flow rate is designed to provide sufficient pressure to exit the perforations without being enough to cause a seroma.
    - Calculate the *total milligrams per hour* for the dog (*kg × 2 mg*).
    - Next check which category this fits most closely from this list:
        - **Five mL/hour of straight lidocaine at 2% provides *100 mg/hour***
        - **Five mL/hour of lidocaine diluted to *1.5%* provides *75 mg/hour***
        - **Five mL/hour of lidocaine diluted to *1%* provides *50 mg/hour***
    - Choose which of these is a best fit for the dog and dilute accordingly.
        - For 1.5% solution remove 3/4 of the volume and replace with the same volume of 2% lidocaine.
        - For 1% solution remove 1/2 the volume and replace with the same volume of 2% lidocaine.
    - Example: Using a 250 mL bag of saline:
        - For 1.5% lidocaine remove 187 mL saline and replace with 187 mL of 2% lidocaine.
        - For 1% lidocaine remove 125 mL saline and replace with 125 mL of 2% lidocaine.

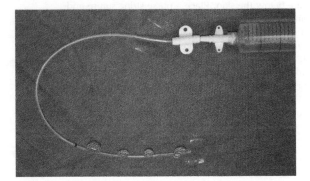

Figure 22.3.   Wound soaker or diffusion catheter showing the perforations that allow local anesthetic to diffuse into the wound or incision bed (available from Mila Int.) The black line on the catheter indicates the start of perforations and the part of the catheter that should be buried.

closely monitored to see whether it can be weaned from oxygen. The pulse oximeter should be watched, along with mucous membrane color, as an oxygen test is done. If the patient cannot tolerate being off of oxygen, desaturation will occur within about a minute. Sometimes these patients just need time to recover a bit more; sometimes they need ongoing oxygen support in the form of nasal O_2 lines or an oxygen cage. These cases often require a great deal of the anesthetist's time and patience in recovery.

Extubating these patients should be done as late as possible, unless the patient is a cat and prone to laryngospasm. Although usually rare, be prepared to reanesthetize and reintubate if needed. Having a clean ET tube, a laryngoscope, and a little induction agent nearby is good planning. Patients should be recovered in sternal position to maximize lung inflation of both lung fields. The head may be supported with a pillow or rolled towels. Once the patient is extubated, pulse oximetry monitoring should continue. Once patients are alert and moving this can be difficult, but if a toe or ear or some other remote area doesn't work, monitor by mucous membrane color, feel for air movement at the nostrils, listen for obstructive sounds, and monitor chest excursions. The experienced anesthetist will know right away whether the patient is going to tolerate being extubated and off of oxygen.

Some patients with extreme trauma, severe complications during surgery, or very radical surgeries may need to be placed on ongoing ventilator support in the ICU if they cannot be successfully weaned from the surgery ventilator.

As always, in any anesthesia case, being prepared and planning for complications can help ensure a successful anesthetic event, even in a challenging patient.

References

Cuvellier, S, Rondenay, Y. 2002. Canine breed specific problems. In Veterinary Anesthesia and Pain Management Secrets, Greene, SA. Philadelphia: Hanley & Belfus, Inc., p.235.

Lemke, K. 2007. Anticholinergics and sedatives. In Lumb and Jones' Veterinary Anesthesia and Analgesia, Ames, IA: Blackwell Publishing, p.208.

McKelvey, D, Hollingshead, KW. 2003. Small Animal Anesthesia, Canine and Feline Practice, 3rd ed. St. Louis: Mosby.

Muir, W, Hubbell, J, Skarda, R, Bednarski, R. 2000. Handbook of Veterinary Anesthesia, 3rd ed. St. Louis: Mosby, pp.236–241, 258–263, 295–296.

Paddleford, R, Greene, S. 2007. Pulmonary disease. In Lumb and Jones' Veterinary Anesthesia and Analgesia, 4th ed., edited by Tranquilli, W, Thurmon, J, Grimm, K. Ames, IA: Blackwell Publishing. 2007.

Robertson, S. 2002. Oxygenation and ventilation. In Veterinary Anesthesia and Pain Management Secrets, Greene, SA. Philadelphia: Hanley & Belfus, Inc.

Anesthesia for Patients with Endocrine Disease

Susan Holland

There are several common diseases connected to the endocrine system that will be encountered in veterinary medicine. The key to a successful anesthetic outcome is knowledge of the presenting disease as well as potential complications. Preventing or being prepared for such complications can be the difference between life and death for the patient. Some of the common endocrine diseases in veterinary medicine include diabetes mellitus, insulinoma, hyperadrenocorticism (Cushing's), hypoadrenocorticism (Addison's), hyperthyroidism, and hypothyroidism. There is no one "silver bullet" anesthesia recommendation that will work for everything. Being familiar with the anesthesia drugs and how they work is the first step toward successfully anesthetizing a patient with endocrine disease. Evaluate every patient to determine the best protocol for that individual. The goal is to return these patients to their normal routines as quickly as possible, so using drugs that are quickly eliminated or easily antagonized is the best plan of action.

Diabetes Mellitus

Diabetes is caused by a deficiency of insulin. There are two types of diabetic patients that may be presented for anesthesia: the unregulated, unstable diabetic or the regulated diabetic patient. Performing anesthesia on an unstable diabetic patient should be avoided unless the patient's life is in immediate danger. Dehydration, polyuria, polydipsia, weight loss, and muscle wasting are common symptoms that may raise a red flag while taking a thorough history. In unregulated cases, increased respirations, a sweet acetone odor to the breath, metabolic acidosis, renal failure, circulatory collapse, coma, and death may occur (Nelson 2007). Acute blindness caused by cataracts is a very common presenting sign in the diabetic dog. In diabetic cats a common presentation is a neuropathy with symptoms such as lack of coordination and rear leg weakness (Nelson 2007). A preoperative CBC, chemistry profile and urinalysis should be performed. A resting glucose of greater than 250 mg/dL with ketones present in the urine is diagnostic for diabetes. On urinalysis the presence of glucose and ketones is diagnostic. Patients should be stabilized, and ketoacidosis corrected and, ideally, regulated prior to anesthesia. For regulated diabetic patients a thorough history is still important. Ask how long the patient has been diabetic, how well it is controlled, whether there are coexisting diseases going on and whether current medications are being administered, as well as any nutritional supplements (Schaer 1995). The well-regulated patient is much easier to manage during and after an anesthetic episode. The goal in the diabetic patient is to keep the anesthesia and recovery time as short as possible so the patient may begin eating again. A common plan is to have the patient fasted overnight and have the owner give ½ dose insulin in the morning prior to arriving at the hospital. Cats that are on oral glipizide should not receive medication the morning of surgery (Schaer 1995). The surgical procedure should be scheduled first in the morning. Blood glucose levels should be monitored preoperatively, perioperatively, and postoperatively. The goal is to maintain the blood glucose level between 150–250 mg/dL. Dextrose may need to be added to IV fluids to maintain this level (Schaer 1995). Most times, 2.5 or 5% dextrose concentrations are used. Remember not to draw the blood glucose sample from the IV catheter that fluids are being administered through because this will result in abnormally high and inaccurate readings (Duncan 2003). Feeding should be resumed as soon as possible after recovery from anesthesia. Ideally, the routine insulin dosing and feeding schedule should be resumed the day after surgery. Due to increased susceptibility to infection of the diabetic patient, aseptic technique is extremely important (Schaer 1995). Clean hands, aseptic catheter placement and maintenance, sterilized endotracheal tubes, and clean and dry incisions are essential. Remember, the most common problem in diabetic dogs is cataract formation, which can lead to acute blindness. Cats are rarely affected by this ocular problem (Basher and Roberts 1995). Surgical correction gives the best prognosis for vision restoration and is a common anesthetic procedure for these patients.

Insulinoma

An insulinoma is a tumor of the pancreas that results in excess insulin production leading to hypoglycemia. Signs of hypoglycemia can include drooling, lethargy, anxiety, ataxia, vocalization, muscle tremors, coma, or seizures, which can lead to death. Insulinoma most commonly occurs in middle-aged dogs, with surgery being the treatment of choice. Like diabetic patients, close monitoring of blood glucose levels is extremely important. Preoperative workup should include CBC, serum chemistries, chest radiographs, and abdominal ultrasound if available. Fasting time should be reduced to 8 hours before surgery. If 24-hour care is available, the patient may be admitted to the hospital the night prior to surgery. An IV catheter can be placed to administer maintenance fluids with the addition of dextrose if indicated by blood glucose readings less than 70 mg/dL. Blood glucose readings can be taken every 30–60 minutes while the patient is under anesthesia. Remember not to draw blood glucose samples from the IV catheter that fluids are being administered through. If patients are on medical management such as prednisone or diazoxide, those medications may be continued until induction (Kerr 2007). The goal before, during, and after anesthesia is to maintain a normal blood glucose level. Hospitalization and surgery can lead to a couple of situations that need to be monitored. Stress, such as the stress of being hospitalized in an unfamiliar environment and being handled by strangers can increase the release of insulin leading to a hypoglycemic episode (Duncan 2003). During surgery, the handling of the tumor itself can cause massive insulin release resulting in severe hypoglycemia. It is not uncommon for patients to have pancreatitis postoperatively. Pancreatitis patients are maintained NPO; therefore, fluid therapy with the addition of dextrose can be necessary for 48–72 hours postoperatively (Kerr 2007). Pancreatitis is also reported (in humans) as being a very painful condition, so appropriate analgesics should be given. A constant rate infusion of dextrose is more effective at managing hypoglycemia than a bolus injection of dextrose. A large bolus of dextrose will temporarily correct the hypoglycemia but will then stimulate further insulin secretion leading to a rebound episode of hypoglycemia (Duncan 2003). Avoid the alpha2 agonists in these patients as well as ketamine and Telazol (Kerr 2007). Alpha-2 agents cause an increase in glucose and a decrease in insulin that can last several hours.

Hyperadrenocorticism— Cushing's Disease

Hyperadrenocorticism, also known as *Cushing's disease*, is caused by a chronic overproduction of adrenal steroids or cortisol in the body (Kintzer et al. 2000). Dogs are more commonly affected than cats (Hill 2007). When taking a history, patient symptoms may include polyuria, polydipsia, excessive bruising, panting, exercise intolerance, muscle atrophy, lethargy, weakness, and the classic potbellied appearance (Fig. 23.1).

In addition to the symptoms above, signs noted on physical examination can include thin skin, bilateral hair loss, hepatomegaly, and hypertension. Cats may present with thin, fragile skin that tears easily (Hill 2007). Cushing's patients commonly also have diabetes. Cortisol antagonizes the actions of insulin leading to a steroid-induced diabetes mellitus (Kintzer et al. 2000). The list of potential complications can be daunting, but having the knowledge of what to watch for and being prepared for potential complications will help aid in a successful anesthetic outcome. Hyperglycemia or hypoglycemia can occur with concurrent diabetes (Kerr 2007). Respiratory compromise can occur for many reasons. Hepatomegaly, or enlarged liver, takes up more space in the abdomen and can press against the diaphragm, compressing the thoracic cavity. Muscle weakness can affect the diaphragm, making ventilation more difficult for the patient. Obesity adds to the difficulties associated with both hepatomegaly and muscle weakness. Cushing's patients are also prone to thromboembolic events (Kerr 2007). The use of capnometry can assist in monitoring ventilation. Hypertension is common due to cortisol's enhancement of epinephrine's vasoconstrictive effect (Pascoe 2006). Hypertension may exacerbate an underlying or unknown cardiac condition.

Preoperative workup should include CBC, chemistry profile, and electrolytes. Clinical signs may also warrant cardiac assessment that includes chest radiographs, ECG, echocardiogram, and blood pressure. The anesthetic plan will depend on the status of the patient, includ-

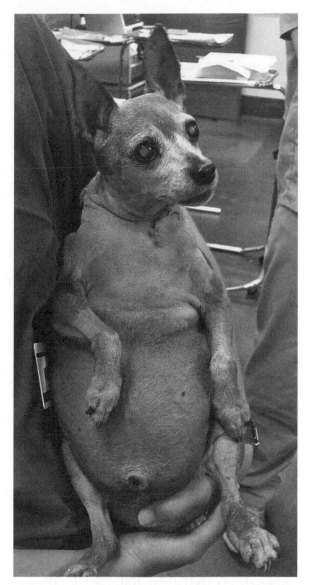

Figure 23.1. Typical potbellied appearance of a dog with Cushing's disease.

ing cardiac function as well as the planned surgical procedure. Corticosteroid supplementation for Cushing's patients during stressful situations is vitally important. Dexamethasone is commonly the steroid of choice for use immediately prior to surgery and for 24–48 hours following surgery (Kintzer et al. 2000). Because these patients have polyuria and polydipsia, water should be available until the time they receive premedication. When placing an IV catheter, care should be taken to decrease trauma as these patients bruise easily (Pascoe 2006). Aseptic technique from IV catheter placement through postoperative care is critical because patients are prone to delayed healing and infection of incisions. If a patient has cardiac compromise, avoid atropine in the preanesthetic plan as well as alpha-2 agonists. For induction, avoid ketamine as well as thiobarbiturates in cardiac patients as these drugs can increase cardiac workload. Propofol can be a good option, although it causes dose-dependent hypotension; adequate premedication drugs should accompany it to reduce the induction dose needed. Etomidate should be avoided if an ACTH test is to be run because it can invalidate the test results (Muir et al. 2000). Preoxygenation is beneficial for the obese patients with a potbellied appearance to help ventilatory compromise. Gas anesthesia should be maintained with isoflurane or sevoflurane. Halothane gas should be avoided because it is commonly associated with arrhythmias.

Hypoadrenocorticism— Addison's Disease

Hypoadrenocorticism, also known as Addison's disease, stems from a deficiency of glucocorticoid and/or mineralocorticoid secretion. The signs of this disease can be vague at first and can mimic many other more common diseases. It occurs most commonly in young to middle-aged dogs and rarely in cats (Bassett 2007). While taking a history, owners may describe waxing and waning that has occurred over weeks or months (Bassett 2007). Other symptoms include weakness, depression, dehydration, abdominal discomfort, and melena. Dogs presenting in an acute crisis are common. Life-threatening clinical signs may include weak pulses, hypothermia, hypotension, hyperkalemia, and hyperkalemia-induced bradycardia. Anesthesia should be avoided in unmanaged patients because cardiovascular collapse is possible.

Preoperative workup should include serum chemistries, blood gases, ECG, and blood pres-

sure. Be sure to correct hypovolemia and electrolyte imbalances prior to anesthesia. Steroid replacement should be started prior to induction of anesthesia and may be repeated every 2–4 hours perioperatively (Kerr 2007). For the patient that is stable on mineralocorticoid and glucocorticoid therapy, the anesthetic protocol depends on the surgical procedure to be performed. The fluid of choice for Addisonian patients is 0.9% NaCl. During anesthesia it is very important to use an ECG to monitor for arrhythmias as well as a blood pressure monitor to watch for hypotension.

Hyperthyroidism

Hyperthyroidism occurs when there is continued excessive secretion of thyroid hormones by the thyroid gland (Graham, 2007). It is a common disease in older cats, either male or female. Ninety-five percent of the time hyperthyroidism occurs in cats older than 8 years of age (Graham 2007). Most feline thyroid masses are benign, with <2% as thyroid carcinomas. On the other hand, canine hyperthyroidism occurs most often with functional thyroid carcinoma (Graham 2007). Either one gland or both glands may be affected. The cause of hyperthyroidism is unknown at this time. Symptoms can include weight loss despite an increased appetite, hyperactivity, polyuria, polydipsia, panting, vomiting, diarrhea, and lethargy. A physical exam may reveal the following: unkempt hair coat, poor body condition, palpable thyroid glands, tachycardia with a heart murmur called a "gallop rhythm," or arrhythmias. An ophthalmic exam may reveal retinal tears, retinal detachment, or tortuous retinal blood vessels. Preoperative workup should include CBC, serum chemistries, urinalysis, and T3 and T4 levels. Thyroid values are not always elevated, and a mild elevation in liver and renal values is common. Thoracic radiographs should be taken prior to surgery in cats to screen for cardiomyopathy or pleural effusion. If cardiac signs are present, a baseline preoperative ECG should be run. The most common arrhythmia is sinus tachycardia, but ventricular arrhythmias and increased QRS voltage can also be seen. Hypertension is common for hyperthyroid patients, so a baseline blood pressure reading prior to anesthesia is a good idea as well. Low stress is the key to handling hyperthyroid cats. They are in a hyperdynamic state and can often be fractious when handled. Restraint or other stressful situations can trigger a "thyroid storm," which is an intense release of thyroid hormone (Graham 2007). The catecholamines released during stress are what predispose these patients to tachycardia, dysrhythmias, hypertension, and hypoxemia due to increased oxygen demand. Respiratory distress, weakness, and cardiac arrest are possibilities. Atropine and glycopyrrolate should be avoided in the preanesthetic protocol (Panciera et al. 2000). Low doses of acepromazine are acceptable either with or without an opioid. The acepromazine will help with hypertension through vasodilation and provide sedation and possible antiarrhythmic effects. An opoid combined with the acepromazine will slow the heart rate and decrease myocardial oxygen consumption. Halothane gas should be avoided due to its tendency to increase cardiac arrhythmias. Isoflurane or sevoflurane are preferred. Perioperative intravenous fluid therapy is necessary to support blood pressure and renal function. In dogs, ECG readings are usually normal, but cats should be closely monitored for arrhythmias and treated as necessary. Postoperative feline patients should be closely monitored for hypothermia. Most times these cats are geriatric and thin. If both thyroid glands are removed, serum calcium monitoring is essential. Signs of hypocalcemia can include facial twitching, ataxia, panting, restlessness, and seizures (Duncan 2003).

Hypothyroidism

Hypothroidism is a syndrome that occurs as a result of decreased circulating serum thyroid hormone levels (Bandt 2007). It is a multisystemic disease in dogs that affects virtually all body systems resulting in a wide array of clinical signs (Panciera et al. 2000). Hypothyroidism

rarely occurs in cats. Clinical signs may occur gradually and include weight gain, obesity, exercise intolerance, lethargy, mental dullness, alopecia, excessive shedding, pyoderma, or a dry, scaly hair coat. Preanesthetic workup should include a CBC, serum chemistries, and T4. If possible, the patient should be euthyroid or adequately treated for 1–2 weeks before being anesthetized. Complications can include decreased ventilation ability, bradycardia, hypotension, and hypothermia. Many of these patients are obese and therefore will not ventilate well on their own due to abdominal and intrathoracic fat. Ventilatory support such as mechanical ventilation or "bagging" the patient may be necessary. Hypothyroid patients may become bradycardic; therefore, ECG monitoring is important to monitor heart rate and to watch for potential arrhythmias. Hypotension is another potential complication during anesthesia. Keep in mind that these patients can have a poor response to vasoconstrictors or positive inotropes (Pascoe, 2006). Temperature should be closely monitored to avoid hypothermia. Preventive steps can be taken by using a warm air blanket during and after surgery. Recovery time can be prolonged in hypothyroid patients and can be attributed to several factors. Obesity and the drug's lack of clearance from adipose tissue, along with decreased metabolism, can prolong the effects of anesthetic drugs. The choice of short-acting drugs can be beneficial or consider reducing doses of longer-acting drugs and tranquilizers.

References

Bandt, C. 2007. Hypothyroidism. In Clinical Veterinary Advisor, Dogs and Cats, edited by Cote, E. St. Louis: Mosby Elsevier.

Basher, AWP, Roberts, SW. 1995. Ocular manifestations of diabetes mellitus: Diabetic cataracts in dogs. In Veterinary Clinics of North America: Small Animal Practice. Volume 25, Number 3. Guest editors Deborah S. Greco and Mark E. Peterson. Philadelphia: WB Saunders Company.

Bassett, CLM. 2007. Hypoadrenocorticism. In Clinical Veterinary Advisor, Dogs and Cats, edited by Cote, E. St. Louis: Mosby Elsevier.

Duncan, J. 2003. Preoperative assessment and preparation of the patient. In Anesthesia for Veterinary Nursing, edited by Welsh, W. Ames, IA: Blackwell Publishing.

Graham, KL. 2007. Hyperthyroidism. In Clinical Veterinary Advisor, Dogs and Cats, edited by Cote, E. St Louis: Mosby Elsevier.

Hill, K. 2007. Hyperadrenocorticism. In Clinical Veterinary Advisor, Dogs and Cats, edited by Cote, E. St. Louis: Mosby Elsevier.

Kerr, C. 2007. Anesthetic Management of Patients with Endocrine Disease. Proceedings from ACVS Conference, 2007.

Kintzer, PP, Peterson, ME, Mullen, HS. 2000. Diseases of the adrenal gland. In Saunders Manual of Small Animal Practice, 2nd ed., edited by Birchard, SJ, Sherding, RG. Philadelphia: WB Saunders Company.

Muir, WW, Hubbell, JAE, Skarda, RT, Bednarski, RM. 2000. Handbook of Veterinary Anesthesia, 3rd ed. St. Louis: Mosby, Inc.

Nelson, R. 2007. Diabetes mellitus. In Clinical Veterinary Advisor, Dogs and Cats, edited by Cote, E. St. Louis: Mosby Elsevier.

Panciera, D, Peterson, ME, Birchard, SJ. 2000. Diseases of the thyroid gland. In Saunders Manual of Small Animal Practice, 2nd ed., edited by Birchard, SJ, Sherding, RG. Philadelphia: WB Saunders Company.

Pascoe, PJ. 2006. Fluid, Electrolyte, and Acid-Base Disorders in Small Animal Practice, 3rd ed., edited by DiBartola, SP. Philadelphia: WB Saunders Company.

Schaer, M. 1995. Surgery in the diabetic pet. In Veterinary Clinics of North America: Small Animal Practice. Volume 25, Number 3. Guest editors Deborah S. Greco and Mark E. Peterson. Philadelphia: WB Saunders Company.

Anesthesia for Patients with Renal Disease

Kristen Cooley

The kidney is a complex organ with three primary functions: filtration, reabsorption, and secretion. The kidney is part of the renal system, which filters blood by removing nitrogenous waste while preventing various solutes, proteins, and blood cells from being excreted. The renal system also maintains the appropriate balance of sodium and water; regulates acid-base balance; upholds and regulates electrolyte homeostasis, bone metabolism, and erythropoiesis; participates in controlling blood pressure and is involved in drug metabolism and excretion (Swan 1999). Understanding the kidney's intricate functions allows the anesthetist to better manage the renal patient by preserving and maintaining kidney function through recovery from anesthesia.

Anatomy

Knowledge of renal system anatomy is integral to understanding its functionality. On gross inspection, each kidney is covered with a capsule consisting of dense fibrous tissue and is surrounded by perirenal fat (in mature animals). These structures serve as shock absorption and protection. The cortex lies beneath the capsule as the outermost layer of the kidney. It consists of reddish-brown granular tissue and contains the majority of the secreting constituents of this organ (Bone 1988). Beneath the cortex lies the medulla; this layer of the kidney is made up of a number of triangular structures called *medullary pyramids*. These pyramids terminate to form the renal calyces, which collect urine before it passes into the renal pelvis on its way out of the kidney by way of the ureter (Fig. 24.1). The medullary pyramids contain nephrons; microscopic coiled tubes that make up the functional part of the kidney. Each kidney is made up of many nephrons: approximately 190,000 in cats and 430,000–580,000 in dogs (Williams 1977).

Each nephron originates with a cup-shaped structure called the *Bowman's capsule*, which surrounds the glomerulus and is designed to filter water and solutes from plasma. The Bowman's capsule continues as follows: the proximal convoluted tubule, the loop of Henle, and the distal convoluted tubule. The blood supply to the nephron begins at the renal artery and enters the hilus of the kidney. The renal artery diverges to form the afferent arterioles, which enter the

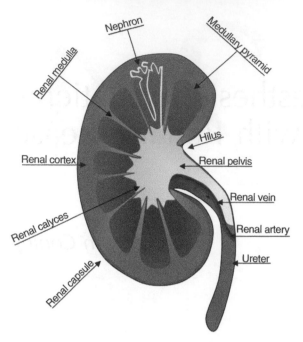

Figure 24.1. Gross anatomy of the kidney. Each kidney is covered with a dense fibrous tissue called a capsule. The cortex is the outermost layer of the kidney and contains the majority of the organ's secreting constituents. Beneath the cortex lie the medulla and the medullary pyramids, which house the nephron. The pyramids terminate to form the renal calyces, which collect urine before it passes into the renal pelvis on its way out of the kidney via the ureter (Bone 1988).

Bowman's capsule and divide to form the capillaries that make up the glomerulus. The capillaries reconvene to form the slightly larger efferent arterioles, which exit the Bowman's capsule and give rise to the vessels that surround and encircle the entire nephron. The capillaries and arterioles surrounding the nephron eventually reunite and ultimately form the renal vein upon exiting the kidney. The proximity of the vessels to the renal tubules facilitates the movement of substances between the two and leads to the formation of urine. The urine that is formed in each nephron drains down the collecting ducts or calyces and into the renal pelvis (Fig. 24.2). The movement of water takes place throughout the nephron and is dependent largely on osmotic pressure within the tubule and in the interstitial fluid. It is associated principally with the

concentration of sodium ions in the interstitial fluid.

Renal Blood Flow and Perfusion Pressure

Most renal functions take place in the nephron. The vascular tone of the afferent and efferent arterioles within each nephron contributes to renal vascular resistance and subsequent renal perfusion pressure. The kidney alters the resistance in the afferent arterioles to protect the delicate glomerular capillaries during hypertension and to conserve their functioning during hypotension. Renal blood flow and glomerular filtration rate tend to remain constant in the face of variations in mean arterial pressures between 80 and 180 mm Hg. This basic essential feature of the kidney is an intrinsic property referred to as *autoregulation*. Autoregulation allows the renal arterioles and arteries to adjust their resistance rapidly and accurately during fluctuations in arterial pressure. Maintenance of adequate systemic blood pressure is significant in any patient, especially those with renal disease, because autoregulation fails when confronted with hypo- and hypertension (Greene and Grauer 2007). Because the kidneys possess inherently unique vasculature, local tissue ischemia and hypoxia may occur regardless of normal organ blood flow. The thick ascending loop of Henle is especially vulnerable to hypoxic injury due to its high metabolic rate and active transport of electrolytes (Merin et al. 1991).

The Renin-Angiotensin System

Renal blood flow and glomerular filtration rate are controlled by a microscopic structure called the *juxtaglomerular apparatus (JGA)*. The JGA is situated where the distal convoluted tubule and the afferent arteriole come into direct contact with each other. This apparatus' function is to control renal blood flow and glomerular filtra-

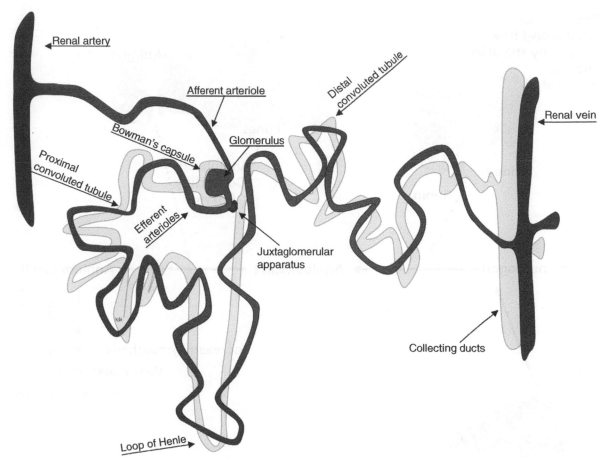

Figure 24.2. The nephron. Each nephron originates with a Bowman's capsule and continues as the proximal convoluted tubule, the loop of Henle, and the distal convoluted tubule. The distal convoluted tubule terminates into the renal calyces and renal pelvis where fluids collect and eventually flow out as urine. The blood supply to the nephron begins at the renal artery, enters the hilus of the kidney, and diverges to form the afferent arterioles. The afferent arterioles enter the Bowman's capsule and divide to form the capillaries that make up the glomerulus. The vessels then form the slightly larger efferent arterioles that exit the Bowman's capsule and become the capillaries and arterioles that surround and encircle the entire nephron. These vessels eventually reunite to ultimately form the renal vein upon exiting the kidney (Bone 1988).

tion rate through the release of renin and the initiation of the renin-angiotensin system. If renal perfusion decreases, the JGA releases the enzyme renin. Renin then splits the inactive peptide angiotensinogen to form angiotensin I. Angiotensin I has little to no biological activity, and it exits solely as a precursor for angiotensin II. Angiotensin I is converted to angiotensin II by the angiotensin converting enzyme (ACE), which is primarily found in the capillaries of the lungs, but is also present in the kidney. Angiotensin II

is a potent systemic vasoconstrictor. It increases renal vascular resistance in both the afferent and efferent arterioles, increases systemic arterial pressure, and decreases renal blood flow, and it may affect the glomerular filtration rate, depending on the physiological state of the animal (Fig. 24.3). Angiotensin II is the major bioactive product of the renin-angiotensin system (DiBartola 2006). Drugs called ACE inhibitors (enalapril, benazapril, etc.) are used to treat hypertension by decreasing the rate of angioten-

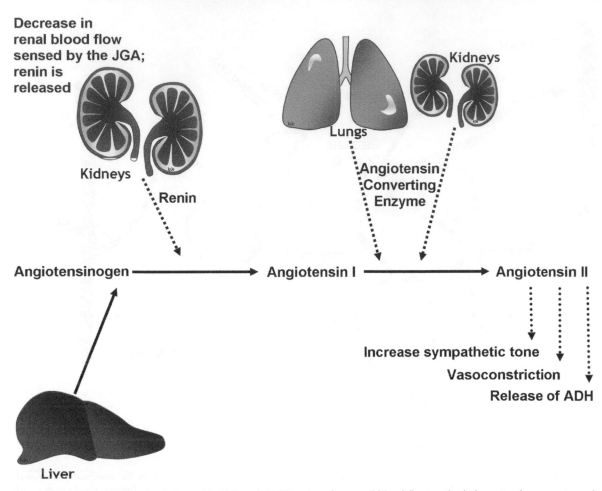

Figure 24.3. The renin-angiotensin system. When the JGA senses decreased blood flow to the kidney, it releases renin and initiates the renin-angiotensin system. Renin splits the inactive peptide angiotensinogen to form angiotensin I. Angiotensin I exists solely as a precursor to angiotensin II and is converted to angiotensin II by the angiotensin converting enzyme (ACE). Angiotensin II is a potent vasoconstrictor that acts to increase renal vascular resistance and increase systemic arterial pressure (DiBartola 2006).

sion II production through inhibition of the ACE enzyme.

Antidiuretic Hormone (ADH)

The kidney helps to maintain the volume and composition of the blood through the utilization of antidiuretic hormone (ADH). The body's water content remains very stable despite wide variations in the amount of fluids taken in and lost each day. This stability can be attributed to

ADH. ADH prevents the production of dilute urine by reducing the amount of water lost as urine and by promoting the reabsorption of water back into the circulation. In the absence of ADH the kidney's collecting ducts are virtually impermeable to water, allowing much of it to flow out as urine (no reabsorption). The release of ADH is triggered by the osmolarity of the blood. Osmolarity refers to the concentration of solutes such as nondiffusible particles, ions, or molecules that are dissolved in a solution such as blood or urine. When the osmolarity of the blood is low (containing few solutes, dilute),

ADH is suppressed and less water is reabsorbed into the blood. When osmolarity is high (containing many solutes, concentrated), ADH is stimulated and more water is reabsorbed into the blood, "diluting" out the high solute concentration. Secretion of ADH can also be stimulated by a decrease in blood pressure or blood volume. This is sensed by baro-receptors located in the heart and large arteries. Changes in blood pressure and volume are not as sensitive as changes in osmolarity. For example, the loss of 15–20% of blood volume is necessary before massive amounts of ADH are excreted.

Acid-Base Balance

The kidney is an important organ in the body's buffer system; however, it is not the most significant organ involved. In this capacity, the renal system operates at a relatively slow rate by eliciting change in blood pH over hours to days (Trim 1979). In contrast, the lungs are able to adjust blood pH in a matter of minutes, and the body's chemical buffering system takes only seconds (Moss and Glick 2005). The renal system functions to maintain acid-base balance in the body by tubular excretion of hydrogen ions and the formation of $NaPO_4$ and ammonium salts. Acids, with the exception of carbon dioxide removed via the lungs, are ultimately eliminated through the kidney by way of metabolic processes. Impaired renal function may mean impaired drug metabolism and excretion as well as acid-base disturbances, making proper drug dosing a challenge.

Tests of Renal Function

There is no single test that is an ideal way of determining renal function. A 70–75% decrease in renal function must be present before abnormalities are noticed on blood chemistry (Kellen et al. 1994). Even a mild increase in blood urea nitrogen (BUN) and serum creatinine (SCr) may indicate severe disease. It is a good rule of thumb

to thoroughly evaluate all middle-aged and older patients and those with suspected renal disease (Paddleford 1988c). Even if renal enzymes are not increased, older patients should be treated with care since there probably exists a degree of renal compromise.

On presentation, renal patients may be dehydrated, anemic, azotemic, and/or anorexic, or they might present with electrolyte abnormalities or acid-base imbalances. An evaluation of the suspected renal patient should include a comprehensive history; a thorough physical exam; a complete blood count (CBC) to assess hematocrit (kidneys produce erythropoietin, a precursor to red blood cells); and a chemistry profile (emphasizing BUN, creatinine, and electrolytes). Ideally, acid/base status, urinalysis with specific gravity, and a urine protein:creatinine ratio (a damaged glomerulus will allow more protein through) should be evaluated prior to anesthesia. Usually, trends are more useful than singular measurements. Plasma creatinine, creatinine clearance, and BUN all look at glomerular filtration rate (GFR). GFR is analogous to the assorted function of the nephrons (Kellen et al. 1994). GFR can be assessed through the use of radioisotopes and nuclear scintigraphy, but it is not readily available and can be technically challenging. In the clinic, we often rely on the results of plasma creatinine, BUN, and urinalysis when evaluating the renal patient.

BUN concentration is influenced by a number of factors. This makes it a potentially misleading test of renal function. Some factors that can elevate BUN in a patient with normal GFR include diet (high protein intake), hepatic insufficiency (decreases BUN), steroid administration, gastrointestinal hemorrhage, and intravascular fluid volume. Serum creatinine (sCr) is similar in that respect because increases in the face of a normal GFR can be seen with protein ingestion, strenuous exercise, and muscle injury.

The above-mentioned blood tests of renal function cannot distinguish between the types or causes of renal disease or determine the magnitude of azotemia (azotemia refers to increased concentration of circulating BUN, creatinine, and other nonprotein nitrogenous compounds in the blood). Renal dysfunction can be broken

Table 24.1.   Categories of azotemia.

Category	Causes	Disease/Condition
Prerenal azotemia	Caused by factors that diminish renal function— kidney is functionally normal prior to insult.	Decreased renal perfusion Heart disease Shock Dehydration Addison's disease
Primary renal azotemia	Diseases affecting the paren- chyma: cortex, medulla, nephrons, etc.	Infection Ischemia Toxins Renal obstruction Congenital abnormalities Polycystic kidney disease Neoplasia
Postrenal azotemia	Disease due to interference with excretion of urine from the kidney Kidneys may be normal initially.	Urinary obstruction Ureter, bladder, or urethral rupture

Source: Paddleford 1988.

down into three categories of azotemia prerenal, primary renal, and postrenal (Table 24.1).

Hyperkalemia is a potentially life-threatening sequela of renal failure, urethral obstruction, or acidemia. Elevated levels of circulating potassium (above 6.5 mmol/L) can lead to decreased myocardial contractility and bradycardia, and may initiate cardiac arrest. The patient with a plasma potassium concentration above 6.5 mmol/L should not be anesthetized unless other processes are concurrently threatening life and must be addressed first. Suspected hyperkalemic patients should have ECG monitoring for the presence of peaked T waves but also for bradycardia, flattening or absence of P waves, and prolongation of QT interval. If left untreated, asystole or ventricular fibrillation often ensues.

Once the physical status of the renal patient has been determined, dosage adjustments may be necessary to prevent cumulative effects of anes-

thetic drugs. Many anesthetic drugs are excreted by the kidney, making a normal GFR important when choosing an anesthetic protocol (Greene and Grauer 2007). It is essential to correct underlying metabolic disturbances and electrolyte abnormalities prior to anesthesia. For example, severe azotemia can reduce the minimal alveolar concentration (MAC) of inhalant anesthetics (Steffey and Mama 2007), hyperkalemia can initiate ventricular fibrillation, and anemia implies a decrease in the blood's oxygen-carrying capacity.

Anesthesia and the Renal Patient

Moderate to severe renal dysfunction poses an increased risk to the patient needing anesthesia. These patients are often debilitated and may present with dehydration, anemia, hypovolemia, or hyperkalemia. Azotemia increases sensitivity and decreases tolerance to all preanesthetic and anesthetic agents and can lessen the liver's ability to metabolize drugs. Animals with chronic renal failure (CRF) often present with subsequent congestive heart failure and/or a decrease in the body's ability to concentrate urine. These disease-states can cause a fluctuation in blood volume, seesawing between hypervolemia and hypovolemia. Metabolic acidosis is also seen with CRF due to the chronic retention of hydrogen ions, sulfates, and phosphates. Regardless of the anesthetic protocol used, adequate renal perfusion cannot always be predicted, and proper monitoring is vital.

Many anesthetic monitors analyze more than one body system. The most complete picture of the anesthetized patient's physiologic status is gained through the utilization of a combination of body system measurements, including cardiovascular, pulmonary, and central nervous system observation. Urinary output (normal 1–2 mL/kg/ hr in the dog) can be monitored as an indirect measure of renal blood flow (RBF). It is possible to increase renal or organ blood flow by optimizing circulating blood volume through delivery of intravenous fluids such as crystalloids and/or with positive inotropes such as dobutamine or dopamine. Fluid administration minimizes hypovolemia, hypotension, and hypoxia.

Specific Drug Classes and Their Effect on Renal Function

Anticholinergics

Anticholinergics such as atropine and glycopyrrolate do not significantly affect renal function at therapeutic doses.

Phenothiazines

Acepromazine is a widely used phenothiazine sedative. Administration of acepromazine may cause intraoperative hypotension because it decreases cardiac output, stroke volume, and mean arterial blood pressure on a dose-dependent basis. Phenothiazines produce hypotension through peripheral vasodilation. This vasodilation may actually improve renal blood flow and increase renal output with normal blood volume and blood pressure. It is also thought that GFR is maintained in dogs given acepromazine and anesthetized with isoflurane (Bostrom et al. 2003). The effects of phenothiazines may be prolonged in the azotemic patient because they are highly protein-bound, and conjugated and unconjugated metabolites are excreted in the urine.

Alpha-2 adrenergic agonists

Alpha-2 adrenergic agonists are the most widely used class of sedatives in veterinary medicine (Lemke 2007). These drugs cause dose-dependent changes in cardiovascular function. After administration, there is an initial peripheral effect that causes vasoconstriction, an increase in arterial blood pressure and a reflex bradycardia. Subsequently, central effects arise with a decrease in sympathetic tone, blood pressure, and heart rate. Despite these decreases in cardiovascular function, blood flow to the heart, brain, and kidney is maintained by way of redistribution of flow from less vital organs and tissues (Lawrence

et al. 1996). In dogs, medetomidine administered at 10–20 μg/kg IV decreases urine specific gravity and increases urine production for approximately 4 hours. Alpha-2 adrenergic agonists interfere with the action of ADH on the renal tubules and collecting ducts. This increases the production of dilute urine and promotes diuresis (Rouch et al. 1997).

Benzodiazepines

This highly protein-bound class of sedatives has minimal effect on renal function at therapeutic doses.

Opioids

The opioids are effective analgesics and are considered to be the foundation of pain management in veterinary medicine. The use of opioids during anesthesia causes minimal effects on cardiovascular function and subsequent renal blood flow at clinically appropriate doses. Morphine is eliminated via glomerular filtration, and very little of it is excreted unchanged in the urine. Persistent clinical effects and an accumulation of morphine's metabolites may be seen with administration of morphine to an animal in renal failure (Mercadante 2004). Administration of pure mu agonist opioids can cause transient oliguria through an increase in the release of ADH (Stoelting 1997). The release of ADH leads to alterations in renal tubular function and decreases urine volume. Kappa agonists have the opposite diuretic effect through the inhibition of ADH secretion.

Epidural opioid administration provides effective analgesia in a variety of cases. This route decreases the negative systemic side effects of opioids, but although controversial, urine retention following epidural administration has been reported. This may occur by way of a dose-dependent suppression of the detrusor muscle (muscle of the bladder wall) contractility as well as a decrease in the sensation of urge (Herpenger 1998). Manual expression of the bladder or urinary catheterization may be necessary until these functions return to normal.

Barbiturates

This class of drugs can have profound effects on cardiovascular function at high doses. Barbiturates decrease renal blood flow and GFR; phenobarbitol and pentobarbitol inhibit water diuresis by stimulating the release of ADH. Azotemia can cause an increase in the amount of circulating active barbiturate and a decreased amount of circulating protein-bound barbiturate.

Dissociative anesthetics

Dissociative anesthetic agents do not have a direct effect on renal function but should be given cautiously in the renal patient. The majority of the drug ketamine is metabolized by the liver in both dogs and horses, and its metabolites are excreted in the urine. In the cat, ketamine is eliminated virtually unchanged by the kidney and is contraindicated for use in cats with primary renal disease (Paddleford 1988b).

Recovery from dissociative anesthesia is achieved through rapid redistribution of the drug from the central nervous system to other tissues in the body such as the fat, lungs, liver, and kidney. Prolonged sleep times after dissociative anesthetic administration are seen in animals with renal disease and those given large doses of ketamine (Short 1987).

Propofol

Propofol administration causes a transitory decrease in renal function secondary to hypotension. The hypotension is a result of vasodilation that depresses arterial blood pressure and cardiac contractility. Quick redistribution of the drug restores these functions to preadministration levels.

Inhalant anesthetics

Commonly used inhalant anesthetics such as isoflurane and sevoflurane are not considered to be nephrotoxic. They provide mild, reversible dose-related changes in renal blood flow and GFR and a release of ADH. The decrease in renal blood flow mirrors the anesthetic-induced decreases in cardiac output commonly seen with vasodilation secondary to inhalant anesthesia (Stoelting 1999). A reduction in GFR is often seen in patients anesthetized with inhalants, leading to reduced volumes of concentrated urine being produced compared to the awake animal. A reduction in renal function is influenced by an animal's hydration level and subsequent intraoperative hemodynamics. Intravenous fluid administration will lessen or counteract anesthesia-induced reductions in renal function. Prolonged inhalant anesthesia can also cause an increase in BUN, creatinine, and phosphorus (Steffey 1993). In most cases, effects of inhalants on renal function are rapidly reversed after anesthesia.

When sevoflurane is degraded by carbon dioxide absorbants like sodalime and baralyme; a nephrotoxic breakdown product called *compound A* is produced. Compound A can cause renal injury and death in rats (Morio et al. 1992). The ultimate importance of this in veterinary patients remains to be established (Driessen et al. 2002). Until such information is available, avoid sevoflurane for prolonged anesthesia utilizing low fresh gas flow rates (promotes compound A accumulation) and in patients with known kidney disease or marginal kidney function.

Nitrous oxide

This adjunctive inhalant anesthetic potentiates the release of ADH produced by other inhalants but is not known to cause renal dysfunction.

Nonsteroidal antiinflammatory drugs

Nonsteroidal antiinflammatory drugs (NSAIDs) should not be given to patients with acute renal insufficiency, dehydration, hypotension, hepatic insufficiency, low circulating blood volume (as seen with congestive heart failure), coagulopathies, and gastric ulceration (Tables 24.2, 24.3). They should also not be used concurrently with steroids. Patient selection should be made

Table 24.2. Quick reference drug chart for the renal patient.

Class	Drugs	Effects on Renal Function	Suggestions for Use in Renal Patients
Anticholinergics	Atropine Glycopyrrolate	No significant effect at therapeutic doses	
Phenothiazines	Acepromazine Chlorpromazine	Dose-dependent hypotension May lead to reduced RBF/GFR	Decrease dose. Monitor blood pressure. IV fluids
Alpha-2 adrenergic agonists	Dexmedetomidine Medetomidine Detomidine Xylazine	↑ urine output ↓ cardiac output Maintains blood flow to main organs by redistribution	Decrease dose. Monitor blood pressure. Do not use in patients with urinary obstruction.
Benzodiazepines	Diazepam Midazolam Zolazepam	No significant effects at therapeutic doses	
Opioids	Morphine Hydromorphone Oxymorphone Fentanyl Butorphanol Buprenorphine Methadone Meperidine Codeine	Transient oliguria Buildup of metabolites with lasting clinical effects May cause urine retention with epidural administration	Morphine is contraindicated in renal failure. Catheterization or manual bladder expression may be necessary in some cases.
Barbiturates	Thiopental Phenobarbital Pentothal	Transient decrease in RBF/GFR Uremia increases sensitivity	Premedicate to decrease induction dose. Titrate to effect.
Dissociative anesthetics	Ketamine Tiletamine (Telazol®)	Majority of drug is eliminated via the kidney in cats Prolonged sleep times possible	Do not use in cats with renal dysfunction.
Intravenous anesthetics	Propofol	Transitory decrease in renal function secondary to hypotension	Use premeds/adjuncts to ↓ amount of propofol needed.
Hypnotic	Etomidate	No appreciable change in renal function	
Inhalants	Isoflurane Sevoflurane	Decrease in RBF secondary to systemic hypotension Prolonged anesthesia may increase BUN, SCr, P Reduction in renal function is influenced by hydration and intraoperative hemodynamics	IV fluids In most cases, the effects of inhalants are reversed after anesthesia. Avoid using sevoflurane for prolonged anesthesia in patients with known renal disease or marginal kidney function.
Nitrous oxide	Nitrous oxide	No known renal dysfunction May potentiate release of ADH initiated by other inhalants	
Nonsteroidal antiinflammatory drugs	Carprofen Ketoprofen Meloxicam Deracoxib Previcoxib Flunixin meglumine		Do not use in conjunction w/ steroids or in patients with acute renal insufficiency, low circulating blood volume, dehydration, coagulopathies, or hypotension.

Sources: Bostrom et al. 2003; Lemke 2007; Lawrence et al. 1996; Rouch et al. 1997; Mercadante and Arcuri 2004; Herpenger 1998; Paddleford 1988; Short 1987; Stoelting 1999; Steffey et al. 1993; Morio et al. 1992; Driessen et al. 2002; Lobetti and Joubert 2000; Lamont and Matthews 2007; Vane and Botting 1995.

Table 24.3. Nonsteroidal antiinflammatory drugs and their COX specificity.

COX-1 and COX-2 Inhibition	Mainly COX-2 Inhibition (Some COX-1)	Exclusive COX-2 (No COX-1)	COX 1,2,3
Aspirin	Meloxicam	Deramaxx	Acetomenophen
Phenylbutazone	Carprofen	Firocoxib	
Ketoprofen	Etodolac		
Flunixin meglumine			

Source: Lobetti and Joubert 2000; Lamont and Matthews 2007; Paddleford 1988.

carefully because NSAIDs may elicit potentially harmful side effects.

These drugs operate by inhibiting the cyclooxygenase (COX) enzyme, which is needed to make prostanoids. Prostanoids are necessary for the mediation of inflammation. Prostaglandins are a type of prostanoid that is derived from an essential fatty-acid called *arachadonic acid*. Prostaglandins participate in a wide range of body functions, such as the contraction and relaxation of smooth muscle, the dilation and constriction of blood vessels, control of blood pressure, and modulation of inflammation.

The prostaglandins (PG) produced by the cyclooxygenase isomers cyclooxygenase-1 (COX-1) and cyclooxygenase-2 (COX-2) are all-pervading in the body. They serve to make possible an array of physiological activities in times of health as well as in times of illness (Lamont and Matthews 2007). COX-1 generates PGs that are responsible for maintaining and defending the gastric mucosa, modulation of renal blood flow, and platelet function. COX-2 enzymes produce PGs that prevent mucosal erosions as well as promote their healing. They possess antiinflammatory effects and they play a role in protection and maturation of the kidney (Vane and Botting 1995). Some evidence also suggests that COX-2 enzymes may be involved in the hyperalgesic state sometimes seen in patients after tissue injury (Paddleford 1988a). Although their specificity is often variable, NSAIDs are frequently said to be either COX-1–specific or COX-2–specific. Those with an affinity for COX-1 inhibition may produce more toxic side effects, such as decrease renal blood flow, gastric ulcers, and reduced platelet function.

All NSAIDs have a narrow safety margin and a host of negative side effects, making accurate dosing and careful patient selection essential.

Summary

The kidney is a multifaceted organ with many essential responsibilities. It filters blood by removing waste while preserving beneficial solutes, maintains appropriate balances of sodium and water, regulates acid-base balance, plays a role in bone metabolism and erythropoiesis and helps to control blood pressure and maintain blood volume. It is important to protect this organ from insult during an anesthetic event so that it can continue to fully perform these vital tasks. Anesthesia can be challenging in the renal patient. When the kidney isn't functioning properly, accurate drug dosing can be a challenge, adequate blood pressure is a high priority, and quality patient management is imperative.

References

Bone, JF. 1988. Animal Anatomy and Physiology, 3rd ed. New Jersey: Prentice-Hall.

Bostrom, I, Nyman, G, Kampa, N, et al. 2003. Effects of acepromazine on renal function in anesthetized dogs. Am J Vet Res 64:590–598.

Dibartola, SP. 2006. Applied renal physiology. In Fluid, Electrolyte, and Acid-Base Disorders in Small Animal Practice, 3rd ed., DiBartola, SP. St. Louis: Saunders-Elsevier, pp.42–43.

Driessen, B, Zarucco, L, Steffey, EP, et al. 2002. Serum fluoride concentrations, biochemical and histopathological changes associated with prolonged sevoflurane anaesthesia in horses. J Vet Med [A];49:337–347.

Greene, SA, Grauer, GF. 2007. Renal disease. In Lumb & Jones' Veterinary Anesthesia and Analgesia, 4th ed, Tranquilli WJ, Thurmon JC, Grimm KA. Ames, IA: Blackwell Publishing, pp.915–919.

Herpenger, LJ. 1998. Postoperative urinary retention in a dog following morphine with bupivacaine epidural analgesia. Can Vet J 39(10):650–652.

Kellen, M, Aronson, S, Roizen, M, et al. 1994. Predictive and diagnostic test of renal failure: A review. Anesth Analg 78:132–134.

Lamont, LA, Matthews, KA. 2007. Opioids, Nonsteroidal anti-inflammatories, and analgesic adjuvants. In Lumb & Jones' Veterinary Anesthesia and Analgesia, 4th ed., Tranquilli, WJ, Thurmon, JC, Grimm, KA. Ames, IA: Blackwell Publishing, pp.241–272.

Lawrence, CJ, Prinzen, FW, de Lange, S. 1996. The effect of dexmedetomidine on nutrient organ flow. Anesth Analg 83:1160–1165.

Lemke, KA. 2007. Anticholinergics and Sedatives. In Lumb & Jones' Veterinary Anesthesia and Analgesia, 4th ed., Tranquilli, WJ, Thurmon, JC, Grimm, KA. Ames, IA: Blackwell Publishing, pp.203–241.

Lobetti, RG, Joubert, KE. 2000. Effect of administration of nonsteroidal anti-inflammatory drugs before surgery on renal function in clinically normal dogs. Am J Vet Res 61:1501–1507.

Mercadante, S, Arcuri, E. 2004. Opioids and renal function. J Pain 5:2–19.

Merin, RG, Bernard, JM, Doursout, MF, Cohen, M, Chelly, JE. 1991. Comparison of the effects of isoflurane and desflurane on cardiovascular dymanics and regional blood flow in the chronically instrumented dog. Anesthesiology 74:586.

Morio, M, Fujii, K, Satoh, N, et al. 1992. Reaction of sevoflurane and its degradation products with soda lime. Anesthesiology 77:1155–1164.

Moss, J, Glick, D. 2005. The autonomic nervous system. In Anesthesia, 6th ed., edited by Miller, RD. Philadelphia: Elsevier, p.617.

Paddleford, RR. 1988a. Analgesia and pain management. In Manual of Small Animal Anesthesia, 2nd ed., edited by Paddleford, RR. Philadelphia: WB Saunders.

Paddleford, RR. 1988b. Anesthetic agents. In Manual of Small Animal Anesthesia, 2nd ed., Paddleford, RR. Philadelphia: WB Saunders.

Paddleford, RR. 1988c. Anesthetic considerations in patients with preexisting problems or conditions. In Manual of Small Animal Anesthesia, 2nd ed., Paddleford, RR. Philadelphia: WB Saunders.

Rouch, AJ, Kudo, LH, Herbert, C. 1997. Dexmedetomidine inhibits osmotic water permeability in the rat cortical collecting duct. J Pharmacol Exp Ther 281:62–69.

Short, CE. Dissociative anesthesia. 1987. In Principles and Practice of Veterinary Anesthesia, edited by Short, CE. Baltimore: Williams and Wilkins, p.158.

Steffey, EP, Mama, KR. 2007. Inhalation anesthetics. In Lumb & Jones' Veterinary Anesthesia and Analgesia, 4th ed., Tranquilli, WJ, Thurmon, JC, Grimm, KA. Ames, IA: Blackwell Publishing, pp.355–395.

Steffey, EP, Giri, SN, Dunlop, CI, et al. 1993. Biochemical and haematological changes following prolonged halothane anaesthesia in horses. Res Vet Sci 55:338–345.

Stoelting, RK. 1997. Opioid agonists and antagonists. Pharmacology and Physiology in Anesthetic Practice. Philadelphia: Lippincott Williams & Wilkins.

Stoelting, RK. 1999. Inhaled anesthetics. In Pharmacology and Physiology in Anesthetic Practice, 3rd ed. Philadelphia: Lippincott-Raven, pp.36–76.

Swan, SK. 1999. Approach to the patient with renal disease. Sci Am Med 1–7.

Trim, C. 1979. Anesthesia and the kidney. Compend Contin Educ 1:843.

Vane, JR, Botting, RM. 1995. New insights into the mode of action of anti-inflammatory drug. Inflamm Res 44:1–10.

Williams, RH, et al. 1977. Autoregulation of nephron filtration rate in the dog assessed by indicator-dilution technique. Am J Physiol 233:F282.

Anesthesia for Patients with Liver Disease

Heather Carter

The liver is located under the diaphragm in the abdominal cavity. It is the largest gland in the body and performs roughly fifteen hundred functions (Pasquini 1995). These include detoxification of drugs and toxins, production and secretion of bile, synthesis of albumin and coagulation (Pasquini 1995). It also plays an important role in digestion by working to prevent changes in blood glucose. The liver's anatomy is arranged into two divisions, right and left (Evans 1993). There are some discrepancies in the divisions of the liver; however, most agree that the liver has six lobes. They are left lateral, left medial, right medial, right lateral, quadrate, and caudate lobe. The caudate lobe is further divided into the caudate process and the papillary process (Evans 1993) (Fig. 25.1).

The gallbladder is a sac that is situated under the right lobe of the liver. It is lined by liver cells, bordered by the quadrate and right medial lobe, and houses and synthesizes bile, which then drains into the bile duct (Evans 1993; Fossum and Duprey 2002).

The caudal vena cava and the portal vein are the two blood supplies present in the liver (Fossum and Duprey 2002). The portal vein brings blood to the liver from the intestines. The nutrients from the digested food pass into the portal vein directly after being absorbed into the bloodstream from the small intestines (Chabner 2004). This gives the liver the first chance to benefit from the nutrients. The portal vein provides roughly 70% of the liver's overall blood supply (Bonagura and Kirk 2000). The hepatic artery supplies 90% of the oxygen and the remainder of the blood supply. Additionally, 20% of cardiac output is continually delivered to the liver (Tranquilli et al. 2007).

An amazing aspect of the liver is its ability to regenerate (Ettinger 2000). It has a large reserve capacity meaning that up to 80% of the liver can be damaged before a patient will exhibit clinical signs or a change in lab values will be noticed (Ettinger 2000). Homeostasis can still be maintained if only 10–20% is functional (Leib and Monroe 1997).

Blood work

The serum enzymes commonly used to evaluate liver function directly are alanine amino transaminase (ALT) and alkaline phosphatase (Alk Phos) (Chabner 2004). Enzymes used to evaluate liver function indirectly are blood urea nitrogen (BUN) and cholesterol. Proteins used to evaluate

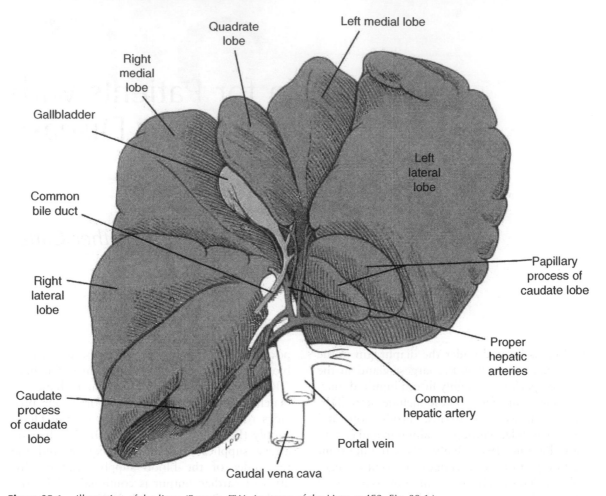

Figure 25.1.   Illustration of the liver. (Fossum, TW, Anatomy of the Liver, p.452, Fig. 22.1.)

liver function are albumin and glucose (Leib and Monroe 1997). Since hypoproteinemia and hypoalbuminemia are common findings in patients with liver disease, special attention should be paid to these test results. Low total protein and albumin can result in decreased drug binding, prolonged recoveries, and relative overdose from highly protein-bound drugs such as barbiturates (Tranquilli et al. 2007). Hypoproteinemia can also predispose patients to developing pulmonary edema and ascites. Blood glucose levels can be affected by liver disease, so monitoring pre-, peri-, and postoperatively is recommended. Appropriate dextrose-containing fluids should be given when indicated to maintain serum levels of glucose. The liver plays a huge role in the production of clotting factors

for the body. Prolonged clotting times should be diagnosed prior to surgery, and arrangements for transfusions of fresh frozen plasma, fresh plasma or whole blood should be made ahead of time. Appropriate tests evaluating liver function should be run prior to any anesthetic event (Table 25.1). Additional diagnostic testing may be indicated, including imaging of the liver through radiographs and ultrasound.

Pharmacology

The liver is important for metabolism and clearance of drugs. Proper drug choice and dosage can help prevent anesthetic complications.

Table 25.1. Blood work to consider prior to anesthesia.

CBC/Chem	Why It's Important	Normal Values	
ALT	Elevations are specific to liver disease. Possible to see no increase if hepatobiliary disease is present.	K9	0–77 IU
		Fel	0–100 IU
Alk phos	It has a short half life and increased levels are seen with cholestasis or bone lysis, or if injections of corticosteroids are present. Increased levels also seen with muscle trauma. Increased levels in cats should be taken seriously. Its half life is 6 hours; a cat's total liver content is 50% less than dogs.	K9	0–400 IU
		Fel	0–193 IU
Glucose	Decreased levels can cause seizures, lethargy, PU/PD, ataxia. Decreased levels can also be associated with portosystemic shunts. Supplement fluids with dextrose.	K9	59–121 mg/dL
		Fel	54–145 mg/dL
Cholesterol	Is required for the production of bile acids.	K9	135–281 mg/dL
		Fel	69–225 mg/dL
Bilirubin	If levels are increased, prehepatic, hepatic, and posthepatic causes should be considered. Elevated levels are indicative of certain diseases. During red blood cell metabolism, hemoglobin is phagocytized and bilirubin is produced. If plasma levels reach 1–2 mg/dL, plasma will appear icteric.	K9	0–0.7 mg/dL
		Fel	0–0.5 mg/dL
GGT	Similar to alkaline phosphatase. Important in amino acid membrane transport. If serum levels are increased, it can be due to cholestatic liver disease. Anticonvulsants and corticosteroids will also elevate GGT, but only in dogs.	K9	1 12 μ/L
		Fel	1–10 μ/L
PCV	Determines patient overall blood status. Important aspect of the CBC. Determines hydration and protein levels. Indicator of anemia.	K9	36–55%
		Fel	29–48%
BUN	Increased levels can indicate dehydration in patients with hepatobiliary disease. Decreased levels are seen with the reduction of converting of ammonia to urea.	K9	5–23 mg/dL
		Fel	14–36 mg/dL
Albumin	Produced entirely in the liver. Maintains oncotic pressure. Half life is 7–10 days, so a severe decrease doesn't correlate to acute liver disease. Decreased levels can cause pulmonary edema. If the liver is diseased, the ability to produce albumin is maintained. Production is decreased only if severe liver disease is present.	K9	2.7–3.8 g/dL
		Fel	2.9–3.9 g/dL
PT/PTT	Associated with liver disease, DIC, sensitive to vitamin K deficiency. Important test to run prior to anesthetizing a patient with neoplasias or biopsies. PT is measured in the extrinsic pathway and PTT is measured in the intrinsic pathway.	K9	12–17 sec
		Fel	15–23 sec
Bile acids	Formed in the liver and excreted in the bile. Most specific test to determine liver function. There will be no increase in bile acids in a patient with a normal liver; a normal liver can clear bile acids by "first-pass extraction."	K9	<25 mmol/L
		Fel	<15 mmol/L

Phenothiazines, benzodiazepines, and alpha-2 adrenergics should be avoided or used sparingly in patients with moderate to severe liver disease. A main concern with phenothiazine tranquilizers is the dose-dependent hypotension that is potentiated due to these drugs. Additionally phenothiazine tranquilizers (acepromazine) have been linked to thrombocytopenia (Tranquilli et al. 2007). These drugs should be avoided in the hepatic patient where clotting factors are a concern. The liver metabolizes phenothiazines (Plumb 2005).

Benzodiazepines can cause prolonged effects in patients with elevated liver enzymes. The prolonged effects are due to diminished biotransformation occurring in the liver (Tranquilli et al.

2007). Diazepam (valium) can cause profound sedation in patients with elevated liver enzymes. Lower doses of diazepam should therefore be used to achieve desired effects. Flumazenil is a reversal agent that antagonizes the effects of benzodiazepines by competitively blocking the receptors in the CNS.

Cats may be especially susceptible to the effects of benzodiazepines. There are reports of cats presenting with liver failure after the administration of oral diazepam. It was reported that these cats presented with anorexia, increased liver values, and hyperbilirubinemia (Plumb 2005).

Alpha-2 adrenergics cause rapid sedation and provide analgesia. They have profound effects on blood pressure and the cardiovascular system. The hepatic effects of alpha-2 agonists are seen more with xylazine versus medetomidine. The administration of xylazine has been shown to augment plasma glucose concentrations by decreasing insulin (Tranquilli et al. 2007). Xylazine activates the alpha-1 receptor, thus stimulating hepatic glucose production by decreasing insulin, which indirectly causes hyperglycemia (Tranquilli et al. 2007). Medetomidine is a more selective drug and has an affinity for the alpha-2 receptor, which causes it to have less hepatic effects. The advantage of these drugs is that any unwanted effects can be reversed with an alpha-2 antagonist. Xylazine is antagonized with yohimbine or tolazoline, and medetomidine is antagonized with atipamezole.

The opioids can be used in patients with hepatic disease. Ideally, doses should be titrated to effect to help control the degree of untoward side effects. Bradycardia can be treated with an anticholinergic in an effort to maintain cardiac output. Opioid-induced respiratory depression may cause reduced oxygenation of the liver and other tissues. Of the mu opioids, morphine and meperidine have been shown to cause histamine release. The release of histamine can cause hypotension, thus causing a reduction in hepatic blood flow. Similar to alpha-2 agonists, unwanted side effects of opioids can be reversed or antagonized. The reversal agent for opioids is naloxone, which can be titrated to effect so as to retain some of the analgesia and sedation provided by the opioid (Tranquilli et al. 2007).

Barbiturates are detoxified by the liver and should be avoided or used sparingly in hepatic patients. A single dose of a thiobarbiturate to facilitate intubation is not necessarily contraindicated due to redistribution. If hypoalbuminemia is present, the length of the anesthesia may be prolonged by these highly protein-bound drugs (Tranquilli et al. 2007). Maintaining a surgical plane by the redosing of barbiturates should never be done in hepatic patients.

Propofol is a nonbarbiturate emulsion, lecithin-based hypnotic that is used for inducing anesthesia and providing maintenance anesthesia as a constant rate infusion. Propofol provides a rapid induction and recovery. Its rapid recovery is due to metabolism in the liver as well as extrahepatic metabolism elsewhere in the body and possibly in the lungs and kidneys (Tranquilli et al. 2007). The metabolites are then excreted in the urine. The rate of hepatic flow is slower than the disappearance of propofol from the plasma making it an ideal drug for hepatic patients (Tranquilli et al. 2007). Cats may experience longer recovery times due to slower metabolism (Plumb 2005). Propofol does cause dose-dependent vasodilation and hypotension. Crystalloid or colloid fluid therapy should be strongly considered.

Etomidate can be a good choice for induction of anesthesia. An advantage of etomidate is that it doesn't cause a decrease in hepatic perfusion (Tranquilli et al. 2007). Metabolism of etomidate is rapid and done by the liver. The metabolism process is done by hydrolysis or glucuronidation, and the metabolites are inactive (Plumb 2005). Etomidate will suppress the adrenal gland, rendering the patient unable to mount a stress response to surgery and so it should not be used in patients with decreased adrenal gland function (Addisonian patients) (Plumb 2005). The main benefit of etomidate is that it does not negatively affect the cardiovascular system. Overall, this can help maintain perfusion to the liver.

Dissociative anesthetics can be used in the hepatic patient. This drug class includes ketamine (Ketaset) and tiletamine (Telazol). The additional component of Telazol is zolazepam, a benzodiazepine. The use of ketamine in a clinical sense has not been shown to cause hepatic dysfunction. The liver metabolizes dissociative anesthetics, which are mostly excreted by the kidneys in cats. Norketamine is a metabolite formed by the liver during metabolism in cats. It is about 1/10 as active as ketamine (Tranquilli et al. 2007).

If hepatic function is impaired, the use of Telazol could cause a longer recovery time due to the benzodiazepine component zolazepam (Tranquilli et al. 2007). As with other benzodiazepines, flumazenil can be used to antagonize any unwanted effects.

The use of inhalant anesthetics has been regarded as "the best choice for maintenance of anesthesia in patients with severe liver disease" (Tranquilli et al. 2007). One caveat is the use of halothane. Halothane will cause a reduction in blood flow to the liver. Roughly 12–20% of metabolism of halothane is done by the liver (Tranquilli et al. 2007; Plumb 2005). The common gas anesthetics used in veterinary medicine today are isoflurane and sevoflurane. Very little of either inhalant is metabolized. Inhalants cause a change in perfusion through vasodilation. Hepatic blood flow and oxygenation appear to be well maintained when inhalants are used to maintain a surgical plane of anesthesia. (Tranquilli et al. 2007).

If severe liver disease is present, the use of local anesthetics should be considered as part of a balanced anesthesia protocol. Drugs from the ester class are preferred because they are hydrolyzed in plasma (Tranquilli et al. 2007). Drugs from the amide class are metabolized in the liver. Lidocaine and bupivicaine are in the amide class, and, although very versatile, drugs are metabolized up to 90% in the liver. The toxic dose of lidocaine may be more apparent in a patient with a severely compromised liver, so doses should be monitored carefully.

Nonsteroidal antiinflammatories (NSAIDs) are a group of drugs that are widely used alone or in combination with opioids to help relieve pain. NSAIDs work by preventing the activity of COX enzymes that function in the production of prostaglandins (Tranquilli et al. 2007). The main disadvantage to NSAID therapy is the effect they can have on the kidneys and gastrointestinal tract. NSAIDs should be used judiciously in patients with hepatic dysfunction because it has been shown that all NSAIDs have the potential to cause harm to the liver (Boothe 2005). Of the six NSAIDs in use, no one drug has been shown to be less hepatotoxic over the others. Risks should be weighed. If the patient could benefit from the NSAID therapy and mild hepatic disease is present, it is possible that the patient can tolerate the drug. Frequent monitoring of liver values should be performed to detect any abnormal change (Boothe 2005).

Conditions That Affect the Liver

Portosystemic shunts are defined as "vessels that allow normal portal blood draining from the stomach, intestines, pancreas and spleen to pass directly into the systemic circulation without first passing through the liver" (Fossum and Duprey 2002). Essentially, toxins that would normally be filtered in the liver are allowed to circulate back through the body. Portosystemic shunts can be intraheptic or extrahepatic. Intrahepatic shunts are within the liver parenchyma and account for roughly 30% of all diagnosed shunts (Leib and Monroe 1997). These shunts are seen more commonly in large-breed dogs. Extrahepatic shunts, occurring outside the parenchyma, occur more commonly in smaller-breed dogs (Fig. 25.2).

The liver can atrophy due to the lack of nutrients from the pancreas and intestines. This atrophy can potentiate liver failure and hepatic encephalopathy (Leib and Monroe 1997).

Hepatic encephalopathy is the inability of the liver to metabolize any nutrients and toxins (Bonagura and Kirk 2000). Because the liver is unable to filter these toxins, they are able to circulate throughout the body and enter the central nervous system. Once the central nervous system is affected, the toxins inhibit neural function and neurotransmission (Leib and Monroe 1997). The effects of hepatic encephalopathy can be reversed; this is done surgically by fixing or attenuating the shunt that is present. Although not completely understood, the main toxin asso-

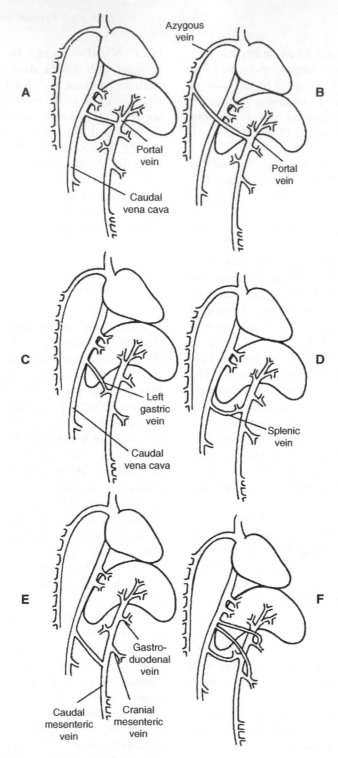

Figure 25.2. Portosystemic shunts described in dogs and cats.

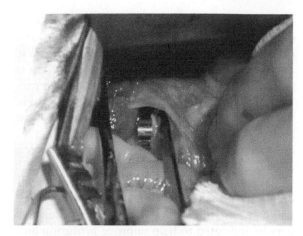

Figure 25.3. Ameroid constrictor.

ciated with hepatic encephalopathy is ammonia (Bonagura and Kirk 2000). Ammonia is produced by a protein that is broken down by the intestinal tract (Leib and Monroe 1997). Because of the shunt, ammonia—a neurotoxin—causes encephalopathy.

Attenuation is done with the use of an ameroid constrictor placed around the abnormal vessel. The ameroid constrictor is a cellophane band that slowly occludes the shunt. As the inner portion of the ameroid constrictor swells, the shunt is constricted. Shunt occlusion continues as fibrosis develops around the abnormal vessel (Fossum and Duprey 2002) (Fig. 25.3).

The animals presenting with portosystemic shunts can show signs of weakness, ataxia, stupor, head pressing, circling, pacing, blindness, dementia, and seizures (Leib and Monroe 1997). Prolonged recovery times after a previous anesthesia experience (i.e., spay or neuter) may be an indicator of an existing portosystemic shunt. This is secondary to the inability of the liver to metabolize the drugs used (Fossum and Duprey 2002).

A common finding in cats affected with extra or intrahepatic shunts is ptyalism (Fossum and Duprey 2002). Ptyalism is defined as an excessive flow of saliva (American 1995). Another finding in cats is a copper color to the iris. As with dogs, cats will also have small atrophied livers and enlarged kidneys (Fossum and Duprey 2002).

Low serum albumin is a common finding in the hepatic patient, but patients with portosystemic shunts tend to have a normal serum albumin. Coagulation panels are usually normal in portosystemic shunt patients. Serum bilirubin is usually within normal limits as well (Fossum and Duprey 2002).

Anesthesia can be uneventful until the shunt is ligated. Portal hypertension is the concern once the shunt is ligated (Tranquilli et al. 2007). Because the ameroid constrictor occludes the vessel slowly, portal hypertension is less common (Fossum and Duprey 2002). IV fluids should be administered during surgery, and intraoperative monitoring should include SpO_2, $ETCO_2$, indirect or direct blood pressure, ECG, and temperature.

Additional surgery that may be required on the liver involves the removal of neoplasias. The tumors seen in the liver are generally metastatic neoplasias; primary tumors are not that common in the liver. Due to its main function as a filter, metastasis is common in the liver. Pancreatic adenocarcinoma, hemangiosarcoma, and insulinoma are seen in the liver with lymphosarcoma being the most common (Fossum and Duprey 2002).

Patients presenting with hepatic neoplasias are generally older dogs. On examination the patient may be weak, anorexic, and lethargic. They may also have pale mucous membranes and a distended abdomen. The distended abdomen may be due to a hemoabdomen or ascites. Patients may also have petechial hemorrhages, be polyuric/dipsic (PU/PD), and be icteric (Tranquilli et al. 2007). Anemia, leukocytosis, and elevated ALT and Alk Phos are common laboratory findings.

Prior to surgery, radiographs, ultrasound, CT, or MRI can be performed to determine the extent of the disease process. Three-view thoracic radiographs should also be evaluated prior to surgery to see whether metastasis is evident.

Surgery performed on the gallbladder also has hepatic considerations. Removal of the gallbladder, or cholecystectomy, is performed when obstruction or neoplasia is present in the extrahepatic biliary system. These obstructions can be extraluminal or intraluminal. Pancreatic disease is extraluminal and is the main cause of hepatobiliary obstruction. An intraluminal example is cholelithiasis (Fossum and Duprey 2002). If the obstruction has been present for an extended period of time clotting factors may become prolonged (Fossum and Duprey 2002). If left untreated, the obstruction can lead to aerobic or anaerobic infection. This will then lead to bacteremia. These patients can be a challenge to anesthetize and maintain during surgery. They must be monitored carefully throughout surgery.

Designing an Ideal Drug Protocol

Patients with hepatic or hepatobiliary disease may require anesthesia for reasons that do not primarily include the liver. Any anesthesia drug protocol should be carefully planned out and any blood work abnormality should be corrected prior to anesthesia. Due to the reduction of liver function, drugs that are metabolized by the liver or are highly protein bound should be avoided, or reduced amounts should be used. These drugs include phenothiazine tranquilizers and benzodiazepines and barbiturates (Fossum and Duprey 2002).

An example of an anesthetic protocol for the hepatic patient includes a mu or kappa opioid, ± anticholinergic and induction with propofol. Anesthetic maintenance would be with either isoflurane or sevoflurane. IV fluid therapy in the form of crystalloids or colloids, if indicated, and inotropic support should be available. Hypotension can be exacerbated by hypothermia and hypoalbuminemia (Tranquilli et al. 2007). Intraoperative monitoring should include SpO_2, $ETCO_2$, indirect or direct blood pressure, ECG, fluids, and temperature. Ideally, packed cell volume (PCV), total protein (TP), electrolytes, and blood gas measurement should be monitored under anesthesia. Clotting times (PT and PTT) should be measured prior to surgery. Pain can be treated with mu or kappa agonists, understanding that adverse effects of any opioid can be reversed with naloxone in an emergency situation. The use of epidurals should be avoided in patients that have extended clotting times. The introduction of the needle can potentiate any coagulopathies that are present.

Antibiotics should be administered when performing surgery on the liver due to anaerobic bacteria that live in the liver. The bacteria can multiply if hepatic ischemia persists. Penicillin derivatives should be used (Fossum and Duprey 2002).

Patient positioning is also a consideration. If ascites is present, the dorsal recumbency may make ventilation difficult. Abdominocentesis may be indicated to help improve profusion and ventilation. Mechanical ventilation may be indicated as well.

References

American Heritage Stedman's Medical Dictionary. 1995. Boston: Houghton Mifflin.

Bonagura, JD, Kirk, RW. 2000. Kirk's Current Veterinary Therapy: Small Animal Practice. Philadelphia: WB Saunders, p.872.

Boothe, DM. 2005. New Information on Nonsteroidal Antiinflammatories: What Every Criticalist Must Know. Veterinary Information Network, p.5.

Chabner, D-E. 2004. The language of medicine: A write-in text explaining medical terms. St. Louis: Saunders pp.147–149.

Ettinger, SJ, Feldman, EC. 2000. Textbook of Veterinary Internal Medicine, Volume 2. Philadelphia: WB Saunders, pp.1272–1277.

Evans, HE. 1993. Miller's Anatomy of the Dog. Philadelphia: WB Saunders, pp.451–457.

Fossum, TW, Duprey, LP. 2002. Small Animal Surgery. St. Louis: Mosby, pp.450–486.

Leib, MS, Monroe, WE. 1997. Practical Small Animal Internal Medicine. Philadelphia: WB Saunders, pp.776–792, 800–802.

Pasquini, C, Spurgeon, T, Pasquini, S, Smith, M. 1995. Anatomy of Domestic Animals: Systemic and Regional Approach. Pilot Point, TX: Sudz Publishing, pp.292–294.

Plumb, DC. 2005. Plumb's Veterinary Drug Handbook. Stockholm, WI: PhrmaVet, pp.340–345.

Tranquilli, WJ, Thurmon, JC, Grimm, DA, Lumb, WV. 2007. Lumb & Jones' Veterinary Anesthesia and Analgesia. Ames, IA: Blackwell Publishing, pp.219, 291, 303, 380, 790, 816, 921–925.

Anesthesia for Pediatric Patients

26

Trish Farry

Canine and feline patients are classed as pediatric until 12 weeks of age and are considered neonatal at less than 4 weeks (Fox 1966a).

When presented with a pediatric patient for anesthesia the veterinary technician must understand the unique anatomical, physiological, and pharmacological differences in these patients to enable them to formulate and provide the most appropriate anesthesia regimen.

Physiology

Pediatric patients are highly dependent on heart rate to maintain cardiac output and blood pressure (Holden 2007). They have less functional contractile tissue, limited cardiac reserve, and low ventricular compliance and therefore a reduced ability to increase stroke volume (Pettifer and Grubb 2007). The sympathetic nervous system is underdeveloped, and these patients may have poor vasomotor control and reduced baroreceptor reflexes, which make them less able to tolerate blood loss and maintain blood pressure (Fox 1966). Bradycardia in the pediatric patient may therefore profoundly affect cardiac output and subsequently blood pressure.

Pulmonary reserve is limited in the pediatric patient. Oxygen consumption is 2–3 times higher than in the adult due to a high metabolic rate (Lukasik 2005). This is accomplished by a high resting respiratory rate and minute volume. Anatomical differences such as a large tongue and less rigid airway cartilage can predispose the pediatric patient to upper airway obstruction. Hypoxia may occur due to low functional residual capacity. These patients are less able to tolerate and compensate should an obstruction or decrease in respiratory rate or depth occur. A more pliable rib cage can result in less efficient ventilation, and respiratory fatigue is common (Haddad et al. 1984).

Both the renal and hepatic systems are underdeveloped in the pediatric patient. One of the main considerations for sedation and anesthesia is the metabolism, biotransformation, and excretion of drugs. An exaggerated effect and prolonged duration of action may be observed, and the technician may need to adjust and reduce dose rates and dosing intervals accordingly. Pediatric patients are prone to hypoglycemia due to minimal glycogen stores and poor gluconeogenesis (Agarwal 2006). Blood glucose monitoring and the administration of glucose-containing fluids may be beneficial during anesthesia.

Renal function is also reduced and these patients are less tolerant of fluid overloading and hypotension.

Preanesthesia Preparation

A complete physical examination is the cornerstone for any animal undergoing sedation or anesthesia. From the observations that are noted during this exam, the technician will be able to formulate the appropriate anesthesia plan.

Due to the minimal glycogen stores in the liver of the pediatric patient, withholding of food should be kept to a minimum. Unweaned puppies and kittens should not be fasted and patients over 6 weeks of age need to be fasted only for a maximum of 3 hours prior to general anesthesia. Prolonged fasting of these patients may result in hypoglycemia and dehydration, and predispose them to hypothermia. Withholding of water is unnecessary.

An accurate weight on all patients is of the utmost importance, particularly in small patients where an overdose of fluids or drugs can have a catastrophic effect. With very small patients it is advisable to use a small scale that can give an accurate weight in grams (Fig. 26.1).

The minimum laboratory evaluations should include a packed cell volume, total protein and blood glucose. Further evaluation of the patient's biochemical and hematological status should be performed if indicated. Any fluid deficits or electrolyte imbalances should be corrected prior to anesthesia where possible.

Avoid repeated blood sampling where possible due to the likelihood of volume depletion in a very small patient.

Premedication

In most cases, with the possible exception of extreme debilitation or illness, premedication is beneficial. The use of a balanced drug combination can alleviate stress and significantly decrease the subsequent amounts of induction and main-

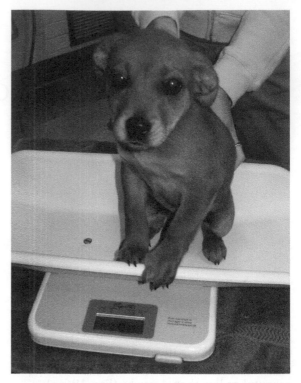

Figure 26.1.   A puppy being weighed on an infant scale for accuracy.

tenance agents required. In the pediatric patient the blood brain barrier is immature, and this increased permeability may result in exaggerated responses to drug administration.

The four main classes of drugs used as premedicants in the pediatric patients are opioids, benzodiazepines, anticholinergics, and tranquilizers. These drugs can be used alone or in combinations.

Opioids

Opioids in general have very little effect on cardiac contractility but may produce a reduction in heart rate. The μ agonists (fentanyl, morphine, methadone, hydromorphone, and oxymorphone) provide the best analgesia but will cause greater cardiovascular and respiratory depression than the partial μ agonists(buprenorphine)and the κ agonist/partial μ agonists(butorphanol). These latter drugs provide only moderate analgesia but may be a more appropriate choice dependent on the procedure and analgesic requirements.

Benzodiazepines

Benzodiazepines usually do not provide reliable sedation in a healthy adult patient, but are often quite effective in the pediatric patient. Midazolam and diazepam cause minimal cardiovascular depression and provide good muscle relaxation. Benzodiazepines do not provide any analgesia, so they are best used in combination with an opioid. Both opioids and benzodiazepines have specific antagonists, naloxone and flumazenil, respectively, which can be administered if undesirable or prolonged effects of these drugs occur.

Anticholinergics

Anticholinergics are indicated in the pediatric patient. Cardiac output in the pediatric patient is dependent on heart rate; thus, care should taken to maintain heart rate. The use of atropine or glycopyrrolate is also indicated in patients with high vagal tone or in procedures that may likely stimulate a vagal reflex.

Acepromazine

Acepromazine, a phenothiazine, is one of the most common drugs used in premedication in the veterinary patient. Acepromazine provides excellent sedation, but its deleterious side effects make it an unwise choice in the pediatric patient. It may cause hypotension and heat loss due to vasodilatation in a patient that is less able to compensate for these effects.

All of these drugs require hepatic metabolism and renal clearance; and with both of these organ systems underdeveloped, prolonged and exaggerated effects may be seen. Care must be taken with drug doses because the pediatric patient is less able to tolerate absolute or relative overdoses.

α_2 adrenergic agonists

Although α_2 adrenergic agonists will provide effective sedation with some analgesia, they can also produce profound bradycardia. This is of particular importance in pediatric patients due to their rate-dependent cardiac output. At higher dose rates respiratory depression may also be an issue due to the high metabolic oxygen demand of the patient. α_2 adrenergic agonists are also extensively metabolized in the liver, so prolonged and more profound effects of these drugs would be expected. Their use is best avoided in the pediatric patient. Table 26.1 lists suggested dosage for pediatric patients.

Induction

Induction of anesthesia is achieved by the administration of injectable drugs or by the use of inhalational agents. Injectable drugs have the benefit of minimizing stress to the patient and a rapid loss of consciousness, which will facilitate rapid control of the airway. Venous access is required for administration, and this may prove challenging in the conscious pediatric patient.

The injectable drugs commonly used as induction agents are propofol, ketamine/diazepam, etomidate, and alfaxalone. All injectable anaesthetics have side effects that need to be considered when selecting the most appropriate drug.

Propofol

Propofol is a short-acting hypnotic agent that can be used for the induction and maintenance of general anesthesia via incremental doses or constant rate infusion. If used in conjunction with opioids and phenothiazines, the use of propofol may cause unwanted cardiovascular effects, including bradycardia and vasodilatation. It can also cause significant respiratory depression and should be titrated to effect. Propofol is highly lipid-soluble and requires hepatic metabolism, though some extra hepatic metabolism does occur (Saint-Maurice 1994).

Table 26.1.   Suggested drug doses (mg/kg) for pediatric small animals.

- Extrapolated from adult doses
- Combining drug groups provides balanced premedication.
- Drug doses should be further reduced for neonatal patients.

Class	Dose mg/kg /Route	Comments—Refer to Text for More Information
Anticholinergics		
Atropine	0.02–0.04 SC IM IV	Anesthetic adjuvant, treatment/prevention of bradycardia
Glycopyrrolate	0.01–0.02 SC IM IV	
Benzodiazepines & tranquilizers		
Diazepam	0.1–0.4 IV	IM, SC uptake unreliable—more effective when used in conjunction with an opioid
Midazolam	0.1–0.3 SC IM IV	More effective when used in conjunction with an opioid—shorter duration of action than diazepam
Flumazenil	0.1 IV	Benzodiazepine antagonist, short duration of action
Acepromazine	0.005–0.02 SC IM IV	Use with caution.
Opioids	(Use lower-end doses in cats.)	
Methadone	0.05–0.3 SC IM IV	Good analgesia
Morphine	0.05–0.25 SC IM	Good analgesia—vomiting may occur.
Buprenorphine	0.005–0.02 SC IM IV	Slow onset of action
Butorphanol	0.1–0.3 SC IM IV	Mild pain only, may provide good sedation
Hydromorphone	0.03–0.07 SC IM IV	Good analgesia
Oxymorphone	0.03–0.07 SC IM IV	Good analgesia
Naloxone	0.01–0.1 IV	Opioid antagonist—all analgesia reversed short duration of action.
Induction agents*		
Propofol	1–4 IV	Hypotension, apnea common
Ketamine ± diazepam	0.15–0.3/1.5–3 IV	
Etomidate	1–2 IV	
Alfaxalone	1–2 IV	

*Induction dose rates are for premedicated patients and should be titrated slowly to effect.

Ketamine

Ketamine, a dissociative anesthetic is often used in combination with a benzodiazepine as an induction agent. Ketamine has a rapid onset of action, causes minimal cardiovascular depression, and provides a short duration of analgesia. Ketamine often produces an increase in blood pressure and cardiac output due to stimulation of the sympathetic nervous system (Wright 1982).

Etomidate

Etomidate is a short-acting, nonbarbiturate intravenous anesthetic agent. It causes minimal adverse cardiovascular effects and is less likely to cause a significant drop in blood pressure when compared to other induction agents. Etomidate produces minimal respiratory depression.

Alfaxalone

Alfaxolone in cyclodextran (Alfaxan®) is a new formulation of the older steroid-injectable anesthetic (Saffan). Alfaxalone is a rapid and noncumulative injectable agent that provides reasonable muscle relaxation, has excellent cardiovascular stability, and causes minimal respiratory depression (Best and Pearson 1997).

All of the injectable drugs require hepatic metabolism and renal clearance. When used in the patient with immature renal and hepatic function, prolonged duration of action and recovery may result, with the possible exception of propofol due to its extrahepatic metabolism.

Accurate dosing of injectable induction agents is important. It is beneficial to dilute the concentration of a particular drug with a compatible diluent to assist in the titration process.

All of the injectable agents have the potential to produce respiratory depression, so the technician needs to be able to take rapid control of the airway, supply oxygen, and ventilate when necessary.

Inhalation agents

The inhalation agents commonly used for induction are isoflurane and sevoflurane. Both agents may cause dose-dependent cardiovascular and respiratory depression. Sevoflurane has a lower solubility in blood than isoflurane, and thus results in a more rapid uptake (induction) and elimination (recovery). A small well-fitting face mask with minimal dead space should be used for an inhalational induction (Fig. 26.2). Wrapping the patient in a warm towel can reduce the stress of restraint.

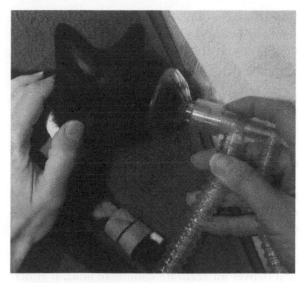

Figure 26.2. Pediatric mask.

When planning to induce anesthesia in the pediatric patient, care must be taken to have the correct equipment available. A selection of endotracheal (ET) tubes of appropriate sizes should be readily accessible, along with a laryngoscope with a good light source and an appropriately sized blade. In very small patients an uncuffed ET tube may be preferable to maximize airway diameter and decrease resistance of breathing. Care must be taken not to overinflate the cuff of an ET tube because the tracheal tissue is very fragile. An oxygen supply and a breathing circuit with a pediatric-sized wye-piece and bag must also be available to assist with ventilation. Oxygenation prior to induction cannot be overemphasized due to the high oxygen demand and increased susceptibility to upper airway obstruction.

Maintenance

All the inhalational agents produce some degree of dose-related respiratory depression, vasodilatation, and hypotension.

A nonrebreathing system is typically used in the pediatric patient due to the lower resistance to breathing and minimal apparatus dead space.

Unfortunately, the fresh high gas flow rate required by these circuits (2–3 times respiratory minute volume) may predispose the patient to hypothermia.

Care must be taken when assisting ventilation because the small tidal volumes of these patients increase the risk of barotrauma from overzealous ventilation. Airway pressures should not exceed 15–20 cm H_2O (10–15 cm H_2O in the open thorax).

Fluid therapy is beneficial to provide hemodynamic support and replace insensible losses. Care must be taken with volumes of fluid administered because pediatric patients have a reduced ability to tolerate acute fluid loading. It is advisable to use a fluid pump or a syringe driver that will deliver an accurate volume of fluid. If either of these is unavailable, a micro drip set with a burette is an acceptable alternative. Fluid rates should not exceed 10 mL/kg/hr (unless faced with acute hemorrhage). Maintenance of adequate serum glucose may require fluids containing dextrose such as 5% dextrose in Ringer's. Care must be taken with some glucose solutions (e.g., 5% glucose) as they are hypotonic in the body. Regular monitoring of blood glucose while the animal is under anesthesia is advisable.

Thermoregulation

Thermoregulation is impaired in pediatric patients and they are extremely vulnerable to hypothermia due to their larger body surface area relative to body weight ratio and minimal fat reserves. Most anesthetic agents affect the thermoregulatory center, and hypothermia may result. This can produce many deleterious effects in the anesthetized pediatric patient, including decreased metabolic rate, increased susceptibility to infection, myocardial depression, respiratory depression, and delays in drug metabolism. Hypothermia significantly reduces the minimum alveolar concentration (MAC) of inhalational agents due to the decrease in metabolic rate. Care must be taken to keep these patients normothermic because they can begin to lose body temperature once they are premedicated. There are many options available to conserve body temperature. The use of temperature-controlled heating mats, hot water bottles, warm air blankets, the wrapping of extremities, and the warming of intravenous and irrigation fluids are all beneficial. Extreme care must be taken to avoid thermal burns, keeping all heating modalities close to body temperature where possible. Airway humidifiers and warmers must be used cautiously in the pediatric patient because they may increase the effort of breathing due to the apparatus dead space.

Skin preparation for surgery should be performed using warmed solutions. Alcohol should only be applied to the animal immediately prior to surgery because the application of alcohol will exacerbate heat loss via evaporation.

Monitoring

The goal of monitoring is to provide information to aid technicians in their ability to assess the physiological status of patients. The veterinary technician then uses this information to provide the most appropriate anesthesia/analgesia plan for each patient.

In veterinary medicine today we have many electronic monitoring devices that can be used, but it must be remembered that all monitors have benefits and limitations and should never replace a skilled, knowledgeable technician. When monitoring, one measurement gives a window into a dynamic situation, whereas repeated measurements provide a better indication of the dynamic picture. Trends have more meaning than single values (Keates 2008).

Tissue perfusion can be assessed subjectively by pulse quality, capillary refill time and mucous membrane color.

Blood pressure can be monitored invasively via an arterial catheter and transducer, but this can be technically challenging in the smaller patient. Noninvasive measurements of blood pressure are taken using a Doppler or oscillometric monitor. The Doppler appears to be more accurate and reliable in smaller animals although some veterinary specific multimonitors provide reliable noninvasive blood pressure measurements in cats and small dogs. Care must be taken to choose the correct size of occlusion cuff. The width of the cuff should be approximately 40% of the circumference of the limb. An incorrectly sized cuff will result in a false high or low reading.

Pulse oximetry gives an indication of the adequacy of circulation and oxygenation. A pulse oximeter indicates the presence of pulsatile blood flow. Peripheral vasoconstriction, decreases in pulse amplitude, or arrhythmias are likely to affect signal quality.

Respiratory function can be subjectively assessed by respiratory rate and depth. Capnography provides a measurement of the CO_2 content of respiratory gases and therefore is a good indicator of the adequacy of respiratory function. Accuracy can be hampered by small tidal volumes in pediatric patients as well as a dilutional effect due to the high fresh gas flow rates. Adapters for a capnograph are usually attached between the endotracheal tube and breathing circuit and thus may contribute significantly to the apparatus dead space in the very small patient. This may be resolved by attaching a needle to the sampling tube and inserting it directly into the endotracheal tube (sidestream sampling) (Fig. 26.3).

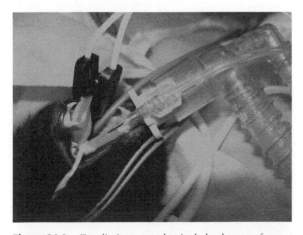

Figure 26.3. To eliminate mechanical dead space from a mainstream adaptor, a surgical needle may be connected to sidestream sampling tubing and inserted directly into the lumen of the endotracheal tube.

Temperature probes placed into either the esophagus or rectum should be used and provide a reliable indication of body temperature.

Postanesthesia

As with any anesthetic recovery, care must be taken to assess the adequacy of respiratory and circulatory function, and support should be provided if necessary.

The hypothermic patient will shiver on recovery, which may increase O_2 demands by up to 300% (Muravchick 2000). It is advisable to supply supplemental O_2 in the shivering patient to maintain tissue oxygenation. Active warming must be instigated in the hypothermic patient.

Appropriate analgesia should always be provided. This can be achieved by systemic administration of analgesic drugs as well as the utilization of local blocks where possible. Pediatric patients may not exhibit overt signs of pain due to survival instincts, and thus the recognition of pain can be more challenging for the technician. Do not assume that the animal is not in pain because it is exhibiting no obvious signs of pain. The opioid analgesics are good choices, but they may cause unwanted respiratory depression, so, as with all drugs in the pediatric patient, doses should be carefully calculated when administered and preferably titrated to effect. Nonsteroidal antiinflammatory drugs require extensive hepatic metabolism; therefore, they may not be the most appropriate choice in the pediatric patient, and repeated doses should definitely be avoided.

Normal feeding should resume as soon as possible and unweaned puppies or kittens should be returned to their mothers as soon they are able to suckle.

With adequate preparation and understanding of the unique physiological and anatomical differences, the anesthetist can provide excellent care for the pediatric patient.

References

Agarwal, R. 2006. Neonatal anesthesia. In Anesthesia Secrets, edited by Duke, J. Philadelphia: Mosby Elsevier, pp.364–380.

Best, P, Pearson, M. 1997. Report on the Safety of Alfaxolone—CD Anaesthetic Compound. On file, Jurox Pty. Ltd.

Fox, MW. 1966a. Developmental physiology and behavior. In Canine Pediatrics, edited by Fox, MW, Himwich, WA. Springfield, IL: Charles C. Thomas.

Fox, MW. 1966b. Canine Pediatrics. Springfield, IL: Charles C. Thomas.

Haddad, GG, et al. 1984. Hypoxia and respiratory control in early life. Ann Rev Physiol 46:629–643.

Holden, D. 2007. Paediatric patients. In BSAVA Manual of Canine and Feline Anaesthesia and Analgesia, 2nd ed., edited by Seymour C, Duke-Novakovski, T. Gloucester: British Small Animal Veterinary Association.

Keates, HL. 2008. Anaesthesia teaching notes provided for undergraduate veterinary students.

Lukasik, VM. 2005. Anesthesia of the Pediatric Patient. Proceedings of the North American Veterinary Conference, pp.53–55.

Pettifer, GR, Grubb, TL. 2007. Neonatal and geriatric patients. In Lumb & Jones' Veterinary Anesthesia and Analgesia, 4th ed., Thurmon, JC, et al. Ames: IA: Blackwell Publishing.

Saint-Maurice, C. 1994. Propofol in pediatric anesthesia. Cah Anesthesiol 39:411–420.

Wright, M. 1982. Pharmacological effects of ketamine and its use in veterinary medicine. J Am Vet Med Assoc 180:1462–1471.

Anesthesia for Geriatric Patients

Trish Farry

Due to continuing developments in veterinary medicine we have seen a marked increase in the number of older patients requiring sedation and general anesthesia. A geriatric patient can be defined as one that has reached 75% of the average life expectancy, dependent on breed and species (Goldston 1995).

Geriatric patients may appear "healthy" for their age, but they can often have underlying multiple organ dysfunctions, which when challenged by general anesthesia can result in a cascade of detrimental events. Although age is not a disease in itself, age related physiological changes must be evaluated and assessed on each individual patient to ensure that the most appropriate sedation and/or anesthesia plan is instigated (Fig. 27.1).

This chapter gives an overview on anesthetizing the healthy geriatric patient. Refer to specific chapters within this book to provide further detail on how to approach a patient with significant organ dysfunction.

Physiology

A decrease in functional cardiac reserve may render the geriatric patient less able to compen-

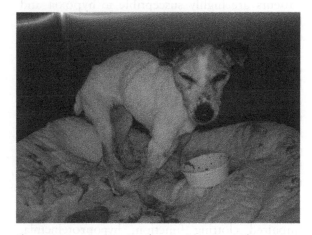

Figure 27.1. An emaciated geriatric patient. This patient will have difficulty thermoregulating under anesthesia because of its body condition.

sate for cardiovascular changes when challenged with sedation or general anesthesia (Neiger-Aeschbacher 2007).

Reduced cardiac output and contractility, decreased blood volume and blood pressure, and decreased ability to autoregulate blood flow and maintain blood pressure all contribute to a reduction in cardiac vascular reserve (Ko and

275

Galloway 2002). An increased circulation time may result in a delayed response to drug administration.

Older patients may have chronic or degenerative valvular disease and may be susceptible to cardiac arrhythmias due to myocardial fiber atrophy and changes in the conduction system (Muravchick 2000). Drugs that are known to potentiate arrhythmias and/or cause extreme changes in heart rate, such as α_2 adrenergic agonists, ketamine, and thiopentone, should be used sparingly or avoided in the geriatric patient (Ko and Galloway 2002).

With increased age there are decreases in respiratory rate as well as tidal and minute volumes. Physical changes include reduced thoracic wall compliance, decreased lung elasticity, and atrophy of the intercostal muscles, and these may contribute to a decreased respiratory reserve in the elderly patient (Paddleford 1995). These patients are highly susceptible to hypoxia and hypercapnia when the respiratory system is depressed by drugs.

Hepatic and renal mass can be significantly decreased in the geriatric patient. A reduction in hepatic and renal blood flow is secondary to a decrease in cardiac output and can result in decreased drug metabolism and clearance. Hypoxia, hypotension, and hypovolemia may exacerbate the reduction of renal blood flow. Due to the reduction of functional organ reserve, these patients have less tolerance for excessive fluid administration, hypovolemia, hypotension, dehydration, and blood loss. Impaired clotting function, hypoproteinemia, and hypoglycemia must also be considered in a patient with reduced hepatic function (Paddleford 1995).

Changes that may be seen in the nervous system of the geriatric patient are altered sensory, motor, cognitive, and autonomic functions. Enhanced effects to anesthetic drugs may occur as a result of decreases in cerebral perfusion, oxygen consumption, thermoregulatory function, and sympathetic responses to stress. Changes in myelination and decreased production of neurotransmitters may also sensitize the elderly patient to local anesthetics (Neiger-Aeschbacher 2007).

Preanesthesia Preparation

All patients must be evaluated on an individual basis. A thorough physical examination, detailed medical history, and laboratory assessment are the bases on which to formulate an anesthesia plan. The animal may present with existing disease—for example, Addison's, Cushing's, diabetes—or may be taking medications that will influence the anesthetist's choice of drugs and supportive therapies. Basic laboratory work should always be performed on the geriatric patient. A complete blood count, biochemistry, and urinalysis may alert the anesthetist to subclinical organ dysfunction, which when challenged by general anesthesia may accelerate the disease process. If cardiac murmurs or arrhythmias are noted on examination, a chest radiograph, electrocardiogram, or echocardiograph may be indicated to rule out existing cardiac disease.

Conservative intravenous fluid therapy may be indicated in the preoperative period to ensure that the patient is in the most stable physiological state prior to general anesthesia. A balanced anesthesia and analgesia plan may necessitate the concurrent use of several drugs at reduced doses to achieve the best outcome for the patient with minimal drug-related side effects.

The patient undergoing elective general anesthesia will need to be fasted. It is recommended that fasting be kept to a minimum, generally 8 hours, due to the risk of hypoglycemia. Water should be withheld only for a short period of time to minimize dehydration (Fig. 27.2).

Premedication

One of the main considerations for drug selection should be minimizing deleterious effects on organ function. All drugs may have exaggerated effects and duration of action may be prolonged in the geriatric patient. Judicious dosing and titration of drugs is advisable until the desired effect is achieved. It is much easier to administer additional drug than to deal with the affects of an overdose.

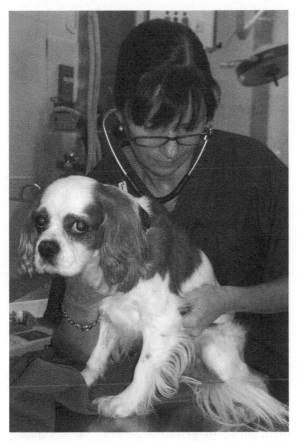

Figure 27.2. Auscultation and examination of the geriatric patient.

The classes of drugs that are commonly used for the sedation of geriatric patients are opioids, phenothiazines, benzodiazepines, and α2 adrenergic agonists. These drugs can be used independently or in combination.

Opioids

Opioids will provide analgesia and sedation in the geriatric patient. They have minimal cardiovascular effects but may cause some respiratory depression. Pure μ agonists (morphine, pethidine, fentanyl, oxymorphone, hydromorphone and methadone) provide better analgesia than the partial μ agonist (buprenorphine) and the κ agonist/μ partial agonists (butorphanol, nalbuphine), but are more likely to cause bradycardia

and a centrally mediated respiratory depression (Ko and Galloway 2002). The use of an anticholinergic may be required to counteract bradycardia (Stoelting 1999). If respiratory depression is evident, this can be exacerbated by a low functional respiratory reserve, and supplemental oxygen should be provided. Some opioids have a relatively short duration of action and this may be beneficial in the geriatric patient. The partial μ agonist and κ agonist/μ partial agonists have a "ceiling effect" on respiratory depression, but do have limited analgesic effectiveness, so are not suitable for severe pain (Ko and Galloway 2002). The perioperative use of opioids may decrease the dose of induction and maintenance agents required. Opioids require hepatic metabolism and should be used judiciously in the patient with severe hepatic disease. A decrease in the dose or frequency of administration may be warranted. If undesirable side effects are seen with the administration of opioids, an opioid antagonist can be administered.

Benzodiazepines

Benzodiazepines (diazepam, midazolam) are popular choices in tranquilization of the elderly patient. They cause minimal cardiovascular and dose-related respiratory depressant effects and have a relatively short duration of action (particularly midazolam). They are commonly used in combination with an opioid for premedication. Benzodiazepines are metabolized by the liver, and a prolonged duration of action may be seen in a patient with hepatic disease. Flumazenil, a benzodiazepine antagonist, can be used as a reversal agent if necessary.

Acepromazine

Acepromazine is one of the most widely used tranquilizers in veterinary practice today. It provides excellent antiemetic, anxiolytic, and antiarrhythmic properties, but should be used with caution on the elderly patient. Hypotension and hypothermia due to peripheral vasodilatation are undesirable side effects seen with the administration of acepromazine. Acepromazine is metabolized by the liver, is not reversible, and has a long duration of action. Blood pressure monitoring and volume support are indicated when acepromazine is administered to a geriatric patient.

Alpha-2 adrenergic agonists

Although alpha-2 adrenergic agonists will provide effective sedation with some analgesia, they will also produce dose-related effects on the cardiovascular, respiratory, and central nervous systems. Alpha-2 adrenergic agonists also require extensive hepatic metabolism. Prolonged and more profound effects of these drugs would be expected in the presence of reduced hepatic function. Their use is best avoided in the geriatric patient.

Anticholinergics

Atropine and glycopyrrolate are anticholinergics commonly used in veterinary medicine. These drugs are used predominantly to treat sinus bradyarrhythmias and decrease respiratory secretions. Anticholinergics should be used judiciously in the geriatric patient because a sinus tachycardia will increase the myocardial oxygen demand and this, complicated by a lack of functional cardiac reserve, can result in myocardial hypoxia and arrhythmias. Sinus tachycardia is poorly tolerated in the geriatric patient with preexisting cardiac disease and may precipitate acute myocardial failure. These drugs should not be used routinely, but as necessary, when bradycardia is exacerbating hypotension. Glycopyrrolate may be a better choice in the elderly patient because it has fewer adverse effects. It does not cross the blood-brain barrier and thus CNS effects are avoided.

Induction Agents

The induction of general anesthesia may be achieved by using injectable anesthetic agents or by delivery of inhalational agents. The commonly used injectable agents are ketamine/benzodiazepines, propofol, etomidate, alfaxolone, and thiopentone.

Hypoproteinemia and decreased protein binding may result in exaggerated effects and prolonged duration of action by highly protein-bound injectable agents (Stoelting 1999; Muravchick 2000).

A delayed response to drug administration may result from an increased circulation time. Adequate sedation will assist in the reduction of the total dose of injectable induction drug required. All of the induction agents have potential to cause significant respiratory depression, so it is vital to be able to take control of the airway and provide oxygen and ventilation if necessary. None of the induction agents, with the exception of ketamine, provide analgesia, so concurrent use of appropriate analgesic drugs should be used when indicated.

Propofol

Propofol is a commonly used injectable anesthetic drug in geriatric patients. It is rapidly cleared from the body, and metabolism is not dependent on the function of a single organ (Saint-Maurice 1991). Propofol can cause significant cardiovascular and respiratory depression and should be administered slowly until the desired effect is achieved. Apnea and cyanosis are relatively common with the administration of this drug. The anesthetist must be prepared to assist ventilation until spontaneous ventilation resumes. Propofol can cause direct myocardial depression and vasodilatation, which may result in arterial hypotension. Recovery from this drug is usually rapid and smooth (Pettifer and Grubb 2007).

Etomidate

Etomidate is another hypnotic induction agent. It has rapid onset of action as well as a rapid recovery due to metabolism. Good cardiovascular stability with minimal changes to heart rate and arterial blood pressure are seen following its administration. This makes etomidate an excellent drug choice for patients with preexisting cardiac disease (Stoelting 1999). As with propofol, it may cause dose-dependent respiratory depression and is best titrated to effect. Etomidate may inhibit adrenocortical function and so should be used with caution in patients with impaired adrenocortical function, for example, a patient with Addison's disease. In unsedated patients, retching, vomiting, and excitation in the early recovery period have been noted (Carpenter et al. 2005).

Ketamine

Ketamine is a rapidly acting dissociative anesthetic agent with a long duration of action. This drug provides good cardiovascular stability due to the stimulation of the sympathetic nervous system (Wright 1996; Kohrs and Durieux 1998). Increased cardiac output and tachycardia may be seen on administration as a result. Tachycardia will increase myocardial oxygen demand, which can result in myocardial hypoxia and subsequent cardiac failure in a compromised patient (Carpenter et al. 2005). Increased airway secretions may produce small airway obstruction and increase the likelihood of laryngospasm in cats. Ketamine does not cause significant respiratory depression. Seizures, muscular tremors, and vomiting have been observed with the use of ketamine as a sole agent, and so this is to be avoided. It is often combined with a benzodiazepine to minimize these undesirable effects (Carpenter et al. 2005).

Alfaxalone

Alfaxalone in cyclodextran (Alfaxan®) is a new formulation of the older steroid injectable anesthetic (Saffan). Alfaxolone is a rapid, noncumulative injectable agent that provides good muscle relaxation and excellent cardiovascular stability. It produces minimal respiratory depression and is rapidly metabolized in the liver. This drug has a wide safety margin (Best and Pearson 1997).

Barbiturates

Barbiturates cause significant cardiovascular and respiratory depression. They are also arrhythmogenic and therefore best avoided in the geriatric patient.

Preoxygenation prior to induction is advantageous

Increasing the oxygen fraction in the lungs will assist in the prevention of hypoxemia during induction and intubation. Table 27.1 summarizes drug dosages for geriatric patients.

Maintenance

Maintenance of general anesthesia is most commonly achieved by the use of inhalational agents. The ideal inhalational agent will have rapid uptake and elimination (i.e., low blood solubility), have little or no deleterious effects on cardiovascular and respiratory function, and require minimal metabolism. All inhalational agents produce dose-dependent cardiovascular and respiratory depression to some degree. Isoflurane, sevoflurane, and desflurane are all appropriate choices for the geriatric patient. These agents require minimal hepatic metabolism and renal elimination. The minimum alveolar concentration (MAC) of inhalational agents is reduced in the geriatric patient, resulting in a decrease in inhalant anesthetic requirements.

A balanced, multimodal anesthesia and analgesia plan utilizing regional blocks and/or opioids will help reduce the amount of the inhalational agent required.

Monitoring

Minimum monitoring for an anesthetized geriatric patient should include pulse oximetry, capnography, noninvasive blood pressure, ECG, and temperature.

Table 27.1.   Suggested drug doses (mg/kg) for geriatric small animals.

- Extrapolated from healthy adult doses.
- Combining drug groups provides balanced premedication.

Class	Dose mg/kg/Route	Comment—Refer to Text for More Information
Anticholinergics		
Atropine	0.02–0.04 SC IM IV	Anesthetic adjuvant, treatment of bradycardia
Glycopyrrolate	0.01–0.02 SC IM IV	
Benzodiazepines & tranquilizers		
Diazepam	0.1–0.4 IV IM	SC uptake unreliable—more effective when used in conjunction with an opioid
Midazolam	0.1–0.3 SC IM IV	More effective when used in conjunction with an opioid—shorter duration of action than diazepam
Flumazenil	0.1 IV	Benzodiazepine antagonist, short duration of action
Acepromazine	0.025–0.05 SC IM IV	Use with caution
Opioids	(Use lower-end doses in cats)	
Methadone	0.05–0.3 SC IM IV	Good analgesia
Morphine	0.05–0.3 SC IM	Good analgesia—vomiting may occur
Buprenorphine	0.005–0.02 SC IM IV	Slow onset of action
Fentanyl	0.005–0.01 IV	Short acting
Butorphanol	0.1–0.3 SC IM IV	Mild pain only, may provide good sedation
Hydromorphone	0.03–0.01 SC IM IV	Good analgesia
Oxymorphone	0.03–0.07 SC IM IV	Good analgesia
Naloxone	0.01–0.1 IV	Opioid antagonist—all analgesia reversed short duration of action
Induction agents*		
Propofol	2–6 IV	Hypotension, apnea common
Ketamine/diazepam	0.15–0.3/1.5–3 IV	
Etomidate	1–3 IV	
Alfaxalone	1–2 IV	

*Induction dose rates are for premedicated patients and should be titrated slowly to effect.

Geriatric patients have decreased thermoregulatory ability. Hypothermia can lead to cardiac arrhythmias, delayed healing, a decrease in anesthetic requirements, increased infection rates, and metabolic acidosis. Hypothermia may also prolong and potentiate the effects of sedative and anesthetic agents (Kaplan 1991).

Additional monitoring as required may include invasive blood pressure, central venous pressure, blood gases, blood glucose, and urine output.

Each patient should have intravenous access and fluid support. Geriatric patients are less tolerant to fluid overload, and overzealous fluid administration may precipitate congestive heart failure or pulmonary edema, particularly in cats or patients with underlying cardiac disease.

Anuria or oliguria during or following anesthesia may indicate renal damage, which may be due to poor renal perfusion or hypotension.

Recovery

Care must be taken to maintain body temperature under anesthesia. Shivering will increase oxygen consumption by up to 300%, and in the elderly patient with limited cardiopulmonary reserve this may lead to hypoxia (Pettifer and Grubb 2008). Supplemental oxygen may be required postanesthesia until the patient is able to maintain adequate oxygenation on room air. Intravenous fluid therapy should be maintained until the animal has adequate intake of food and water and is hemodynamically stable.

Appropriate analgesia should be provided by the systemic administration of analgesic drugs as well as the utilization of local blocks where possible. Analgesia should never be withheld from a geriatric patient due to concerns about unwanted side effects of drugs. The anesthetist needs to be aware of the potential beneficial and detrimental effects of drugs and then choose the most appropriate analgesic protocol for each patient. NSAIDS should be used with caution in all elderly patients, particularly those with coagulopathies, or renal, hepatic, or gastrointestinal disease.

The geriatric patient may have sensory deficits such as impaired vision or hearing, which can result in increased levels of anxiety. Elderly animals often require extra attention and respond well to regular positive interactions with staff. Hospitalization should be kept to a minimum because these patients will often do better at home with their owners.

Appropriate nutrition must be instigated as soon as feasible in the recovery period. Each patient should have an individual diet plan based on its current disease status and metabolic requirements.

Comfortable bedding and diligent nursing care should always be provided. Special care needs to be taken with providing support with the positioning of the recumbent or anesthetized patient. Extra padding and support for arthritic joints should be provided when positioning these patients on the surgery table. Geriatric patients with minimal body fat and decreased muscle mass often have bony prominences (hips, hocks, elbows, and sternum), that may be susceptible to the formation of decubital ulcers if they are not padded and protected appropriately.

Safely dealing with a geriatric patient requires the veterinary technician or nurse to approach the case well informed and aware of potential complications. A thorough history and workup cannot be overemphasized for these patients. Drug doses should be reduced, slower response times may be seen, and drugs that have long durations of action are best avoided. The anesthetist needs to be vigilant and prepared to respond to a variety of situations. An understanding of the physiological and anatomical differences in the geriatric patient will ensure that the anesthetist is well prepared for the successful management of these often complex and difficult cases.

References

Best, P, Pearson, M. 1997. Report on the safety of Alfaxolone-CD anaesthetic compound. On file, Jurox Pty, Ltd.

Carpenter, RE, Pettifer, GR, Tranquilli, WJ. 2005. Anaesthesia for geriatric patients. In Veterinary Clinics of North America Small Animal. St. Louis: Elsevier, pp. 571–580.

Goldston, RT. 1995. Introduction and overview of geriatrics. In Geriatrics and Gerontology of the Dog and Cat, edited by Goldston, RT, Hoskins, JD. Philadelphia: WB Saunders.

Kaplan, RF. 1991. Hypothermia/Hyperthermia. In Manual of Complications during Anesthesia, edited by Gravenstein, N. New York: JB Lippincott, pp. 121–150.

Ko, JCH, Galloway, DS. 2002. Anesthesia of geriatric patients. In Veterinary Anesthesia and Pain Management Secrets, edited by Greene, SA. Philadelphia: Hanley & Belfus, Inc.

Kohrs, R, Durieux, ME. 1998. Ketamine: Teaching an old drug new tricks. Anesth Analges 87:1193–1198.

Muravchick, S. 2000. Anesthesia for the elderly. In Anesthesia, 5th ed., edited by Miller, RD. Philadelphia: Churchill Livingstone.

Neiger-Aeschbacher, G. 2007. Geriatric patients. In BSAVA Manual of Canine and Feline Anaesthesia and Analgesia, 2nd ed, edited by Seymour, C, Duke-Novakovski, T. Gloucester: BSAVA.

Paddleford, RR. 1995. Anesthesia. In Geriatrics and Gerontology of the Dog and Cat, edited by Goldston, RT, Hoskins, JD. Philadelphia: WB Saunders.

Pettifer, GR, Grubb, TL. 2007. Neonatal and geriatric patients In Lumb & Jones' Veterinary Anesthesia and Analgesia, 4th ed, edited by Thurmon JC. et al. Ames, IA: Blackwell Publishing.

Saint-Maurice, C. 1991. Propofol in pediatric anesthesia. Cah Anesthesiol 39:411–420.

Stoelting, RK. 1999. Pharmacology and Physiology in Anesthetic Practice, 3rd ed. Philadelphia: Lippincott Williams & Wilkins.

Wright, M. 1996. Pharmacologic effects of ketamine and its use in veterinary medicine. J Am Vet Med Assoc 209:967–968.

Cesarean Section Techniques

28

Christopher L. Norkus

Patients presenting during the periparturient period may require anesthesia for elective or emergency cesarean section necessitated by dystocia. The primary objective when providing anesthesia for the cesarean section patient is to supply ample maternal analgesia, muscle relaxation, and restraint to facilitate adequate surgical conditions while concurrently avoiding morbidity and mortality to either the mother or fetus. In observing this principle, the anesthetist strives to prevent maternal and fetal hypoxia and hypotension, minimize fetal central nervous system (CNS) depression, diminish post anesthetic maternal depression, and minimize changes in uterine contraction and blood flow. The selection of an appropriate protocol for cesarean section should take into account safety of the mother and fetus, patient comfort, and the anesthetist's familiarity with the anesthetic technique.

Physiological Alterations in Pregnancy

The demands for successful gestation and parturition are met by significant alterations in physiological function.

Hemodynamic changes during pregnancy include varying degrees of increased stroke volume, heart rate, and cardiac output. Increases in estrogens result in decreased systemic vascular resistance (Tranquilli et al. 2007). Maternal blood volume (cardiac preload) increases during gestation although central venous pressure (CVP) and arterial blood pressure (BP) remain mostly unchanged until labor. Cardiac reserves are decreased and oxygen consumption is increased. Increased uterus weight can cause significant compression to the caudal vena cava and aorta, especially if the patient is placed in dorsal recumbency, resulting in dramatic compromises in venous return and cardiac output. Vascular engorgement can result in a decreased epidural space size and therefore necessitate a small volume of drug for epidural anesthesia (Tranquilli et al. 2007).

Progesterone increases during pregnancy induce sensitivity in the respiratory centers to carbon dioxide (Tranquilli et al. 2007). Respiratory rate is increased and $PaCO_2$ becomes decreased. However, as a compensatory mechanism, respiratory alkalosis does not dramatically affect arterial pH. Changes to PaO_2 and SaO_2 are not observed in pregnancy; however, decreases in hemoglobin concentration are seen. Functional residual capacity (FRC) is decreased in the pregnant patient. Cranial displacement of the uterus reduces FRC, causes respiratory depression, and may diminish effective ventilation. Patients are at risk for greater ventilation perfusion mismatch and secondary decreases in oxygenation. Increases in alveolar ventilation allow for rapid changes in alveolar anesthetic inhalant rate. Additional increases in progesterone and circulating endorphins decrease inhalant anesthetic requirements (Tranquilli et al. 2007). Both of these factors increase the potential occurrence of an inhalant anesthetic overdose.

The pregnant patient experiences cranial displacement of the stomach as a result of the enlarged uterus. Lower esophageal sphincter tone is also decreased and gastric motility decreases. Hydrochloric acid and enzyme concentrations in gastric sections are increased with gestation and intragastric pressure is increased (Tranquilli et al. 2007). These factors result in increased risk of regurgitation and aspiration pneumonia. Patients undergoing anesthesia for cesarean section should therefore always have their airway rapidly secured and protected via a cuffed endotracheal tube. An H_2 antagonist drug (famotidine, ranitidine, or cimetidine) and metoclopramide could be considered in the preoperative period.

There are minor alterations to hepatic function as a result of pregnancy in the veterinary patient. Drug biotransformation and elimination are not generally affected. Decreases in plasma cholinesterase may increase the action of succinylcholine and ester type local anesthetics (e.g., procaine). This may not be of clinical consequence. Physiological changes to the renal system include increased renal blood flow (RBF) and glomerular filtration rate (GFR) (Tranquilli et al. 2007). Serum blood urea nitrogen and creatinine are generally decreased as a result. Normal or increased levels may indicate renal pathology. Urine specific gravity should be evaluated.

Sodium and water balance are unaffected by pregnancy. Packed cell volume and plasma protein levels are generally decreased during gestation. A physiological leukogram may also be observed during labor. Hypoglycemia, hypocalcemia, dehydration, and exhaustion are frequent occurrences observed in the emergency cesarean section patient.

Uterine vasoconstriction may occur by endogenous sympathetic discharge via excitement, pain, or fear or through exogenous sources such as sympathomimetic drugs with alpha 1 adrenergic agonist effect (epinephrine, norepinephrine, phenylephrine, etc). Situations that decrease circulating maternal blood flow will decrease placental perfusion and result in fetal hypoxia and lactic acidosis.

Common factors that cause decreases in maternal perfusion include maternal dehydration from prolonged labor or concurrent disease, surgical hemorrhage, poor venous return from patient positioning or drug selection, drug or endotoxemic induced peripheral vasodilation, and anesthetic-induced negative inotropy. Administration of large and repeated doses of oxytoxcin may also lead to maternal vasodilation and decreases in fetal perfusion.

Cesarean section patients are at a greater anesthetic risk than are healthy nonpregnant cases because of said physiological alterations. Maintaining normotension, adequate ventilation, and patient oxygenation are top priorities in case management.

Anesthetic Drug Selection

In general, most drugs used in the anesthetic process affect the fetus and typically have longer and more pronounced effects on the fetus than on the mother. Ideally, drugs that cross the placental barrier slowly, for a short duration, or not at all are preferred when possible. Factors that increase drug diffusibility across the placenta include high lipid solubility, high nonpolarity, low molecular weight, and decreased degree of ionization and protein binding.

Preanesthetic agents

Preanesthetic drug options include neuroleptics (tranquilizers), sedatives, and analgesics. These drugs have the benefit of reducing induction and maintenance of anesthetic drug doses, minimizing patient and anesthetist stress, and providing patient analgesia. However, many of these drugs also have profound cardiovascular, respiratory, and fetal CNS depressant qualities. In general, this author limits or excludes their use in the majority of cesarean patients that are not markedly apprehensive or excited.

Phenothiazine tranquilizers such as acepromazine rapidly cross into fetal blood. As a result of acepromazine's alpha-1 and beta-1 adrenergic antagonism, the drug may cause vasodilation and negative inotropy, resulting in maternal hypotension and secondary alterations in fetal blood flow and oxygen delivery. Acepromazine has an unpredictable duration of action and its irreversibility makes it a poor choice for the cesarean section patient.

Although reversible, alpha-2 adrenergic agonists such as xylazine, romifidine, and dexmedetomidine can result in profound respiratory depression to the mother and fetus. Their cardiovascular effects can also significantly decrease perfusion via negative inotropy and decrease cardiac output. Their use in the cesarean patient, especially in combination with ketamine, has been shown to cause significant and potentially life-threatening cardiopulmonary changes and decreases to tissue perfusion in the canine patient (McDonnel et al. 1982). These drugs are also potent CNS depressants to the newborn (Moon et al. 2000).

Opioids are a mainstay of most small animal preanesthetic protocols. They typically provide solid sedation and excellent analgesia. In the small animal cesarean section patient, they rapidly cross the placenta and can rapidly rise in concentration. Low to moderate doses of opioids may be used with care. The main concern with their use is fetal respiratory and CNS depression.

If selecting an opioid for premedication, either a mixed agonist/antagonist such as butorphanol or nalbuphine, or a partial mu agonist such as buprenorphine may be preferred to minimize respiratory depression. If a pure mu agonist is selected, a shorter-duration agent such as fentanyl or remifentanil is preferred. If the newborn shows adverse affects to an opioid, the drug can

be reversed with sublingual, intratracheal, intraosseous, or intravenous naloxone. Newborns can become renarcotized from an opioid, however, as the short effects of the naloxone wear off. Careful nursing and observation for CNS and respiratory depression in the postoperative period is paramount, and redosing of naloxone may be necessary.

Due to the short duration of action, if a mixed opioid agonist/antagonist (e.g., butorphanol) is used in the preanesthetic period, a perioperative dose of a longer-acting pure mu agonist (e.g., morphine, hydromorphone, oxymorphone) can be safely administered upon fetus removal to provide maternal analgesia and avoid significant newborn depression.

Benzodiazepine tranquilizers such as diazepam and midazolam are reversible agents that typically yield minimal respiratory and cardiovascular depression in the adult. High concentrations can be seen in fetal blood, and they result in fetal CNS depression. If they are used in the premedication phase, their dose should be kept low (e.g. <0.15 mg/kg). Adverse effects in the newborn can be reversed with flumazenil.

Anticholinergic drugs are not routinely administered to cesarean section veterinary patients in most preanesthetic situations. These drugs will effectively block vagal stimulation that may occur with uterus traction. However, they may additionally cause fetal tachycardia, fetal CNS excitement, maternal tachycardia, arrhythmias, or hypertension. Atropine is a tertiary antimuscarinic, is widely distributed, and readily crosses the placenta. Glycopyrrolate is a quaternary antimuscarinic that does not cross the placenta. As a result, glycopyrrolate is generally considered the drug of choice if an anticholinergic drug is to be routinely selected for maternal support of heart rate. Atropine remains the drug of choice in emergency situations and must be used to treat fetal bradycardia.

Induction agents

Induction of anesthesia in the cesarean section patient should be a rapid and smooth process that strives to minimize physiological alterations.

The dissociative anesthetic ketamine and drug combinations such as tiletamine/zolazepam generally provide rapid and smooth anesthetic induction in the adult. They also have the added analgesic benefit of N-methyl-D-aspartate (NMDA) antagonism. However, these agents are poor muscle relaxants alone, effectively cross the placenta, and can result in fetal depression. Ketamine may also increase uterine tone. Respiratory and CNS depression, along with increased mortality at birth, has been reported with their use (Lunda et al. 2004; Moon et al. 2002). In general such agents are not preferred for use in the cesarean section patient.

Barbiturates are known to cause respiratory and cardiovascular depression in the adult dog and cat. Their use is typically reserved for the young and healthy. In the cesarean section patient, these risks are of significant concern. Thiopental, an ultra–short-acting thiobarbiturate, quickly crosses the placenta but then undergoes rapid redistribution. Still, severe fetal respiratory depression may be observed. Additionally, newborns often experience decreased sucking and CNS activity after removal from the uterus (Lunda et al. 2004; Moon et al. 2002). In general, it is best to avoid this class of drug in cesarean section patients.

Neuroleptanalgesic drug combinations (e.g., fentanyl/diazepam, hydromorphone/midazolam) are often used to induce anesthesia in the elderly or sick dog. They provide excellent cardiovascular and respiratory stability for these cases. However, larger doses of these agents are often required for induction, and their depressant qualities to the fetus are generally seen as less than ideal. The time to induce patients with this technique is also generally noticeably longer than with alternative intravenous drugs.

Propofol, a unique sedative hypnotic agent, has gained significant popularity in small animal cesarean sections in recent years. Although the drug may cause respiratory depression and cardiovascular changes (predominantly through vasodilation), the drug's effects are generally short because the agent is rapidly redistributed. Fetal effects are also generally short, and newborns and mothers typically do well with the agent. Propofol followed by isoflurane anesthesia in dogs resulted in newborn survival rates comparable to epidural anesthesia and superior to general anesthesia induced with thiopental (Funkquist 1997). In the majority of cesarean section cases, this is the induction agent of choice. The drug should be avoided in the very sick cesarean section case because patients will not likely tolerate the adverse effects of the drug well.

Both etomidate and alfaxalone are two additional agents that produce mild respiratory and cardiovascular changes in the adult. Side effects of etomidate typically necessitate the coadministration of a benzodiazepine. Still, these drugs appear to have little effect on the fetus and mother and are excellent choices to use in the ill cesarean section. Etomidate is likely the drug of choice in the sick and unstable cesarean section case. Alfaxalone appears to be a solid choice in the healthy and sick cesarean case alike.

Mask induction with isoflurane or sevoflurane was once seen as commonplace in veterinary medicine. Today, numerous concerns and liabilities limit its regular use. Its use is associated with increased patient stress, increased arrhythmic risk, and unnecessary staff exposure to anesthetic agents. Time required for complete induction of anesthesia is also longer than that for intravenous agents. Mask induction therefore promotes a prolonged period of an unsecured airway with an increased risk of airway compromise, obstruction, and aspiration. Perhaps most importantly, high concentrations of inhalant agents are required to achieve mask induction. Higher inhalant doses produce more cardiovascular and respiratory depression than seen with comparable doses of intravenous induction agents. Many safer options than mask inhalant induction presently exist. Table 28.1 lists drugs for the canine and feline cesarean section patient.

Maintenance agents

Once anesthesia is achieved, maintenance can be provided through a variety of different means.

Table 28.1.   Drug selection for the canine and feline cesarean section patient.

Drug Option	Canine Dose	Feline Dose	Considerations
Preanesthetic Agent			
None			Not in nervous, excited, or painful cases
Butorphanol	0.1–0.4 mg/kg IV/IM	Same	Mild and brief analgesia provided
Nalbuphine	0.1–0.4 mg/kg IV/IM	Same	Mild and brief analgesia provided
Buprenorphine	0.01–0.03 mg/kg IV/IM	Same	Slow (45 minutes) onset of analgesia
Fentanyl	0.002–0.005 mg/kg IV/IM	Same	May cause fetal respiratory depression
Diazepam	0.1–0.2 mg/kg IV/IM	Same	Rarely required
Midazolam	0.1–0.2 mg/kg IV/IM	Same	Rarely required
Induction			
Local/opioid epidural			May cause hypotension
Propofol	1–6 mg/kg IV slowly	Same	May cause hypotension
Etomidate	0.5–2 mg/kg IV	Same	Administer benzodiazapine prior to use.
Alphaxalone	2 mg/kg IV slowly	2–5 mg/kg IV slowly	
Maintenance			
Sevoflurane			Vigilant attention to anesthetic depth
Isoflurane			Vigilant attention to anesthetic depth
Propofol CRI	0.1–0.4 mg/kg/min	Same	Intubate and place on oxygen
Alphaxalone CRI	6–11 mg/kg/hr	Same	Intubate and place on oxygen
Patient Support			
Balanced crystalloid (LRS, 0.9% NaCl)	10–20 mL/kg/hr	Same	Adjust rate accordingly
Ephedrine	0.03–0.1 mg/kg IV slowly	Same	Dilute & titrate to effect
Phenylephrine	0.5–3 mcg/kg/min	Same	Not for prolonged use

CRI = Constant rate induction.

Inhalant agents such as isoflurane and sevoflurane produce dose-dependent respiratory and cardiovascular depression in the healthy adult. Geriatric or ill patients routinely tolerate their effects poorly. Minimum alveolar concentration (MAC) in the pregnant patient will be dramatically reduced (Tranquilli et al. 2007). When using an inhalant for maintenance, ensuring the shortest and most limited exposure of the patient to the agent is preferred. Careful monitoring must be observed.

Inhalants rapidly cross the placenta due to their lipid solubility. CNS, cardiovascular, and respiratory depression of the newborn are typically correlated to the depth and duration of maternal anesthesia. Speed and quality of anesthetic recovery are generally smooth and similar between isoflurane and sevoflurane (Polis et al.

2001). Total intravenous anesthesia (TIVA) with propofol or alphaxalone is an alternative to the use of an inhalant. When using such a technique, patients should still be intubated and provided with supplemental oxygen.

Additional drug considerations

Amide local anesthetics such as lidocaine, bupivicaine, and ropivicaine can be utilized safely in the pregnant patient for local anesthesia or epidural anesthesia. These agents cross the placental barrier but result in little clinically significant fetal depression. When administering epidural anesthesia to the pregnant female, there is risk for sympathetic blockade, which could result in maternal hypotension and decreased uteroplacental perfusion. Ephedrine and phenylephrine have been shown to be effective in correcting this problem in human women (Ngan Kee et al. 2008). A slow titrated ephedrine bolus of 0.03–0.1 mg/kg IV is often chosen in veterinary patients (Plumb 2008).

Neither nondepolarizing (e.g., vecuronium, pancuronium, and atracurium) nor depolarizing (e.g.. succinylcholine) neuromuscular blocking agents cross the placental barrier. These agents can be selected to supplement anesthesia in the cesarean section patient. Ventilation support must be provided, and it is important to note that analgesia is not provided by these agents. The nondepolarizing agents can be reversed by neostigmine or edrophonium to ensure prompt maternal recovery.

Anesthetic Technique

When presented with a cesarean section case, a complete physical exam and baseline laboratory work should be performed. Such cases should, at a minimum, have a complete blood count, chemistry panel, and electrolyte panel performed. Plasma lactate monitoring is also recommended in any ill patient.

An intravenous catheter should be placed and intravenous fluids started. Every effort should be

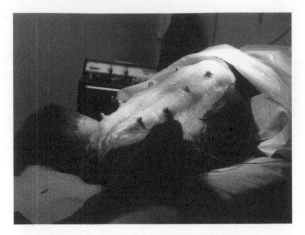

Figure 28.1. To minimize anesthesia duration, patients should be surgically clipped and briefly prepped prior to drug administration.

made to have patient electrolyte and metabolic derangements fully stabilized prior to anesthesia. Cases in a state of hypoperfusion (e.g., hypovolemic shock) or that have significant fluid deficits (e.g., dehydration) should be fully volume-resuscitated and stable prior to anesthesia.

Patients should be surgically clipped and briefly prepped prior to drug administration (Fig. 28.1). The operating room and surgical equipment should be fully ready, and the surgeon should be available for incision as soon as the patient is on the operating room table.

Restraint should be kept to a minimum. Apprehensive, excited, or painful patients can receive butorphanol at 0.01–0.04 mg/kg IV, IM or buprenorphine 0.01–0.03 mg/kg IV, IM (Plumb 2008). Diazepam or midazolam can also be included at 0.1–0.2 mg/kg IV if absolutely needed (Plumb 2008). Most patients, however, will already be quiet and will not require preanesthetic treatment. Preoxygenation of the patient with 3–6 L/min oxygen via face mask should be performed for 5 minutes before induction.

Epidural opioid/local anesthetic combinations can be a highly effective tool and dramatically reduce or eliminate the need for general anesthesia. However, their use should be considered only if they can be performed quickly. In some circumstances, it may be faster to avoid their use. In nonpregnant patients, a local anesthetic (e.g.,

2% lidocaine or 0.5% bupivicaine) is administered at 1 mL/4.5 kg combined with preservative-free morphine at 0.1 mg/kg (Tranquilli 2004). Drug doses should be reduced by 50–75% in pregnant patients due to engorgement of the venous plexus, which makes the epidural space smaller.

Hemodynamically stable cats and dogs can be induced with propofol 1–6 mg/kg IV slowly titrated to effect (Plumb 2008). An alternative drug option is a slow titrated induction with alphaxalone 2–5 mg/kg IV in the cat or 2 mg/kg IV in dogs (Alfaxan Product Insert). Inhalant mask induction is not routinely recommended. Unstable patients can be induced with etomidate 0.5–2 mg/kg IV slowly (Plumb 2008). Diazepam or midazolam at 0.1–0.2 mg/kg IV should be administered prior to the etomidate if not already used as a premedication (Plumb 2008).

Following induction, patients should be immediately intubated with a cuffed endotracheal tube and placed on 100% oxygen. If inhalant anesthesia is not used, a propofol 0.1–0.4 mg/kg/min constant rate infusion (CRI) or alphaxalone 6–11 mg/kg/hr CRI is selected (Plumb 2008; (Jurox Pty Ltd 2006)). Patients should be placed in dorsal recumbency as little as possible. For many cases, this equates to the cesarean section being performed in lateral or dorsal-lateral recumbency. A line block with 0.5% bupivicaine or 2% lidocaine can be performed to help further reduce MAC and the need for additional anesthetics.

Once the neonates are removed, maternal analgesia must be provided if no analgesia was previously administered or if the drug has worn off (e.g., butorphanol). A dose of a pure mu agonist such as hydromorphone 0.1 mg/kg IV, IM will provide excellent analgesia for approximately 2–6 hours (Plumb 2008). If no contraindications exist, a single dose of a non-steroidal antiinflammatory drug (NSAID), such as meloxicam 0.2 mg/kg IV, is considered safe in an otherwise healthy dam (Plumb 2008). Postoperative analgesia can consist of buprenorphine 0.01–0.03 mg/kg IV, IM, q6–8h (Plumb 2008). Patients can be sent home with tramadol or transmucosal buprenorphine for small dogs and feline patients.

Resuscitation of the Newborn

For optimal support, a trained individual should be designated for each anticipated newborn. Upon removal from the uterus, puppies and kittens should initially have their airways cleared with gentle suction from a suction bulb to remove meconium and secretions. Oxygen should then be delivered by face mask; each newborn should be wrapped in warm dry towel and gently rubbed to stimulate breathing.

Puppies should never be swung because of the potential for cerebral hemorrhage from concussion and unintentional removal of pulmonary surfactant from the lungs (Figs. 28.2, 28.3). If breathing is labored or stridorous, the airway should be suctioned again. Newborns who are not breathing should be intubated with a 20–22 red rubber feeding tube or a 14–18 g IV catheter

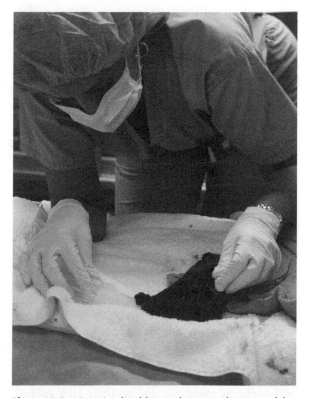

Figure 28.2. Puppies should never be swung because of the potential for cerebral hemorrhage from concussion and unintentional removal of pulmonary surfactant from the lungs.

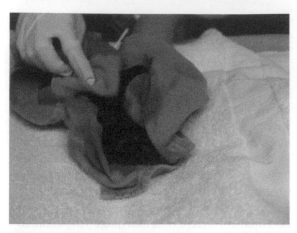

Figure 28.3 Upon removal from the uterus, each newborn should be wrapped in a warm dry towel and gently rubbed to stimulate breathing.

(stylet removed). If initial orotracheal intubation proves difficult, a retrograde intubation can be performed. Two initial breaths are then given. This is often sufficient to begin respirations. If it is not, intermittent positive pressure ventilation is continued at a rate of 8–12 breaths per minute. If the mother received opioids prior to uterus removal, newborns should receive 0.02 cc (1 drop) of naloxone sublingually (Tranquilli et al. 2007). Because it has been shown to increase cerebral oxygen demand, doxapram is no longer recommended for use in the newborn (Dani et al. 2006, Roll and Horsch 2004).

The acupuncture point GV26 (Jen Chung) can also be useful to stimulate respiration and may increase cerebral oxygen (Davies et al. 1984; Janssens et al. 1979). This point can be stimulated by inserting a regular 25 g needle or acupuncture needle into nasal philtrum and performing jabs in a hen-pecking motion.

Newborns with no palpable pulse should have their airway suctioned again and have external chest compressions started at a rate of 100–120/minute. If there is still no detectable heart beat, epinephrine 1:1000 can be considered sublingually every 3–5 minutes. Unlike in adult dog and cat resuscitation, atropine is unlikely to be of benefit in neonates due to their lack of full cardiac autonomic development (Fox 1966; Mace et al. 1983). Drugs such as vasopressin or

terlipressin may prove to be of additional benefit in neonatal resuscitation in future years (Matok et al. 2007).

Once newborns are stable, the umbilicus is ligated and disinfected and the puppies or kittens are placed in warm comfortable bedding until the mother is fully awake and able to nurse.

References

Dani, C, Bertini, G, Pezzati, M, et al. 2006. Brain hemodynamic effects of doxapram in preterm infants. Biol Neonate 89(2):69–74. Epub 2005 Sep 12.

Davies, A, Janse, J, Reynolds, GW. 1984. Acupuncture in the relief of respiratory arrest. NZ Vet J 32:109–110.

Fox, MW. 1966. Developmental physiology and behavior. In Canine Pediatrics, edited by Fox, MW, Himwich, WA. Springfield, MO: Charles C Thomas, pp. 22–25.

Funkquist, PM, Nyman, GC, Lofgren, AH, et al. 1997. Use of propofol-isoflurane as an anesthetic regimen for cesarean section in dogs. JAVMA 1 221(3):313–317.

Janssens, L, Altman, S, Rogers, PA. 1979. Respiratory and cardiac arrest under general anesthesia: Treatment by AP of the nasal philtrum. Vet Rec 105(12):273–276.

Jurox Pty Ltd, June 2006. Alfaxan drug insert, Rutherford, Australia.

Lunda, SP, Cassu, RN, Castro, GB, et al. 2004. Effects of four anesthetic protocols on the neurological and cardiorespiratory variable of puppies born by cesarean section. Vet Rec 27:154(13):387–389.

Mace, SE, Levy, MN. 1983. Neural control of heart rate: A comparison between puppies and adult animals. Pediatr Res 17:491–495.

Matok, L, Vardi, A, Augarten, A, et al. 2007. Beneficial effects of terlipressin in prolonged pediatric cardiopulmonary resuscitation: A case series. Crit Care Med 35(4):1161–1164.

McDonnel, W, Van Corder, I. 1982. Cardiopulmonary effects of xylazine/ketamine in dogs [Abstract]. In Annual

Scientific Meeting American College of Veterinary Anesthesiologist, Las Vegas, Nevada, 1982.

Moon, PF, Erb, HN, Ludders, JW, et al. 2000. Perioperative risk factors for puppies delivered by cesarean section in the United States and Canada. JAAHA 36(4):359–368.

Moon-Massat, PF, Erb, HN. 2002. Perioperative factors associated with puppy vigor after delivery by cesarean section. JAAHA 38(1):90–96.

Ngan Kee, WD, Khaw, KS, Lau, TK, et al. 2008. Randomized double-blinded comparison of phenylephrine vs ephedrine for maintaining blood pressure during spinal anesthesia for nonelective cesarean section. Anesthesia 63(12):1319–1326.

Plumb, DC. 2008. Veterinary Drug Handbook, 6th ed. Stockholm: PharmaVet Inc.

Polis, I, Gasthuys, F, Van Ham, L, Laevens, H. 2001. Recovery times and evaluation of clinical hemodynamic parameters of sevoflurane, isoflurane and halothane anesthesia in mongrel dogs. Am J Vet Res 62(4):555–560.

Roll, C, Horsch, S. 2004. Effects of doxapram on cerebral blood flow velocity in preterm infants. Neuropediatrics 35(2):126–129.

Tranquilli, WJ. 2004. Pain Management for the Small Animal Practitioner, 2nd ed. Jackson: Teton NewMedia, p. 37.

Tranquilli, WJ, Thurmon, JC, Grimm, KA. 2007. Lumb & Jones' Veterinary Anesthesia & Analgesia, 4th ed. Ames, IA: Wiley-Blackwell. pp. 955–965.

29
Anesthesia for Emergency Trauma Patients

Katy W. Waddell

This chapter is broken down into multiple sections as there are many different types of trauma patients that present to our hospitals in need of emergency anesthesia/analgesia support.

As with any trauma patient presented to triage, a thorough preoperative assessment must be performed and patient assessment begins with the first step inside the door. The traumatized patient will have altered physiological responses that will in turn alter the pharmacokinetics of the agents commonly used to provide anesthesia. Never labor under the assumption that the trauma patient was a previously healthy patient or that the patient arrives with an empty stomach. Many patients are presented with underlying preexisting physical conditions.

Trauma caused by any means creates pain, and each patient should be evaluated and managed as an individual due to the site/severity of injury received (Fig. 29.1). Trauma patients are unfortunate in the fact that administration of analgesics cannot be done preemptively for the original trauma, thus laying the course for developing "windup" pain. Always presume the trauma patient to be in pain and respect and handle your patient accordingly during the assessment and surgical preparatory period.

Ideally, anesthesia should not be initiated until vital organ function has been stabilized. Patients who have undergone severe trauma should be considered candidates for developing some type of shock. If possible, the goals of the triage team and nurse anesthetist should be the following:

1. Ensure that the airway is patent. Supplemental oxygen can be administered by flowby or via tight-fitting mask IF *it* does not cause stress and excitation.
2. Ventilation should be assessed by observing respiratory effort and chest excursions. Mucous membranes can be evaluated for color. Pulse oximetry can be used, if possible, to evaluate oxygen saturation. Frequently, multiple injuries to the respiratory system occur during thoracic trauma, but not all are immediately evident (pulmonary contusions).
3. Optimizing the physiological function of the cardiovascular system includes normalizing cardiac function and maintaining circulating volume in order to provide tissue perfusion and oxygen delivery to all vital organs. At least one large-bore catheter should be placed immediately for resuscitation pur-

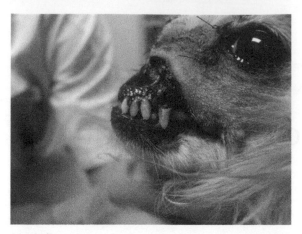

Figure 29.1.   A facial degloving injury.

poses. Administration of shock volume IV fluids should be with the goal of resuscitation of systolic blood pressure to a minimum of 90 mm Hg (Devey 2003). Attempts to stop blood loss must be made; losses should be replaced; and transfusions of whole blood, packed red blood cells, and/or plasma may be indicated. Once volume has been reestablished, the use of a positive inotrope may be considered to maintain cardiac output during anesthetic administration if necessary.

Monitoring patient vital signs should begin during triage and continue well through the postoperative recovery phase. Each patient will require continued evaluation based on its affected organ system or systems.

Types of Trauma

Ocular trauma

Common ocular traumas include proptosed globes, corneal lacerations, or foreign bodies. It is essential for any trauma patient that the cardiovascular system be stabilized prior to having general anesthesia induced. In addition, normal intraocular pressure must be preserved to avoid further damage to the affected eye. (Techniques

for ophthalmological procedures are discussed in Chapter 19.)

Tracheal trauma

Tracheal trauma, although not very common in small animals, can be caused by bite wounds, impaled objects, vehicular accidents, diagnostic procedures such as transtracheal wash, misguided jugular venipuncture attempts, over inflation of and/or excessive movement of endotracheal tubes while in the trachea (especially in the feline patient and during dentistry procedures), and improper use of rigid stylets during endotracheal intubation (Fig. 29.2).

Crushing or nonpenetrating wounds may be caused by blunt force trauma or choke collars. These patients may present with subcuticular emphysema or in a state of collapse and cyanosis if there is sufficient obstruction of the airway. While a rapid prep is performed for a tracheostomy, oxygen may be delivered by inserting a large-bore catheter or needle directly into the lumen of the trachea distal to the obstruction. Injuries not causing life-threatening obstructive compromise may be stabilized and supplemented with oxygen via a tight-fitting mask or oxygen hood if the patient's overall assessment indicates that there is no current or preexisting organ dysfunction and if the patient is not in an anxious state due to the stress of attempting to ventilate adequately.

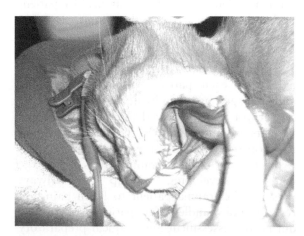

Figure 29.2   A cat with an impaled object in the pharynx.

Thoracic trauma

Approximately one-third of the patients with blunt forelimb or hindlimb trauma additionally incur thoracic injury. Pulmonary lesions usually continue to worsen within 24–36 hours. Thoracic traumas include the following:

1. **Pulmonary contusions:** Hypoxia often results from severe contusions as a result of ventilation/perfusion (V/Q) mismatch. Overzealous treatment of blood volume restoration may lead to pulmonary edema and a further decrease of lung function (Clutton 2007; Tello 2006).
2. **Emphysematous bulla:** These lesions should be suspected and ventilation should be with low tidal volumes with peak inspiratory pressure (PIP) <12 cm H_2O and a higher rate to maintain minute volume.
3. **Hemothorax:** Hemothorax indicates blood in the pulmonary spaces. Aspiration of the thoracic cavity can/should be performed to get the fluid off of the lungs. These patients often desaturate as the blood impedes lung space. Hemothorax may result from rib fractures.
4. **Pneumothorax:** Aspiration of the thoracic cavity should be performed to allow for normalization of intrapleural pressure. Nitrous oxide should not be used with patients with known pneumothorax. Ventilation should be of lower tidal volume and a higher frequency.
5. **Diaphragmatic hernia:** A diaphragmatic hernia vastly reduces the available space for proper lung inflation due to abdominal organs entering the chest cavity. If possible, elevate the patient to at least a 30° incline to help relieve lung compression and provide oxygen supplementation, especially while anesthetized and during recovery. Placing the patient in dorsal recumbency often exacerbates desaturation—be prepared. These patients often need intensive ventilatory support under anesthesia depending on the severity of the lesion.
6. **Fractured ribs:** Caution must be taken to prevent additional injury to the lungs by patient manipulation. Intercostal blocks using bupivicaine will provide analgesia and aid in hypoventilation due to pain postoperatively.

Preoxygenation of any patient with known or suspected pulmonary lesions can be achieved with a tight-fitting mask and should ideally be left on for 5 minutes prior to induction. Even flow by oxygen is advantageous if the patient is stressed by a mask. Small dogs and cats in severe respiratory distress may decompensate even with minimal handling. The use of an oxygen cage or an induction chamber while gathering the necessary supplies to immediately capture the airway will provide an oxygen rich environment.

Burn injuries/smoke inhalation

The presence of soot in the nostrils, facial burning and dyspnea should hasten the responder's effort to initiate lifesaving measures. The immediate concerns with these patients will be protection of the airway, venous access, fluid resuscitation, and pain management. A sterile endotracheal tube (low pressure high volume cuff) lubricated with sterile lidocaine gel should be used. Propofol, thiopental, etomidate, benzodiazepines, and inhalant agents do not provide any analgesia. Patients should be provided with 100% oxygen at the earliest possible moment. Pain management could include adjunctive agents such as lidocaine and ketamine along with an opioid. Opioids can cause dose-dependent respiratory depression so careful monitoring is necessary following administration.

Burn patients are often presented with the additional trauma of smoke inhalation. Dermal burns seen in human medicine appear to have inflammatory cells sequester in the lungs thus causing more pulmonary edema than simple smoke inhalation (Carrol and Martin 2007). Regardless of the extent and severity of the burns, once the primary patient survey has been completed analgesia should be provided (Fig. 29.3). These patients should always be assessed while providing supplemental oxygen, and the

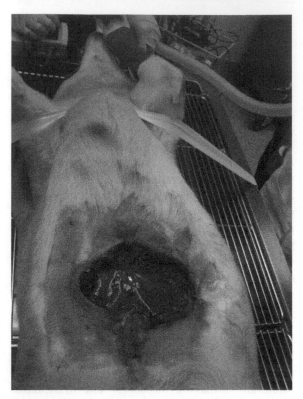

Figure 29.3 Full body wall thickness burn. This injury could have been caused by a surgery light with the wrong type of bulb installed.

necessary equipment to capture the airway should be nearby in case sudden need arises.

Hypovolemia in these patients is due to the fluid loss at the site of injury as well as vasoconstriction. Keep in mind that with the fluid loss, decreased protein contributes not only to decreased oncotic pressure but renders greater availability of the analgesic agents because the majority of the agents used are protein bound. It is ideal to start with 1/4 to 1/2 dose of the agent and titrate to effect.

Blunt force trauma

Blunt force abdominal trauma may involve several organs as in splenic/liver ruptures, kidney/ bladder rupture or avulsion or bowel perforation.

Penetrating wounds are more easily recognized but do not always reveal the damage to underlying body systems. Impaled objects should be stabilized until the patient has been fully evaluated, and body systems should be supported until diagnostics have been performed.

Bite wounds can cause penetrating wounds as well as crushing/tearing injuries. Bite wounds may actually penetrate a body cavity, thus allowing a portal for bacterial infection.

Before premedicating any trauma patient, take into consideration the analgesic agents previously administered during the triage/assessment period, the cardiovascular stability of the patient and the effect of the agent on all body systems. As previously mentioned, the trauma patient may require decreased dosages of analgesics due to altered physiological response. Titrating to effect is usually the best plan. Consider the procedure to be performed and the anticipated pain associated with the surgery when making drug selections. Anesthesia should be designed to incorporate multiple agents, thus decreasing the adverse effects of any sole agent. Ideally, these agents should have the ability to be antagonized or reversed should the need arise. The goal with premedication should be to provide analgesia as well as decrease the amount of induction agent required.

Anticholinergics may or may not be indicated and should not be "routine" because there is no "routine" with a traumatized individual. Anticholinergics will increase heart rate, thus increasing cardiac workload and oxygen consumption. If there is an underlying systolic dysfunction, an anticholinergic can decrease myocardial perfusion by decreasing diastolic filling time due to an increased heart rate.

Agents capable of increasing intracranial/ intraocular pressure such as ketamine should be avoided in those patients with cranial and or ocular trauma.

Induction Agents

In many fragile trauma patients a neuroleptanalgesic may be the best option for induction (Table 29.1). Combining an opioid with a benzodiazepine tranquilizer provides a safe, titratable pro-

Table 29.1. Induction agents.

Drug	Dosage	Route	
Thiopental	18–20 mg/kg	IV	Unpremedicated
	6–12 mg/kg	IV	Premedicated
Propofol	6–10 mg/kg	IV	Unpremedicated
	4–6 mg/kg	IV	Premedicated
Etomidate	3 mg/kg	IV	Unpremedicated
	1–2 mg/kg	IV	Premedicated

Paddleford 1999; Clutton 2007.

tocol that is gentle on the cardiovascular and pulmonary systems. Many critical patients can be intubated under this protocol in a calm, quiet atmosphere. Both the opioid and the benzodiazepine can be antagonized if necessary. At the very least, a neuroleptanalgesic technique will drastically reduce the amount of additional induction agent needed to get the patient intubated. If additional drug is needed, a low dose of propofol may be added to allow for intubation. Propofol can cause profound respiratory depression and/or apnea and can cause myocardial depression and subsequent decrease in cardiac output and arterial blood pressure. Propofol's side effects must be considered prior to its use.

In patients where increased intracranial pressure and /or tachycardia is not a concern, ketamine/diazepam can provide some indirect cardiovascular support as well as some adjunctive analgesic from the ketamine.

An ultra–short-acting thiobarbiturate, thiopental does not provide any analgesia, can cause profound respiratory depression, decreases myocardial contractility, and is not recommended in patients with existing volume depletion, cardiovascular disease, or hemodynamically unstable patients.

Etomidate, an ultra–short-acting hypnotic agent, does not provide any analgesia; does not depress myocardial activity; maintains heart rate, contractility, and blood pressure; and produces only a mild to moderate respiratory depression which is dose-dependent. Recovery in unpremedicated patients may be accompanied by excitation and myoclonus (twitching, tremors). It is advisable to combine a benzodiazepine or opioid with etomidate for induction to reduce such adverse reactions for short procedures and reduce the volume of etomidate required for induction. Table 29.2 summarizes dosages for parenteral opioids.

Case Report

Signalment: Dexter, a 4.9 kg, 2-year-old, intact male Chihuahua

Presenting complaint: HBDT (hit by dump truck)

Pertinent history: previously healthy dog, current on vaccinations and heartworm negative.

Current medications: None.

Physical examination: Dexter was presented with tachycardia (HR 202), tachypnea (RR70), and a body temperature of 97 °F. His femoral pulses were of poor quality, mucous membranes were pale with a capillary refill time (CRT) of 3 seconds. Three disruptions of the ventral abdominal body wall were noted. Crepitus was palpated in the pelvic limbs.

Initial assessment: Presumed pulmonary contusions, pelvic limb fractures, ruptured bladder and/or urethral avulsion, strangulated testicle, and hypotension. Anemia was presumed and probably due to hemorrhage in the multiple trauma sites.

Interventions: IV access with a peripheral venous catheter, crystalloid resuscitation at shock dose (90 mL/kg), oxymorphone to start, and fentanyl CRI for analgesia. Dexter's vital signs were monitored hourly and active rewarming was provided with a forced warm air blanket.

Diagnostics: Pelvic radiographs revealed left femoral head and neck fracture, ilial fracture, and a right-sided sacroilial luxation. Thoracic radiographs revealed no immediately apparent pulmonary contusions, pneumothorax, or bulla, and an intact diaphragm. Abdominal radiographs showed a small liver, small bladder, and a fluid line within the abdomen. An abdomino-

Table 29.2 Parenteral opioids.

Drug	Dosage	Route	Frequency
Butorphanol	0.2–0.4 mg/kg	IV, IM, SQ,	2–3 hr
	1 mg/kg	PO	2–3 hr
Buprenorphine	7–14 mcg/kg	IV, IM, SQ	4–6 hr
Hydromorphone	0.05–0.2 mg/kg	IV, IM, SQ	4 hr
Oxymorphone	0.05–0.2 mg/kg	IV, IM, SQ	4–6 hr
Fentanyl	2–5 mcg/kg	IV, IM	20–40 min
	2–5 mcg/kg/hr	CRI	
Nonopioid adjunctive parenteral drugs			
Ketamine	0.5–2 mg/kg	IV	20–30 min
	2–10 mcg/kg/min	CRI	
Lidocaine 2%	2 mg/kg	IV	10 min half life
w/o epi	20–50 mcg/kg/min	CRI	
Midazolam	8 mcg/kg/min	CRI	

Grubb 2008; Clutton 2007; Devey 2003; Paddleford 1999.

centesis was performed and the fluid was determined to be urine. A lead II ECG revealed a normal sinus rhythm with an increased rate. Stat lab work revealed a decrease in packed cell volume, normal white blood cell count and platelets. The chemistry panel showed values within normal limits.

Anesthesia plan: Dexter was currently receiving a fentanyl CRI at 3 mcg/kg/hr in the ICU. Due to Dexter's continued elevated heart rate, I added lidocaine as a CRI preoperatively at 25 mcg/kg/min as an adjunct to analgesia. The lidocaine CRI was started an hour prior to his induction because he was scheduled to be started on a fresh frozen plasma infusion due to an abnormal coagulation profile. If there had not been a delay in induction, a lidocaine bolus would have been administered calculated at 1–2 mg/kg to be given IV over a 2-minute period just prior to administering his induction agents. As it was, I considered the two CRIs (fentanyl and lidocaine) to be his premedicants. An arterial catheter was placed in the dorsal pedal artery to monitor direct blood pressure. This was achieved

comfortably in Dexter's cage after a 0.1 mL lidocaine "bleb" was injected over his metatarsal area following the initial clip and prep of the area. Induction and intubation was achieved using a combination of diazepam at 0.2 mg/kg IV, followed by etomidate calculated at 1 mg/kg IV and titrated to effect. He was then placed on oxygen and sevoflurane inhalant for anesthetic maintenance.

Intraoperative intervention: Dexter was placed on a ventilator to provide intermittent positive pressure ventilation (IPPV) to protect against hypoventilation and control tidal volume. Active warming was provided by a forced warm air blanket. A positive inotrope (dobutamine) was prepared to provide blood pressure support and administered dependent on arterial blood pressure readings. Packed red blood cells were administered at a rate of 8 mL/kg/hr to compensate for blood loss into the abdomen, scrotum, and muscle tissue due to trauma. Fresh frozen plasma was continued at a rate of 4 mL/kg/hr to assist in supporting oncotic pressure as well. Dexter's blood pressure continued to be low;

vasopressin was started calculated at 0.0015 mcg/kg/min CRI, the fentanyl CRI was increased from 3 mcg/kg to 4 mcg/kg in order that the inhalant agent sevoflurane could be decreased from 2.5% to 1.5% (MAC in the canine being 2.35%) to help allay the potent peripheral vasodilation effects of the inhalant. Analgesia continued to be a challenge despite intermittent boluses of oxymorphone, as was evidenced by Dexter's repeated "bucking" of the ventilator. An arterial blood gas sample done at this time showed adequate ventilation was being provided: pH—7.31, $PaCO_2$—43.0, and PaO_2—423.9. Midazolam was added as a CRI calculated at 8 mcg/kg/min. The addition of midazolam as a CRI in conjuction with fentanyl will assist with the multimodal approach of anesthesia and analgesia. A combination of a benzodiazepine and an opioid is considered a neuroleptic combination.

Intraoperative monitoring: ECG, arterial blood pressure, end-tidal CO_2, SpO_2, body temperature, esophageal stethoscope. Vital signs were recorded every 5 minutes with the exception of body temperature, which was noted every 15 minutes.

Body systems supported: Pulmonary function (pulmonary contusions presumed), renal perfusion protected based on arterial blood pressure to be no lower than a mean of 60 mg with dobutamine and vasopressin support. Vascular support was provided by administration of crystalloids, packed red blood cells, fresh frozen plasma. Initial fluid rate of 10 mL/kg/hr the first hour and decreasing to 5 mL/kg/hr the second hour. All products were calculated in the total fluid volume to prevent volume overload.

Anesthetic drug choices were dictated by Dexter's ASA status of IV/emergency:

1. Diazepam is a Class IV controlled substance, which acts as an anxiolytic, muscle relaxant, hypnotic and anticonvulsant. It provides no analgesia unless used with an opioid to produce neuroleptanalgesia.
2. Etomidate is an ultra–short-acting hypnotic. It undergoes rapid hepatic metabolism, resulting in rapid recovery and lack of accumulation when used as repeated boluses. It also produces no change in heart rate, arterial blood pressure or myocardial performance. It can induce transient respiratory depression/apnea, sneezing, retching, and myoclonic twitching as side effects. *Note*: it inhibits adrenocortical function for up to 6 hours postadministration (Plumb 2005).
3. Sevoflurane was selected as the inhalant because of the rapidity of induction and recovery. It does cause myocardial depression and vasodilation. It also causes respiratory depression. The severity of the myocardial depression, vasodilation, and respiratory depression are dose-dependent.
4. Fentanyl is a Class II controlled substance and a short-acting pure opiate agonist. It possesses minimal cardiovascular effects except a vagally mediated bradycardia that is responsive to anticholinergics. It causes profound respiratory depression at high doses. It has a rapid onset (within 1 minute) and short duration of 15–30 minutes. It can be given by bolus or as a CRI. The sedative effects can be reversed if necessary by administering nalbuphine or butorphanol, or it may be totally reversed by using naloxone. Recent studies have shown fentanyl administered as a CRI for greater than 60 minutes can have a cumulative effect (Clutton 2007).
5. Lidocaine 2% as a CRI has been shown to be a useful adjunct to anesthesia by having a MAC-sparing effect, reported to range between 19 and 43% reductions in the canine, thereby allowing the anesthetist to decrease the amount of inhalant (Clutton 2007; Pascoe 2007). I have had good success in abdominal procedures giving an initial bolus of 1 mg/kg IV and starting a CRI of 25 mcg/kg/min. It has rapid onset and a short half-life of 20 minutes to 2 hours. In abdominal procedures it is also used as a prokinetic to enhance gut motility (Devey 2003). It is metabolized by the liver and excreted by the kidneys. Use cautiously in those patients with liver disease, shock, or hypovolemia. Lidocaine provides protection against cytokines and free radials during reperfusion injuries. Do not use in patients with severe SA or AV heart block or in patients with other bradyarrhythmias with VPCs. Toxic

IV dose for most species is 10–20 mg/kg. Any bradycardic rhythm showing premature ventricular beats may actually be unrecognized junctional or escape beats. These may be thought of as rescue beats in those patients with SA or AV blocks (Clutton 2007).

6. Midazolam, a benzodiazepine, was used in addition to the fentanyl as a CRI to produce neuroleptanalgesia.

Surgical procedures included in the exploratory laparotomy included repair of three ventral abdominal wall hernias, reattachment of the avulsed urethra, indwelling urinary catheter placement, and castration due to the devitalized testicle. The pelvic limb fractures were scheduled to be addressed 3 days post–soft-tissue repair to give Dexter a chance to stabilize as they were not considered to be life threatening.

Recovery: Even though at this time there were no definitive signs of pulmonary contusions radiographically, due to Dexter's small size and the extent of his injuries, it was deemed advisable to provide oxygen supplementation by a single nasal cannula. Analgesia was continued with fentanyl and lidocaine CRIs. ICU continued crystalloid fluid therapy utilizing lactated Ringer's® solution with potassium supplementation. The arterial catheter was maintained to monitor ventilation via arterial blood gases during the first 24 hours.

References

Carroll, GL, Martin, DD. 2007. Veterinary Anesthesia and Analgesia, 3rd ed., Lumb & Jones' Veterinary Anesthesia and Analgesia, edited by Tranquilli, W, Thurmon, J, Grimm, K, Ames, IA: Blackwell Publishing.

Clutton, RE. 2007. BSAVA Manual of Canine and Feline Anaesthesia and Analgesia, 2nd ed., edited by Seymour, C, Duke-Novakovski, T. Gloucester: BSAVA.

Devey, JJ. 2003. Trauma Surgery and Pain Management. Proceedings of the 9th IVECCS, 2003.

Grubb, Tamara. 2008. Small Animal Anesthesia and Analgesia, edited by Carroll, G. Ames, IA: Blackwell Publishing.

Paddleford, RR. 1999. Manual of Small Animal Anesthesia, 2nd ed. Philadelphia: WB Saunders Company.

Pascoe, PJ. 2007. BSAVA Manual of Canine and Feline Anaesthesia and Analgesia, 2nd ed, edited by Seymour, C, Duke-Novakovski, T. Gloucester: BSAVA.

Plumb, DC. 2005. Plumb's Veterinary Drug Handbook, 5th ed. Ames, IA: Blackwell Publishing.

Tello, LH. 2006 Clinical Management in Thoracic Trauma. Proceedings of the 2006 World Congress WSAVA/FECAVA/CSAVA.

Anesthesia for Nontrauma Emergency Patients

30

Ami Gilkey

In the case of dogs and cats presented to emergency care for nontraumatic conditions, initial assessment of the patient should be quick but thorough to address any immediate stabilization requirements. The veterinarian first evaluates cardiovascular and respiratory function to determine whether the patient has adequate circulation, oxygenation, ventilation, and tissue perfusion. Neurological status should also be evaluated, but this can be difficult depending on the patient's mentation on initial presentation. The veterinary team then can perform a more meticulous physical examination, gather a detailed history, and collect blood samples to analyze following stabilization of the patient (Syring and Drobatz 2000; Ford and Mazzaferro 2006). Analyzed blood results will indicate the patient's acid-base status, any electrolyte imbalances, and other abnormalities that need to be corrected. With this information and other indicated diagnostic tests, the veterinarian can make an initial diagnosis and proceed with a treatment plan. Many of these emergency patients will require anesthesia for a surgical procedure or other diagnostic test to address their current disease or condition.

The patient must be stabilized as much as possible before an anesthetic event due to the fact that anesthetic agents do have profound effects on an already debilitated animal (Battaglia 2001). An anesthetic regimen needs to take into consideration the current condition of the animal as well as the procedure to be performed.

This chapter focuses on anesthetic considerations of several diseases that require emergency procedures.

Shock

Shock is a condition of poor tissue perfusion from inadequate circulating blood volume. The result is decreased oxygen delivery to the tissues; ultimately, the oxygen requirements of the cells are not met (Ford and Mazzaferro 2006; Day and Bateman 2006). Patients can exhibit signs of tachycardia, tachypnea, pale mucous membranes, prolonged capillary refill time, hypothermia, hypotension, and depressed mentation. Laboratory blood work findings can include hypoglycemia, hypoalbuminemia, azotemia, acid-base disorders, and electrolyte imbalances. Types of shock include cardiogenic, hypovolemic, and septic (Ford and Mazzaferro 2006; Macintire et al. 2005).

In cardiogenic shock, the heart is no longer an effective pump because of heart disease or arrhythmias, thus leading to decreased cardiac output. Hypovolemic shock occurs due to acute hemorrhage, severe dehydration, or third space loss of fluids (Day and Bateman 2006). Septic shock with systemic inflammatory response syndrome results from known infections or the presence of toxins in the bloodstream. Early signs of septic shock can include dark pink to red mucous membrane color and decreased capillary refill time (Macintire et al. 2005).

Resuscitation of shock patients must include restoration of tissue perfusion and oxygen delivery (Syring and Drobatz 2000). Intravenous fluids are an important part of this process, but the type of fluid (crystalloid, blood product, or synthetic colloid) and rate of delivery are dependent upon the type of shock and the underlying disease present (Day and Bateman 2006). Once the veterinary team begins to stabilize the patient, the anesthetist can proceed with an anesthetic protocol.

Debilitated shock patients may not require any premedications. Acepromazine should be avoided because it causes vasodilation and hypotension, further compromising the animal's cardiovascular status (Plumb 2005). The patient should receive oxygenation via face mask or flowby prior to anesthetic induction to offer some protection against hypoxia (Ford and Mazzaferro 2006; Carroll 2003). Rapid induction may be done with an opioid and benzodiazepine combination, where the anesthetist initially gives a low dose of an opioid (oxymorphone 0.05 mg/kg IV or fentanyl 5–10 µg/kg IV) followed by either midazolam or diazepam (0.2 mg/kg IV). If intubation is not possible, additional amounts may be given to facilitate intubation. Etomidate (1.0–2.0 mg/kg IV titrated to effect) is also suitable as an induction agent because of its cardiovascular sparing properties (Kruse-Elliott 2008). One side effect seen with etomidate is myoclonus, but this can be minimized by first administering diazepam (0.1–0.2 mg/kg IV) (Carroll 2003). Ketamine (5 mg/kg IV) combined with diazepam (0.25 mg/kg IV) titrated to effect may also be used for induction. Once intubated, the patient is transitioned to inhalant anesthesia with isoflurane or sevoflurane. An anticholinergic is administered if bradycardia is present (glycopyrrolate 0.01 mg/kg IV or atropine 0.02 mg/kg IV); however, it should be noted that increasing the heart rate will increase the oxygen demand of the myocardial tissue (Carroll 2003).

Monitoring of the patient during anesthesia should include blood pressure, blood gas and electrolyte analysis, pulse oximetry, capnography, and ECG. The anesthetist evaluates pulse quality, mucous membrane color, and capillary refill time (CRT) as well. If available, direct arterial blood pressure measurements will provide the anesthetist with continuous readings; otherwise, blood pressure can be measured by indirect methods every 2 to 3 minutes. Hypotension is addressed by providing fluid replacement to restore intravascular volume or by giving inotropic support (dopamine or dobutamine 2–10 µg/kg/min IV). If the patient is hypoalbuminemic, a colloid such as hetastarch or plasma can provide intravascular volume expansion with oncotic and blood pressure support (Day and Bateman 2006).

For animals with hyperkalemia, 0.9% sodium chloride is an appropriate fluid choice because it does not contain any additional potassium (Fossum 2007). If the patient is hypokalemic, addition of potassium to the IV fluids may not be necessary during surgery, but if administered, it should be given with fluids through a separate IV catheter from the main fluid line and delivered via infusion pump. If potassium is administered too quickly, as when giving a bolus of fluids, the patient could die. Postoperative maintenance fluid therapy with addition of potassium (not to exceed 0.5 mEq/kg/hr) and with concurrent electrolyte monitoring is another treatment option (Pettifer 2003).

Metabolic acidosis may occur in the patient with shock. If it is due to poor perfusion, fluids given to restore perfusion may resolve the acidosis (Day and Bateman 2006). If the pH is less than 7.2, sodium bicarbonate may be given to increase the pH. The calculation used is: sodium bicarbonate needed (mEq) = 0.3 × base deficit × body weight (kg). Slowly give approximately one-quarter to one-half of the calculated dose intravenously, and repeat a blood gas analysis in 30 minutes to evaluate the effect on blood pH (Carroll 2003).

It is important to monitor the patient's ventilatory status as well. End-tidal carbon dioxide (ETCO$_2$) measured with a capnograph can help approximate the level of partial pressure of arterial blood carbon dioxide (PaCO$_2$) (Kruse-Elliott 2003). Increases in PaCO$_2$ can result in respiratory acidosis, so the anesthetist must be sure adequate ventilation is provided by either manual or mechanical means (Muir et al. 2007).

Electrolyte imbalances, poor perfusion, hypoxemia, and anemia can contribute to cardiac arrythmias. Ventricular tachycardia and ventricular premature contractions (VPCs) can be associated with severe shock (Day 2003). Continuous ECG analysis is invaluable during resuscitation and during the anesthetic period and displays any life-threatening changes that may require intervention.

Patients in shock should receive adequate analgesia to counter any detrimental responses to pain such as decreased ventilation or tachycardia. Providing heat to the hypothermic animal is crucial throughout the perianesthetic event and can be accomplished by using a forced-air warming blanket (Bair Hugger®, Arizant Inc., Eden Prairie, MN), circulating warm water blanket (Carroll 2003), and IV fluids warmed to body temperature before administration. Avoid electrical heating blankets due to the potential for severe thermal burns.

Postoperatively, good nursing care and diligent monitoring of the patient is essential so that any potential problems can be detected and treated as quickly as possible.

Gastric Dilatation-Volvulus (GDV)

GDV is a syndrome that affects mostly large-breed, deep-chested, older dogs. The exact cause is unknown, but contributing factors can include eating only one large meal daily, exercising shortly after eating, and gulping its food, and thus air along with it (Hedlund and Fossum 2007; Monnet 2003). GDV is characterized by stomach distention and clockwise rotation. This disease is considered a surgical emergency. The stomach fills with air, becoming increasingly enlarged (dilatation) with concurrent clockwise rotation around the distal esophagus (volvulus) (Rasmussen 2003). The animal is commonly presented with nonproductive retching, restlessness, pain, ptyalism, dyspnea, and distention and tympany of the abdomen. It also may be depressed (Aronson et al. 2000). Because of the many physiological parameters this disease can affect, the GDV patient is commonly presented in severe cardiovascular shock (Macintire et al. 2005; Monnet 2003). Members of the veterinary team commonly place a large-bore cephalic or jugular vein catheter and begin fluid therapy immediately. Fluids administered through a catheter in a lateral saphenous vein are not recommended prior to stomach decompression because the distended stomach occludes the caudal vena cava thus venous return is restricted (Aronson et al. 2000; Macintire et al. 2005). A combination of crystalloids and synthetic colloids are given for fluid resuscitation and hemodynamic stability (Monnet 2003). Abdominal radiographs taken of the patient will show the gas filled stomach and the dorsal displacement of the pylorus (Aronson et al. 2000).

The stomach must be decompressed, and this process can be facilitated by two preoperative methods. The first involves passing an orogastric tube to release the trapped gas. The tube is first measured against the dog for length from the nose to the xiphoid process or last rib. The tube is then well lubricated and passed into the esophagus (Aiello 1998; Ford and Mazzaferro 2006). If the dog is resistant or in pain, it can be sedated with butorphanol (0.2–0.4 mg/kg IV) or hydromorphone (0.05–0.1 mg/kg IV) in combination with diazepam or midazolam (0.1–0.2 mg/kg IV) to facilitate the passing of the tube. Because side effects of morphine include vomiting and histamine release resulting in possible hypotension (Paddleford 1999), it should be avoided in the GDV patient. If tube placement is unsuccessful, the veterinarian can place a trocar or large bore needle through the abdominal wall into the stomach to release some gas. The spleen may be engorged or displaced by the distended stomach,

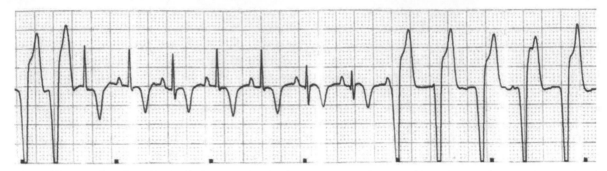

Figure 30.1.   Lead II, speed 25 mm/sec. ECG showing VPC and sinus rhythm with transition to slow ventricular tachycardia.

so careful palpation of the abdomen before tro-carization is essential to avoid splenic puncture (Aiello 1998). The veterinarian will then perform an exploratory celiotomy to decompress and reposition the stomach, and perform a perma-nent gastropexy (Hedlund and Fossum 2007).

Many possible complications need to be con-sidered when formulating an anesthetic regimen for the animal with GDV. The abdomen is dis-tended and restricts movement of the diaphragm and thorax. As a result, functional residual capacity and tidal volume are decreased, causing hypoventilation and hypoxemia (Jacobson et al. 1995). It also results in an increase of CO_2 leading to respiratory acidosis, further com-pounding the metabolic acidosis already present (Rasmussen 2003). The $PaCO_2$ is monitored with blood gas analysis or approximated with capnographic $ETCO_2$ readings (Haskins 1999). Manual or mechanical ventilation is necessary to improve the ventilatory status of the patient (Rasmussen 2003).

The bloated and torsed stomach compresses the caudal vena cava and the portal vein, which decreases the amount of venous blood returned to the heart. This in turn can negatively affect cardiac output and arterial blood pressure (Rasmussen 2003). Tissue perfusion is ultimately compromised, including perfusion to the already compromised organs (Hedlund and Fossum 2007). The anesthetist must monitor arterial blood pressure to ensure adequate tissue perfu-sion during surgery. Blood pressure can also decline during surgical manipulation of the spleen and torsed stomach. Aggressive fluid

administration combined with inotropic agents such as dobutamine or dopamine (2–10 μm/kg/min IV) are used to support blood pressure.

Gastric ischemia can lead to the breakdown of the gastric mucosa, leading to tissue necrosis of the stomach. Bacteria and endotoxins can enter the circulation through the compromised tissue precipitating septic shock to an already cardiovascular-compromised patient (Monnet 2003). If gastric perforation occurs, peritonitis may exacerbate the problem.

Electrolyte imbalances, hypoxemia, and inad-equate myocardial perfusion can lead to cardiac arrythmias in the patient with GDV (Evans and Wilson 2007). The most common arrythmias observed are ventricular tachycardia and ven-tricular premature complexes (VPCs) (Rasmussen 2003). Multifocal VPCs and sustained ventricu-lar tachycardia should be addressed and often respond to lidocaine (2.0 mg/kg IV bolus fol-lowed by 25–75 μg/kg/min IV CRI) (Fig. 30.1). Procainamide (2–10 mg/kg IV given slowly, fol-lowed by 20–50 μg/kg/min IV CRI) is used if the arrythmias are unresponsive to lidocaine. Arrythmias may persist for many hours postop-eratively and must be monitored and corrected if they result in decreased cardiac output and poor tissue perfusion (Hedlund and Fossum 2007).

Regurgitation and aspiration of stomach con-tents are complications of the treatments for GDV dogs. When passing the orogastric tube pre- or intraoperatively and when the surgeon manipulates the stomach during surgery, fluid and food material can drain around the orogastric tube into the pharynx and into the trachea. The contents can be accidentally aspirated or even leak past the inflated cuff of the endotracheal tube. Aspiration leads to infection, edema, and inflammation of the airways. If this happens during anesthesia, the anesthetist must check the cuff to be sure it is properly inflated. The oropharyngeal area is flushed with water or saline and suctioned until all fluids are clear and no stomach contents remain. This can be done during surgery as well as recovery to assure that all fluids are removed prior to extubation (Rasmussen 2003).

Rapid induction and intubation of the patient for anesthesia can be facilitated by different drug protocols. Ketamine (5 mg/kg) combined with diazepam (0.25 mg/kg) can be titrated intravenously to effect. Diazepam (0.1–0.2 mg/kg IV) followed by etomidate (1.0–2.0 mg/kg IV) can also be used. Another induction option is lidocaine followed by thiopental. Lidocaine (2.0 mg/kg IV) is given first, and then thiopental (9 mg/kg IV) is titrated to effect. Either isoflurane or sevoflurane is used as the inhalant to maintain a surgical plane of anesthesia.

Intraoperative and postoperative analgesia is provided by hydromorphone or oxymorphone (0.05–0.1 mg/kg IV for either drug), administered as needed (usually every 4–6 hours). If arrhythmias persist following extubation, the ECG should be monitored and a lidocaine or procainamide CRI is continued. Postoperative monitoring and correction of electrolyte, fluid, and acid-base imbalances are also recommended (Aronson et al. 2000; Hedlund and Fossum 2007). Oxygen therapy via nasal cannula or face mask is used if the patient becomes hypoxic during recovery (Jacobson et al. 1995).

Foreign Bodies and Obstructions

Dogs and cats indiscriminately eat objects such as bones, rocks, sticks, strings, clothing, carpet, fish hooks, needles, and coins. These objects can become lodged in the pharynx or trachea; under the tongue; or in the esophagus, stomach, or small intestine, causing partial or complete obstructions. Systemic toxicities can also develop from ingested objects containing lead or zinc. In addition, intraluminal intestinal obstructions can also be the result of an intussusception or neoplasia (Macintire et al. 2005).

Airway obstructions can cause severe respiratory distress and anxiety. The increased respiratory effort and decreased heat exchange through respiration can lead to hyperthermia, and inadequate ventilation can lead to hypercapnia (Perkowski 2000). Inflammation of tissues surrounding the object can cause further complications. The administration of acepromazine (0.005–0.05 mg/kg IV, IM) can decrease anxiety and sedate the patient in order to provide oxygen via face mask or with flowby oxygen (Ford and Mazzaferro 2006). Be aware that acepromazine causes vasodilation, which can affect blood pressure, especially in patients under anesthesia. It is also not reversible.

Establishing a patent airway is top priority when presented with a patient having an upper airway obstruction. This is achieved by endotracheal intubation or by emergency tracheostomy, if required, in order to bypass the obstruction (Ludwig 2000; Syring and Drobatz 2000). Thiopental (12–15 mg/kg IV) or propofol (4–6 mg/kg IV) is given slowly in small, incremental doses to allow intubation and visualization of the foreign body.

Once the airway is secured and oxygen is delivered, the clinician can locate and remove the object and further evaluate any tissue damage via tracheoscopy. It is important to monitor the patient's oxygen saturation and ventilatory status throughout this procedure and provide manual ventilation if the oxygen saturation level drops below acceptable reference ranges (Ford and Mazzaferro 2006).

Recovery complications include possible respiratory distress due to occlusion of the airway secondary to tissue swelling (Hedlund 2007b). The anesthetist should monitor the patient for signs of respiratory depression and, if painful during recovery, butorphanol (0.2–0.4 mg/kg IM) or buprenorphine (5–15 µg/kg IM) is administered.

Animals with esophageal foreign bodies can show signs of retching, gagging, ptyalism, and food regurgitation (Aronson et al. 2000). Thoracic radiographs and contrast esophagrams are used to locate the foreign body and identify thoracic complications (i.e., pneumothorax or pneumomediastinum) secondary to an esophageal perforation. An esophagoscopy is performed to identify the foreign body and attempt to remove it. If the patient requires initial sedation, the anesthetist can administer acepromazine (0.02–0.05 mg/kg IV, IM). For rapid induction, thiopental (12–15 mg/kg IV) or propofol (6 mg/kg IV) is titrated to effect to allow for intubation followed by inhalant anesthesia (isoflurane or sevoflurane) (Kyles 2003).

The clinician should attempt to pull out the object with grasping forceps or, if necessary, advance the object into the stomach for dissolution by gastric acid or retrieval via gastrotomy (Macintire et al. 2005). If bradycardia develops during the endoscopy, glycopyrrolate (0.01 mg/kg IV) or atropine (0.02 mg/kg IV) can be given.

If endoscopic extraction of the object is successful, the patient will have discomfort or pain from the manipulation of the esophagus. Butorphanol (0.2 mg/kg IV, IM) is administered before or after extubation as needed for pain control. A potential complication of endoscopy is regurgitation with possible aspiration. The clinician can suction the esophagus with the endoscope during the procedure, but the oropharynx must be examined during recovery and suctioned if any fluids remain.

During the procedure, the esophagus is evaluated for any perforations that may have been caused by the foreign body or by attempts to retrieve it. Changes in respiration rate and effort, oxygenation, and ventilatory status can indicate a possible tension pneumothorax caused by air escaping through an esophageal tear (Kyles 2003). If a large perforation is present or if the object is firmly lodged and cannot be retrieved during endoscopy, a thoracotomy is necessary to access and repair the esophagus (Macintire et al. 2005).

Gastric and intestinal foreign bodies can obstruct the outflow of ingesta or cause perforations of the wall, allowing contents to leak into the abdominal cavity. The dissolution of the object in the stomach can lead to systemic illness if toxic chemicals are absorbed (Rasmussen 2003). Septic peritonitis and shock result from gastrointestinal leakages through intestinal perforations into the abdomen (Aiello 1998).

Vomiting is the most frequent clinical sign associated with gastric and intestinal obstructions, but it varies from acute to chronically intermittent, depending on the location of the foreign body in the intestinal tract (Brown, D.C. 2003; Macintire et al. 2005; Rasmussen 2003). Other clinical signs include dehydration, lethargy, diarrhea, abdominal distention, and pain (Aiello 1998). Anemia as a result of bleeding or toxicity may be present along with abnormal electrolyte and acid-base values (Macintire et al. 2005; Rasmussen 2003).

Abdominal radiographs help locate the obstruction or suspected foreign bodies, and should be repeated just prior to anesthesia to evaluate whether the foreign body has moved (Hedlund and Fossum 2007). Radiographs can reveal enlarged loops of bowel with trapped gas or fluids just proximal to the obstruction (Macintire et al. 2005). The small intestine may appear plicated if a linear foreign body is present (Brown, D.C. 2003).

The location and duration of the obstruction or foreign body will influence the anesthetic plan. Animals that are presented to the clinic soon after ingesting foreign material may be otherwise healthy. Electrolyte and acid-base disturbances may be profound with obstructions of the small intestine and require medical therapy. Appropriate intravenous fluid therapy is initiated prior to anesthesia in debilitated animals (Macintire et al. 2005). Patients exhibiting signs of toxicity, such as from zinc or lead, may require medical management in addition to the removal of the object (Ford and Mazzaferro 2006).

If the object is in the stomach or just past the pylorus, the veterinarian can use an endoscope to examine the foreign body and possibly retrieve it with grasping forceps or other endoscopic tools. Surgical removal of a foreign body is required if endoscopic retrieval is not possible or if the obstruction is in the small intestine (Macintire et al. 2005). The veterinarian performs an exploratory laparotomy to gain access to the stomach and small intestine to remove the object and evaluate the organs for signs of perforation, ischemia, and necrosis (Hedlund and Fossum 2007).

The anesthetic plan must address any fluid, electrolyte, or acid-base disturbances throughout the perioperative period. When ischemic necrosis is likely or intestinal contents have leaked into the abdominal cavity, surgery should not be delayed (Macintire et al. 2005). The anesthetist can collect intraoperative blood samples to be analyzed for changes in arterial blood gas values. The choice of fluids to be administered (crystalloids, colloids, blood products) will be based on serum chemistry and complete blood count values prior to anesthesia.

For sedation, the anesthetist can administer acepromazine (0.02–0.05 mg/kg IV, IM) only if the patient is stable. The compromised or hypovolemic patient may not require sedation, but if necessary, diazepam or midazolam (0.2–0.4 mg/kg IM, IV) can be given instead of acepromazine. Cats may also receive ketamine (5 mg/kg IM) for preoperative restraint if indicated. Analgesics include hydromorphone (0.1–0.2 mg/kg IM, IV) or oxymorphone (0.05–0.1 mg/kg IM, IV) that can be included with premedications or can be administered intravenously after anesthetic induction. Additional doses of intraoperative opioids are administered as needed.

For rapid induction, thiopental (12–15 mg/kg IV), propofol (6 mg/kg IV), or ketamine (5 mg/kg IV) combined with diazepam (0.25 mg/kg IV) are titrated to effect to allow for intubation, followed by inhalant anesthesia (isoflurane or sevoflurane). If bradycardia develops during the exploratory celiotomy, glycopyrrolate (0.01 mg/kg IV) or atropine (0.02 mg/kg IV) can be used for treatment.

Once the patient is anesthetized, the oral cavity and tongue are examined for linear foreign bodies (i.e., string) that may be anchored underneath the tongue (Macintire et al. 2005). If the animal requires surgery, direct arterial blood pressure should be monitored because manipulation of abdominal viscera can cause a profound hypotensive crisis. Colloids (hetastarch or plasma) or inotropic drugs can be administered to elevate blood pressure and improve tissue perfusion (Muir et al. 2007). If the surgeon elects

for open abdominal drainage, the anesthetist needs to provide appropriate amounts of compensatory IV fluids and needs to keep the patient warm with circulating hot water pads or forced-air blankets (Rasmussen 2003).

Prior to extubation, any regurgitated fluid in the oropharynx needs to be suctioned out to avoid aspiration pneumonia (Rasmussen 2003). If endoscopic extraction of the object is easily performed, the patient may only require an analgesic such as butorphanol (0.2–0.4 mg/kg IM, IV) or buprenorphine (5–15 μg/kg IM, IV, also buccal in cats) for postoperative pain.

Animals undergoing exploratory celiotomies require postoperative analgesics. The surgeon can infiltrate the subcutaneous and muscle layers around the incision with bupivicaine (0.5–1.0 mg/kg for cats; 1.0–2.0 mg/kg for dogs) just prior to surgical closure for local pain management (Carroll 2008). Postoperative hydromorphone (0.1–0.2 mg/kg IV, IM) or oxymorphone (0.05–0.1 mg/kg IV, IM) are administered as needed after extubation.

Intervertebral Disk Disease (IVDD)

Intervertebral cartilaginous disks are pads that lie between two adjacent vertebrae, which absorb shock and assist in vertebral movement. A disk consists of an outer layer of fibrocartilaginous material (the annulus fibrosus) surrounding a center of gelatinous material (the nucleus pulposus) (Toombs and Waters 2003). Degenerative changes in the disk can result in its herniation dorsally into the vertebral canal, compressing and injuring the spinal cord. The type of change and the resulting extrusions or protrusions of the disk are classified as either a Hansen type I or Hansen type II degeneration (Kapatkin and Vite 2000; Toombs and Waters 2003).

A common emergency presentation of a thoracolumbar disk rupture is a dachshund or other chondrodystrophoid breed having progressive signs of back pain, then loss of proprioception and motor function, and superficial and potentially deep pain. A complete neurological examination allows the veterinarian to localize the lesion, but survey radiographs followed by a myelogram, a computed tomography (CT) scan, or magnetic resonance imaging (MRI) of the area is needed to provide a definitive diagnosis (Toombs and Waters 2003).

Spinal imaging and decompressive surgery of the lesion require the patient to be anesthetized. These dogs are usually metabolically stable (Kapatkin and Vite 2000), and owners describe them as healthy just prior to the acute onset of the back pain or paraparesis. For preoperative analgesia and sedation, diazepam or midazolam (0.2–0.4 mg/kg IM, IV) in combination with hydromorphone (0.1 mg/kg IM, IV) or oxymorphone (0.05–0.1 mg/kg IM, IV) can help reduce anxiety and pain. For rapid induction, use thiopental (12–15 mg/kg IV) or propofol (6 mg/kg IV) titrated to effect to allow for intubation followed by inhalant (isoflurane or sevoflurane) anesthesia. Intravenous fluids are initiated following intubation to maintain intravascular volume and blood pressure (10 mL/kg/hr for the normovolemic patient) (Pascoe 2006).

Survey radiographs and myelogram require that the patient be repositioned frequently to obtain several views. The anesthetist must be attentive to accidental extubation of the patient, dislodgement of the intravenous catheter and fluid lines, and detachment of the various monitoring instruments. The clinician injects an iohexol contrast agent through a spinal needle into the subarachnoid space following the completion of survey radiographs. The flow of the contrast agent in the spinal canal is evaluated with the aid of fluoroscopy to determine the exact location of the lesion (Seim 2007). During the subarachnoid injection of iohexol, severe bradycardia can develop due to vagal stimulation (Jacobson et al. 1995). If the patient's heart rate is low or drops rapidly during the injection, the anesthetist can administer glycopyrrolate (0.01 mg/kg IV) or atropine (0.02 mg/kg IV) to prevent or correct bradycardia. Iohexol may flow intracranially as well, creating the risk of seizures at recovery (Harvey et al. 2007).

If CT or MRI is available for spinal imaging, the contrast media used to highlight the lesion (i.e., Ultravist® or Magnevist®, Berlex, Montville, NJ) is injected intravenously as needed and can

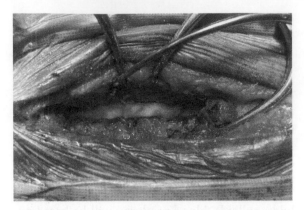

Figure 30.2. Gelatin sponge soaked with preservative-free morphine placed at the laminectomy site.

cause temporary hypotension or an increased heart rate, rarely requiring intervention.

If surgical decompression (i.e., via hemilaminectomy) is performed, intraoperative pain control can be accomplished by giving hydromorphone (0.05–0.1 mg/kg IV), oxymorphone (0.05 mg/kg IV), or fentanyl (2–5 µg/kg IV followed by 2–10 µg/kg/hr IV CRI). Local analgesia to the spine can be applied by the surgeon before closing. A small piece of gelatin sponge is soaked with preservative-free morphine (Duramorph®, Baxter Healthcare Corp., Deerfield, IL) (Gibbons et al. 1995) at a dose of 0.1 mg/kg and then placed at the laminectomy site (Figure 30.2). Bupivicaine (1–1.5 mg/kg) can then be injected into the paraspinal musculature of the operative field by the surgeon prior to closing the incision to further assist in postoperative pain control (Al-Khalaf et al. 2003) (Figure 30.3).

Urinary bladder function may be impaired in the paraplegic patient (Toombs and Waters 2003); the bladder is emptied by manual expression or urinary catheterization before anesthetic recovery. During recovery, the patient who received subarachnoid contrast agent (i.e., iohexol) for myelography must be monitored for seizures once the inhalant has been discontinued. Elevation of the head during recovery is important to reduce any intracranial contrast agent that may cause seizures (Jacobson et al. 1995).

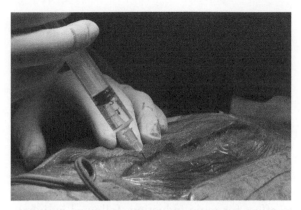

Figure 30.3. Bupivicaine injected into the paraspinal musculature of the operative field.

Hypothermia is a common complication in IVDD patients receiving imaging and surgery. Providing heat throughout the perianesthetic event using a forced-air warming blanket (Bair Hugger®, Arizant Inc., Eden Prairie, MN), a circulating warm water blanket, and IV fluids warmed to body temperature before administration is essential.

Any postoperative pain control may be addressed by administration of additional doses of oxymorphone (0.05 mg/kg IM, IV), hydromorphone (0.1 mg/kg IM, IV), or morphine (0.25–0.5 mg/kg IM) as needed.

Urethral Obstruction

Urethral calculi prevent or severely restrict the outflow of urine from the urinary bladder. The animal often strains to urinate and makes frequent attempts to do so. This condition can become very painful as the bladder is increasingly distended with urine (Ford and Mazzaferro 2006). Urinary bladder rupture is possible. The patient can develop azotemia and present with vomiting, dehydration, and lethargy (Syring and Drobatz 2000).

Hyperkalemia is a common finding in obstructed animals and can profoundly affect cardiac function. Bradycardia; large, peaked T waves; widening of the QRS complex; and absent

or flat P waves can often be seen on the ECG (Fossum 2007). In addition, metabolic acidosis may be present on blood gas analysis (Grubb 2008).

Treatment begins with the initial goal of relieving the obstruction and correcting the electrolyte imbalances. Heavy sedation or general anesthesia may be required while the clinician proceeds with urinary catheterization and urohydropropulsion to unblock the urethra (Ford and Mazzaferro 2006). Concurrently, intravenous fluid therapy with 0.9% NaCl is started to promote hemodynamic stability and renal perfusion (Fossum 2007). Hyperkalemia and acidosis may require additional drug therapies, such as sodium bicarbonate, insulin given with dextrose, or calcium gluconate (Perkowski 2000). To decrease the risk of complications, severe hyperkalemia with significant ECG changes needs to be corrected before anesthesia (Greene and Grauer 2007).

Analgesia can be provided by giving the animal butorphanol (0.2–0.4 mg/kg IM), buprenorphine (5–15 μg/kg IM), or hydromorphone (0.1–0.2 mg/kg IM for dogs; 0.05 mg/kg IM for cats). Urethral spasms may be reduced with opioid administration, facilitating urinary catheter placement. For sedation, ketamine (2.5–5.0 mg/kg IM) can be used in cats along with diazepam or midazolam (0.2–0.4 mg/kg IM) if the patient is stable during the early stages of the disease (Grubb 2008).

If surgery (i.e., urethrotomy, urethrostomy, or cystotomy) is indicated, general anesthesia is needed. Use propofol (4–6 mg/kg IV) titrated to effect to allow for intubation followed by isoflurane inhalant anesthesia. If the animal is in shock or hypovolemic, use diazepam (0.2 mg/kg IV) followed by etomidate (1–2 mg/kg IV) for induction to help maintain cardiovascular function (Fossum 2007). Epidural administration of preservative-free morphine (Duramorph®, Baxter Healthcare Corp., Deerfield, IL) before surgery is beneficial to reduce pain. It should also allow for a lower vaporizer setting to decrease the vasodilation effects of isoflurane and ultimately support blood pressure and tissue perfusion (Muir et al. 2007). If urinary catheter placement is possible, urine output should be measured intraoperatively to evaluate renal perfusion and function.

Additional analgesics can be provided during recovery as needed. Urinary retention caused by epidural administration of morphine is possible; thus urine output should be measured postoperatively as well (Mason 2003).

It is important to monitor the patient postoperatively for electrolyte imbalances and hypovolemia because postobstruction diuresis can lead to hypokalemia and fluid losses. Maintenance intravenous fluids can be switched to a balanced electrolyte solution; rates may need to be increased to support the patient (Fossum 2007).

Pyometra

Pyometra is the result of a bacterial infection within the uterus. This disorder develops during diestrus if the bitch or queen has an abnormally high progesterone influence or response. Secretions that collect within the uterus along with tissue that has become cystic and thickened provide an ideal environment for bacterial growth leading to pyometra. Purulent and sometimes bloody vaginal discharge can indicate an open pyometra. If the cervix is closed, purulent fluid is retained within the uterus and can lead to septicemia, endotoxemia, and possible uterine rupture (Hedlund 2007a).

Clinical signs associated with pyometra include uterine enlargement and abdominal distention, vaginal discharge, lethargy, anorexia, polyuria and polydipsia, vomiting, and dehydration. Fever, sepsis, and shock may also be present. Laboratory blood work findings may include hypoglycemia, hypoalbuminemia, azotemia, and neutrophilia. Electrolyte values and acid-base status may also be abnormal, with metabolic acidosis being the most important concern (Hedlund 2007a; Macintire et al. 2005).

Aggressive intravenous fluid therapy to correct any electrolyte imbalances, dehydration, and acidosis, if present, is initially used to stabilize the patient prior to surgery (Macintire et al. 2005).

Ovariohysterectomy is the surgical treatment for pyometra (Hedlund 2007a). The animal that is stable can be premedicated with hydromorphone (0.1–0.2 mg/kg IM) and midazolam or diazepam (0.2–0.4 mg/kg IM) to provide analgesia and sedation. Ketamine may be used in cats if no renal abnormalities are present. Suggested premedication doses for cats are ketamine (5–10 mg/kg IM) and diazepam (0.2–0.4 mg/kg IM) along with butorphanol (0.2–0.4 mg/kg IM), oxymorphone (0.05 mg/kg IM), or buprenorphine (5–15 µg/kg IM).

The stable patient can receive thiopental (10–15 mg/kg IV) or propofol (4–6 mg/kg IV) titrated to effect for rapid induction, followed by inhalant anesthesia (isoflurane or sevoflurane). Ketamine (5 mg/kg IV) mixed with diazepam (0.25 mg/kg IV) titrated to effect is another option. Severely debilitated patients may be induced using oxymorphone (0.05 mg/kg IV) or fentanyl (5–10 µg/kg IV) followed by either midazolam or diazepam (0.2 mg/kg IV) incrementally until intubation is possible (neuroleptanalgesia technique). Additionally, the patient may require a small amount of etomidate (0.5 mg/kg IV) to allow for intubation.

During surgery, appropriate monitoring is essential to identify and correct any anesthetic complications. Hypotension can be managed with appropriate vaporizer settings and fluids or inotropic support. Hetastarch (5–10 mL/kg IV given over the first hour of surgery) may be beneficial to the hypoalbuminemic patient with hypotension (Hedlund 2007a). Bradycardia can be treated with glycopyrrolate (0.01 mg/kg IV) or atropine (0.02 mg/kg IV) if necessary.

Intra- and postoperative doses of opioids (hydromorphone 0.1 mg/kg IV, IM or oxymorphone 0.05 mg/kg IV, IM) are administered for pain management. The surgeon can infiltrate the subcutaneous and muscle layers around the incision with bupivicaine (0.5–1.0 mg/kg for cats; 1.0–2.0 mg/kg for dogs) during surgical closure for local pain control as well (Carroll 2008).

During recovery, fluid therapy is continued to provide adequate tissue perfusion and correct any continued acid-base or electrolyte abnormalities. Good nursing care and diligent monitoring of the patient is essential so that any potential problems can be detected and treated as quickly as possible.

References

Aiello, S, ed. 1998. The Merck Veterinary Manual 8th ed. Whitehouse Station, NJ: Merck & Co.

Al-Khalaf, B, et al. 2003. Prospective comparative study of the effectiveness of epidural morphine and ropivicaine for management of pain after spinal operations. Acta Neurochirurgica 145:11–16.

Aronson, LR, Brockman, DJ, Brown, DC. 2000. Gastrointestinal emergencies. Vet Clin North Am Small Anim Pract 30(3):555–579.

Battaglia, AM. 2001. Small Animal Emergency and Critical Care: A Manual for the Veterinary Technician. Philadelphia: WB Saunders.

Brown, DC. 2003. Small intestines. In Textbook of Small Animal Surgery, 3rd ed., edited by Slatter, D. Philadelphia: WB Saunders, pp. 644–664.

Carroll, GL. 2003. Anesthesia and analgesia for the trauma or shock patient. In Textbook of Small Animal Surgery, 3rd ed., edited by Slatter, D. Philadelphia: WB Saunders, pp. 2538–2545.

Carroll, GL. 2008. Local anesthetic and analgesic techniques. In Small Animal Anesthesia and Analgesia, edited by Carroll, GL. Ames, IA: Blackwell Publishing, pp. 107–122.

Day, TK. 2003. Shock: Pathophysiology, diagnosis, and treatment. In Textbook of Small Animal Surgery, 3rd ed., edited by Slatter, D. Philadelphia: WB Saunders, pp. 1–17.

Day, TK, Bateman, S. 2006. Shock syndromes. In Fluid, Electrolyte, and Acid–Base Disorders in Small Animal Practice, 3rd ed., edited by DiBartola, SP. Elsevier Inc.: St. Louis, pp. 540–564.

Evans, AT, Wilson, DV. 2007. Anesthetic emergencies and procedures. In Lumb & Jones' Veterinary Anesthesia and Analgesia, 4th ed., edited by Tranquilli, WJ, Thurmon, JC, Grimm, KA. Ames, IA: Blackwell Publishing, pp. 1033–1048.

Ford, RB, Mazzaferro, EM. 2006. Kirk and Bistner's Handbook of Veterinary Procedures and Emergency Treatment, 8th ed. St. Louis: Saunders Elsevier.

Fossum, TW. 2007. Surgery of the bladder and urethra. In Small Animal Surgery, 3rd ed., edited by Fossum, TW. St. Louis: Mosby Elsevier, pp. 663–701.

Gibbons, KJ, et al. 1995. Lumbar discectomy: Use of an epidural morphine sponge for postoperative pain control. Neurosurgery 36(6):1131–1136.

Greene, SA, Grauer, GF. 2007. Renal disease. In Lumb & Jones' Veterinary Anesthesia and Analgesia, 4th ed., edited by Tranquilli, WJ, Thurmon, JC, Grimm, KA. Ames, IA: Blackwell Publishing, pp. 915–919.

Grubb, TL. 2008. Anesthesia for patients with special concerns. In Small Animal Anesthesia and Analgesia, edited by Carroll, GL. Ames, IA: Blackwell Publishing, pp. 193–238.

Harvey, RC, Greene, SA, Thomas, WB. 2007. Neurological disease. In Lumb & Jones' Veterinary Anesthesia and Analgesia, 4th ed., edited by Tranquilli, WJ, Thurmon, JC, Grimm, KA. Ames, IA: Blackwell Publishing, pp. 903–913.

Haskins, SC. 1999. Equipment and monitoring. In Essentials of Small Animal Anesthesia & Analgesia, edited by Thurmon, JC, Tranquilli, WJ, Benson, GJ. Baltimore: Lippincott Williams & Wilkins, pp. 269–291.

Hedlund, CS. 2007a. Surgery of the reproductive and genital systems. In Small Animal Surgery, 3rd ed., edited by Fossum, TW. St. Louis: Mosby Elsevier, pp. 702–774.

Hedlund, CS. 2007b. Surgery of the upper respiratory system. In Small Animal Surgery, 3rd ed., edited by Fossum, TW. St. Louis: Mosby Elsevier, pp. 817–866.

Hedlund, CS, Fossum, TW. 2007. Surgery of the digestive system. In Small Animal Surgery, 3rd ed., edited by Fossum, TW. St. Louis: Mosby Elsevier, pp. 339–530.

Jacobson, JD, et al. 1995. Introduction to Veterinary Anesthesiology. Blacksburg, VA: Brush Mountain Publishing.

Kapatkin, AS, Vite, CH. 2000. Neurosurgical emergencies. Vet Clin North Am Small Anim Pract 30(3):617–644.

Kruse-Elliott, KT. 2003. Patient monitoring. In Textbook of Small Animal Surgery, 3rd ed., edited by Slatter, D. Philadelphia: WB Saunders, pp. 2516–2520.

Kruse-Elliott, KT. 2008. Induction agents and total intravenous anesthesia. In Small Animal Anesthesia and Analgesia, edited by Carroll, GL. Ames, IA: Blackwell Publishing, pp. 83–94.

Kyles, AE. 2003. Esophagus. In Textbook of Small Animal Surgery, 3rd ed., edited by Slatter, D. Philadelphia: WB Saunders, pp. 573–592.

Ludwig, LL. 2000. Surgical emergencies of the respiratory system. Vet Clin North Am Small Anim Pract 30(3):531–553.

Macintire, DK, et al. 2005. Manual of Small Animal Emergency and Critical Care Medicine. Baltimore: Lippincott Williams & Wilkins.

Mason, DE. 2003. Urinary system. In Textbook of Small Animal Surgery, 3rd ed., edited by Slatter, D. Philadelphia: WB Saunders, pp. 2545–2552.

Monnet, E. 2000. Gastric Dilatation-Volvulus Syndrome in Dogs. Vet Clin North Am Small Anim Pract 33(5):987–1005.

Muir, WW, Hubbell, JAE, Bednarski, RM. 2007. Handbook of Veterinary Anesthesia, 4th ed. St. Louis: Mosby-Elsevier.

Paddleford, RR. 1999. Preanesthetic agents. In Manual of Small Animal Anesthesia, 2nd ed, edited by Paddleford, RR. Philadelphia: WB Saunders, pp. 12–30.

Pascoe, PJ. 2006. Perioperative management of fluid therapy. In Fluid, Electrolyte, and Acid-Base Disorders in Small Animal Practice, 3rd ed., edited by DiBartola, SP. St. Louis: Elsevier Inc., pp. 391–419.

Perkowski, SZ. 2000. Anesthesia for the emergency small animal patient. Vet Clin North Am Small Anim Pract 30(3):509–530.

Pettifer, G. 2003. Fluids, electrolytes, and acid-base therapy. In Textbook of Small Animal Surgery, 3rd ed., edited by Slatter, D. Philadelphia: WB Saunders, pp. 17–43.

Plumb, DC. 2005. Plumb's Veterinary Drug Handbook, 5th ed. Ames, IA: Blackwell Publishing.

Rasmussen, L. 2003. Stomach. In Textbook of Small Animal Surgery, 3rd ed., edited by Slatter, D. Philadelphia: WB Saunders, pp. 592–640.

Seim III, HB. 2007. Fundamentals of neurosurgery. In Small Animal Surgery, 3rd ed., edited by Fossum, TM. St. Louis: Mosby Elsevier, pp. 1357–1378.

Syring, RS, Drobatz, KJ. 2000. Preoperative evaluation and management of the emergency surgical small animal patient. Vet Clin North Am Small Anim Pract 30(3):473–489.

Toombs, JP, Waters, DJ. 2003. Intervertebral disc disease. In Textbook of Small Animal Surgery, 3rd ed., edited by Slatter, D. Philadelphia: WB Saunders, pp. 1193–1209.

31

Anesthesia for Small Exotics: Ferrets, Rodents, and Rabbits

Jennifer Stowell

Ferrets

The ferret comes from the Mustelidae family, the same family as badgers, wolverines, skunks, weasels, and polecats. The ferret's anatomic structure is a long, thin, and tubular-shaped body. They have poor eyesight but a very good sense of smell and hearing. They also experience seasonal changes in weight, and males are typically bigger than females. Ferrets may undergo seasonal molting and possess a strong odor, which is caused by sebaceous secretions from their skin. Their life span averages about five to eight years (Quesenberry and Carpenter 1997).

Preparation for anesthesia

Complete a thorough physical examination prior to anesthesia. Observe the ferret's attitude and alertness. Attention should be paid to coat condition, lymph nodes, mucous membrane color, and size of the abdomen. This will provide clues to the ferret's overall health. Poor coat condition or symmetrical thinning head to tail may indicate adrenal or other endocrine disease. Evaluate the heart and lung sounds, because cardiomyopathy

is not uncommon. Pursuing further workup of any irregularities or murmurs is recommended. A detailed history is very important. The anesthetist should know how the ferret has been acting regarding activity level, appetite, water intake, urination, and defecation. Any changes in the normal behavior can be a good indicator of how critically ill the ferret may be.

It is recommended that ferrets be fasted for 4 to 6 hours prior to anesthesia, but not longer due to their high metabolic rate and the concern for hypoglycemia. Vomiting or regurgitation during anesthesia can lead to aspiration and pneumonia. Ferrets also tend to hypersalivate, which can be minimized if appropriate fasting times are met. Ferrets can be difficult to properly restrain for medical procedures. Improper restraint can lead to stress and injury of the animal and anesthetist. One restraint technique is to scruff the animal with one hand and with the other hold the hips and stretch the ferret out on a table or flat surface. Take care not to pull on the legs, because joint trauma may occur. Avoid stress during handling, if the ferret appears overly stressed by restraint it is best to take a break and try again in a few minutes. The caudal lumbar muscles located on either side of the spine can be used for intramuscular (IM) injection sites.

Care should be taken to not move laterally and risk injection into a kidney. IM injections into the caudal thigh risk damaging the sciatic nerve. Use the intrascapular region for subcutaneous (SC) injections because the skin is loose and large volumes may be given here compared to other sites. Obtaining a blood sample for analysis can be difficult. Areas to draw from include jugular, lateral saphenous, and cephalic veins. The use of alcohol swabbing prior to a blood draw on a ferret that is not premedicated or under anesthesia is not recommended because they are extremely sensitive to the alcohol smell and it tends to make them salivate or vomit.

With help from an attending veterinarian, determine whether the thorough exam indicates that the patient needs additional workup or stabilization. Depending on the ASA status of the patient, consider radiographs, ultrasound, echocardiogram, electrocardiogram, and perhaps a more detailed blood work evaluation. These key diagnostic tests will help prepare the patient for anesthesia and may significantly impact the plan, care and support throughout surgery.

Anesthesia induction, care, and support

The setup for anesthesia should be done prior to premedication. The following items are useful to have on hand for ferret anesthesia:

- Cuffed endotracheal tubes (CETT), sizes 2–4 mm with a Murphy eye
- Intravenous (IV) catheters 24–22 g with injection cap (fill injection cap with saline flush to prevent air emboli)
- T-Connector with 0.5 mL volume and 15.2 cm length supplied by Baxter or small-volume IV extension tubing
- Several 1 mL heparinized saline flushes
- Tape for securing the CETT tube (Hy-Tape® (a specialty tape used for epidural catheters in humans) is invaluable for exotic anesthesia use; however, the use of umbilical tape or leftover IV fluid lines is adequate).
- 0.1 mL of 2% lidocaine to desensitize larynx for intubation

- EMLA® cream or other topical local anesthesia preparation (see below)
- Small anesthesia mask or rodent mask
- Three additional injection caps and three 25–22 g needles for ECG placement (described below)
- Cotton swabs for removing oral secretions
- Tongue depressors
- Stylet (cat size) may be useful in some cases.

Premedicating ferrets prior to catheter placement helps reduce the stress of handling and facilitate the process. The lateral saphenous and cephalic veins are good locations for IV catheter placement. The topical local anesthetic, Emla® cream may be used 45 minutes to 1 hour before IV catheter placement. Cover the Emla® cream with a bandage after application to ensure that it is not ingested. This is to be used only under constant observation. Catheters such as the Insyte® over the needle intravenous catheters have a sharper stylet, which is good for getting through the ferret's unusually tough skin. Other catheters may be less sharp and a vascular cutdown may be warranted by using a needle with a gauge one size bigger than the IV catheter to make a small skin incision or entry hole over the vein. Heparinized 1 mL saline flushes are helpful to gently flush the IV after placement or drug administration. Sometimes preflushing the IV catheter prior to placement is helpful because the blood flash is seen sooner once the vein is hit. This can help prevent pushing the catheter "through" the vein, which causes hematoma formation and often renders the vein unusable. Care should be taken to minimize the amount of flush used to prevent inadvertent fluid overload and heparinization. A T-connector and a small-volume extension set (preferably <1 mL volume) can be attached to the catheter after placement to provide an easily accessed port to administer drugs or fluids. Once again, the total volume of IV tubing used should be kept to a minimum so that any drug that is injected does not require excessive amounts of saline flush to reach the vein.

Picking an anesthesia protocol can be complicated. The goal is to provide good sedation and analgesia to allow for smooth transition to general anesthesia. A pure agonist opioid, such as oxymorphone, is preferable for most painful surgeries (laparotomy, fracture repair, etc.) because it provides the best analgesia and is easily reversed with naloxone if necessary in an emergent situation. The duration of action of oxymorphone is not yet determined in ferrets, but in other similar species, such as the cat, its duration is between 4–6 hours. If oxymorphone is not available, other opioids such as butorphanol or buprenorphine can be used, and although butorphanol provides good sedation at 0.2–0.3 mg/kg IM, it does not appear to be as potent an analgesic and its duration of action is much shorter than that of oxymorphone. Buprenorphine may not cause good sedation; however, it is a better analgesic than butorphanol and is more often available than oxymorphone. It does have a longer onset time. If the animal is relatively healthy, low doses of ketamine can be added to the premedication (2 –8 mg/kg) to restrain feisty and strong ferrets. This can benefit the analgesic protocol as well. Depending on the length and invasiveness of the surgical procedure, additional intravenous doses of opioid may be necessary. Midazolam, a benzodiazepine tranquilizer, provides good muscle relaxation. Midazolam is also easily reversed with flumazenil, if necessary in an emergent situation. Glycopyrrolate, an anticholinergic, counteracts hypersalivation, which is commonly seen, but it is not generally needed in ferrets to counteract bradycardia. For induction, the combination of ketamine and midazolam; 1 mL per 20 pounds of a 50:50 mixture by volume works very well. This combination provides additional muscle relaxation, adequate time for intubation, and indirect support of the cardiovascular system due to the ketamine. Prior to induction, preoxygenation by mask is recommended if the patient allows. If the ferret is not sedate enough to permit easy placement of a catheter, a light plane of anesthesia can be induced by mask. Lubrication for the end of the CETT, taking care not to occlude the Murphy's eye, provides a less irritating intubation. A laryngoscope with a 3 mm Miller blade is very useful in helping to visualize the larynx. A drop of 2% lidocaine (0.1 mL) on the larynx helps to decrease laryngospasm. The oral cavity can be gently cleared of salivation with cotton swabs prior to intubation if needed. If excess salivation or regurgitation is observed, mechanical suction may be used with an 8 French suction catheter to rid the area of debris before intubation is performed (be careful not to desaturate the patient by sucking all of its oxygen away). A guide wire made of 20 g wire and an 8 French polypropylene urinary catheter may be needed when intubation is difficult or visualization of larynx is compromised by salivation or other oral structures. The guide wire is passed through the end of the CETT by 2 or 3 mm. This can be fed through the arytenoids first and the CETT fed over it and into the trachea. Hy-Tape® is optimal in securing the CETT, but umbilical tape or adhesive tape may be used. After placing the middle of the tape over the CETT the tape is then crisscrossed over the tube and around the patient's head sticking it to itself in a modified figure eight. The Hy-Tape® is extremely sticky and works well to prevent the tube from sliding out of place and extubating the patient. Place sterile eye lubrication in the eyes frequently throughout the procedure.

For maintenance of anesthesia, the inhalant anesthetic sevoflurane in a precision vaporizer allows for quick onset and recovery from anesthesia. If sevoflurane is not available, isoflurane is an acceptable maintenance inhalant. Inhalant anesthetic in 100% oxygen should be administered through a non-rebreathing system such as a Bain modified Mapleson D that is connected and pressure-checked before anesthesia begins. Depending on the patient parameters, premedication, and degree of illness, the vaporizer setting is adjusted to keep the ferret in a surgical plane of anesthesia. It is easy to overdose inhalant anesthetic and this may result in renal compromise or death. Ferrets rely on the diaphragm for ventilation, and for some surgical procedures this may be difficult because of positioning. Ventilatory support may be necessary either manually or mechanically to provide adequate oxygenation to tissues and vital organs. This can be initiated with intermittent positive pressure breaths, either manually or via a mechanical ventilator. Positive pressure ventilation should be done carefully to prevent barotrauma.

The fluid therapy plan

The complexity and nature of the procedure can influence the fluid therapy plan. Using a balanced electrolyte solution, such as lactated Ringer's®, at a maintenance rate of 10 mL/kg/hr is generally adequate unless otherwise contraindicated by preexisting disease. Fluids can be administered via syringe with intermittent injections of 1 mL or less, infusion pump, or buretrol to avoid potential fluid overload. In the event that crystalloid therapy is inadequate due to blood loss or hypotension, consider the need for colloid support using hetastarch. Hetastarch is a synthetic polysaccharide that increases colloid osmotic pressure. As with any patient presenting for surgery, considerations for blood loss should be made. It is ideal to have a healthy blood donor ferret in the hospital in the event a transfusion is required. Oxyglobin, a solution made from purified bovine hemoglobin in modified lactated Ringer's® maximizes oxygen-carrying capacity in the blood but does not supply red blood cells. This also provides support to the hypotensive patient by scavenging nitric oxide, a substance in the blood that causes vasodilation. Monitor for transfusion reactions as necessary.

Monitoring during anesthesia

Monitoring during anesthesia is crucial to the life of the patient. Multiparameter monitors, such as the Cardell or Datascope Passport, can be beneficial. The Cardell has been reported to reliably measure oscillometric blood pressure in the small exotic patient. However, the use of several separate monitors can be just as effective. Ferrets can be especially difficult to monitor due to their small size and anatomy. Having multiple monitoring sources (e.g., pulse oximetry, esophageal stethoscope, ECG, Doppler blood pressure) is beneficial in ferrets because of the tendency for one type of monitoring to fail during anesthesia. Use a lead II electrocardiogram (ECG) to measure heart rate and assess for arrhythmias. Placement of 25 g or 22 g needles poked through the skin with an injection cap to cover the tip of the needle is a nice way to provide ECG clips without having the skin trauma from alligator clips.

A pulse oximeter estimates hemoglobin oxygen saturation and heart rate. Placement of a clip Y-probe on the tongue may cause harm or damage to delicate nerves because the probe is meant for larger species. Placement of the probe on the footpad secured with tape or over the skin in the axilla can give a good reading.

A Doppler blood pressure instrument and size 1 occlusion cuff are great for monitoring blood pressure. The probe can be placed in the brachial artery above the carpus and secured with tape. This is a good area for measurement, and the Doppler also supplies audible heart sounds. If assistance is needed for securing the Doppler probe, use a tongue depressor. Break the tongue depressor in half and use tape to pad the ends. Acting as a splint for the leg, it assists placement and may enhance sound.

The esophageal stethoscope is another means to evaluate heart and lung sounds and can be a valuable tool during an emergent situation. Temperature may fluctuate dramatically during anesthesia. Methods for warming include circulating hot water blanket, forced-air warmer with blanket, heat lamp, and IV fluid warmer. Snuggle Safe microwavable disc is a commercially available warming device for small exotics that also works well. As with all warming devices, take precautionary measures to prevent burns. Place a towel, drape, or several layers between items that are too hot to leave on your own skin for a long duration of time. It is imperative to monitor temperature via rectal or esophageal probe continually throughout anesthesia. In addition to these monitors a hands-on evaluation of the patient is necessary by assessment of jaw tone, palpebral reflex, toe pinch response, anal sphincter, and muscle tone. All are similar to that of the feline patient under anesthesia. Determine the depth of the patient as well as the anticipated response to surgical stimulation. To achieve the best outcome, ferrets should have limited anesthesia time. Only extremely quick procedures should be attempted in critically ill patients.

Anesthesia recovery

The recovery period is a very critical time. Place the patient in a quiet area near oxygen if needed. Monitoring during this period is imperative. Keep the IV catheter in place until unable to do so due to activity level. Encourage the patient to eat and regain normal activity as soon as possible. Check blood glucose if the recovery is prolonged. A dextrose solution of 2.5–5% can be given IV or administer (0.5 mL) sublingual dextrose. Hypothermia is common, and shivering increases oxygen consumption and demand for the body. Hypothermia can also slow recovery because it decreases the rate in which drugs are excreted. Ensure that heat is continued until body temperature returns to normal. Due to their small body size ferrets can overheat very rapidly, so they should be monitored quite frequently when heat is being supplied. Frequent observation of ferrets is crucial, because they may remove their IV or chew at their incision. Assessment of pain requires that the observer be familiar with normal ferret behavior. Signs indicative of pain or other abnormal conditions include a hunched posture with tension in affected muscle groups, lethargy, self trauma, stiff gait, and anorexia (Mayer 2007). Use of analgesics in the perioperative period is essential. For invasive procedures such as an abdominal explore with adrenalectomy, opioids with kappa receptor activity (butorphanol, oxymorphone) may cause a significant amount of sedation in ferrets. However, oxymorphone can be used for severe pain (e.g., invasive abdominal surgery, fracture repair) prior to surgery and for several doses every 4–6 hours postoperatively without complication. Buprenorphine acts at the opioid mu receptor and thus may represent a good alternative for pain of lesser magnitude or when oxymorphone-induced sedation is not desired. Multimodal analgesia can be achieved by adding a nonsteroidal antiinflammatory drug (NSAID), such as carprofen or meloxicam, to lessen opioid requirements and produce a better overall effect on controlling pain in the postoperative period. However, NSAIDs must be used with care in sick, dehydrated, or debilitated animals due to the risk of gastric ulceration and renal impairment.

Rodents

Rodent species include mice, rats, squirrels, chinchillas, porcupines, beavers, hamsters, and guinea pigs. In this chapter, the discussion is limited to mice and rats.

Small rodents have bulging eyes and tails longer than their bodies. Rats normally have poor eyesight and do not have a gallbladder. Thermoregulation is difficult because they do not have sweat glands and are unable to pant. Heat is dispersed via the ears and tail, and some rodents excessively salivate in response to hyperthermia. They have a high metabolic rate and rarely regurgitate. Male mice produce a musty odor and are typically bigger than the females. Mice average a life span of 1–3 years. Comparatively, rats average a lifespan of 2–4 years (Quesenberry and Carpenter 1997).

Preparation for anesthesia

Conduct a physical examination of the rodent prior to anesthesia. Observe attitude and movement around the cage or enclosure. Consider coat condition, lymph nodes, mammary region, and respiratory system. It is important to decrease stress in the clinical setting. As a prey species, rodents hide illness well, and thus additional stress or pain can result in shock or collapse and death. Disease of the respiratory system is common, and the small rodent may present with signs of sniffling, sneezing, or teeth chatter. When exhibiting signs of respiratory distress, limit handling during physical examination. A high incidence of death is reported in respiratory-compromised patients placed under anesthesia. Further workup or cancellation of the procedure is required.

With use of proper restraint techniques, a complete physical examination, obtaining a blood sample, or injections can be accomplished. IM injections can be given in the caudal lumbar muscles, on either side of the spine. SC injections can be given over the neck, abdomen, or lumbar region. Blood samples may be difficult to obtain in these patients because the amount you are able to safely remove is limited. The tail vein is an acceptable location to obtain a blood sample. Because of the small volume of blood in rodents, extensive blood sampling cannot be recommended. Due to the rodent's high metabolic rate and inability to vomit, fasting is not recommended prior to anesthesia.

After a thorough exam, determine—with help from an attending veterinarian—whether the patient needs any additional workup or stabilization. Depending on the ASA status of the patient, consider radiographs, ultrasound, echocardiogram, electrocardiogram, and perhaps a more detailed blood work evaluation. These key diagnostic tests will help to prepare the patient for anesthesia and may significantly impact the plan, care, and support throughout surgery.

Anesthesia induction, care, and support

Setup for anesthesia is completed prior to premedication. See setup for ferrets for an all inclusive list of materials. Intubation of the rodent is an advanced technique that is extremely difficult and may necessitate expensive light sources, small ridged endoscopes, and time. Although in theory an intubated patient is best, the ability to intubate rodents requires an injectable anesthesia technique (which may kill sick rodents) and specialized training and equipment. Therefore, intubation of rodents is seldom used in practice and they are usually maintained with inhalant anesthesia.

Picking an anesthesia protocol for the rodent patient can be complicated. Many protocols published for laboratory rodents involve large doses of anesthetics that, although suitable for the healthy young laboratory rodent, will overwhelm the homeostatic capability of the older or sick pet rodent. The goal of premedication is to provide good sedation and analgesia to allow for smooth transition to general anesthesia and reduce the amounts needed for maintenance. Butorphanol, a partial agonist antagonist opioid, provides good sedation with mild analgesia. When combined with acepromazine, a phenothiazine tranquilizer, the combination provides sedation and chemical restraint. Glycopyrrolate,

an anticholinergic, counteracts bradycardia, vagal-induced bradycardia and hypersalivation. Pain control can be achieved with the addition of buprenorphine, an agonist-antagonist opioid, with less sedative effects. IV catheter placement in rodents can be very challenging due to the small size of the patient and veins. Most often the patient needs to be masked with inhalant to allow catheter placement. Before masking, place sterile eye lubrication in eyes. One technique is to place a small face mask over the entire rodent on a flat, nonporous surface. The mask should be at least twice the size of the rodent. The inhalant anesthetic agents sevoflurane or isoflurane can be administered via precision vaporizer in 100% oxygen. Once the patient is sleepy enough, trade out the large induction mask for a small, tight-fitting mask that covers the muzzle. Use a 24 g–22 g Insyte catheter in the lateral saphenous or tail vein. Do not spend a lot of time attempting IV access. Time becomes a critical factor during anesthesia, risking life-threatening complications as time progresses. Intraosseous (IO) catheters may be placed in the femoral head if necessary. If the patient is critically ill, take into consideration the length of anesthesia time and type of procedure. Placement of the IO catheter may increase anesthesia time, which can severely affect morbidity. An acceptable and faster technique is the use of a rodent mask specifically designed to fit their pointy faces. Secure the rodent mask with Hy-Tape® or other available means (Fig. 31.1). Continue maintenance anesthesia on a non-rebreathing delivery system. Be familiar with the non-rebreathing circuit. Follow the patient's vitals and trends throughout anesthesia. If any parameters change drastically, troubleshooting both the equipment and the patient is necessary. If respirations are diminished, evaluate chest movement during inspiration and expiration by palpating the chest. It is important to position the head so that the neck is not hyperextended or flexed, allowing an unobstructed pathway for ventilation. The fluid therapy plan depends greatly on whether an IV or IO catheter is placed. Lactated Ringer's®, a balanced electrolyte solution, can be infused at a maintenance rate of 10 mL/kg/hr. See the ferret section for additional types of fluids that can be

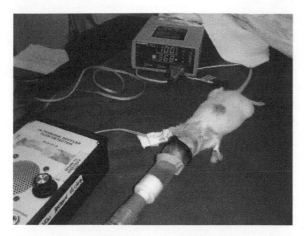

Figure 31.1. Rat instrumented with monitors. Note rodent mask, Doppler, and SpO$_2$.

used in the small-animal exotic patient. SC fluids may be administered; however, uptake and distribution is limited during anesthesia, and this method will not be helpful in an emergent situation. Monitoring during anesthesia is complicated in the small animal exotic patient, but it is crucial to ensuring life.

For a detailed explanation see the ferret section. Additional suggestions for Doppler placement in the rodent include use of the tail artery. Blood pressure measurements may be limited due to the size of the tail and limited space for cuff placement. When masking a patient, complications may occur. Watch respirations and pulse oximetry closely to ensure adequate ventilation. If parameters are decreased, consider suctioning the oral cavity, and repositioning of the head and neck.

Anesthesia recovery

The recovery period is a very important time to continue monitoring. Assess vital signs during this time to ensure adequate recovery from anesthesia. See the ferret section for specifics on the recovery period because most objectives are similar for the rodent. It is important to monitor and evaluate for pain in the postoperative period. Indicators of pain include, but are not limited to, decreased appetite, self trauma, increased time to

normal activity, and flinching, biting, or moving away from the gentle palpation of incision. To decrease the chances of a stress response, provide adequate analgesia. Because of pain this stress response leads to increased cardiac output, cardiac work, and oxygen consumption, which can be detrimental to the life of the patient. Using multimodal analgesia with an opioid and nonsteroidal antiinflammatory medication provides an overall better effect on relieving pain.

Rabbits

The rabbit's anatomical structure is a round body made for agility and speed with powerful hindquarters, back legs, and large feet. They have a large abdominal cavity comprised mostly of stomach and cecum. Comparatively, the thoracic cavity is small with lungs and heart size-proportional to the size of the body. Rabbits have a good sense of smell and are obligate nose breathers, using their diaphragm to ventilate. They have exceptionally long ears and good hearing for detecting predators. Being coprophagous, they get necessary vitamins, minerals, and proteins through their feces. Rabbits are also physiologically unable to vomit and possess sweat glands only on their lips. The water requirements of rabbits are much higher than that of other species, averaging 50–150 mL/kg/day. Rabbits are territorial, nocturnal, and do not tend to hibernate. To sound alarm or show aggression rabbits sound a loud foot thump. Well-developed scent glands and urine marking are a primary means of communication among rabbits. Rabbits are exceptionally vulnerable to stress. They do not adapt well in stressful situations and thus can be very challenging patients in the hospital. The life span of the rabbit averages about 6–9 years (Quesenberry and Carpenter 1997).

Preparation for anesthesia

Every rabbit presenting for surgery and anesthesia should be given a thorough physical examination. Conduct a normal exam, starting at the nose and working backward. Pay special attention to the respiratory system, teeth, and hocks. Rabbits are prone to respiratory diseases and further workup or precautions are recommended in these patients. Weight loss or decreased appetite may be caused by malocclusion of the teeth. Improper housing may cause abscess or infection to form in the hock region (Thurmon et al. 1996). Assess overall health and condition of the rabbit to determine how critical its illness might be.

Rabbits have a high metabolic rate and inability to vomit; they normally require only 1 hour fasting time before anesthesia. This time allows stomach contents to empty somewhat and thus reduces the pressure placed on the diaphragm and lungs, facilitating better ventilation in the supine rabbit.

Proper restraint of the rabbit during physical examination or blood draw is imperative. The body structure and flight response combination makes rabbits subject to fractures of the back and legs when they attempt to flee their restrainer. It is important to limit stressful or harmful situations to decrease the chances of creating a dangerous situation for the rabbit. Extreme caution should be taken to handle rabbits appropriately. Do not use ears as a means to catch the rabbit. The scruff of the neck can be used if necessary; take care to support the hind end. For excitable rabbits or for IM or SC injections, snugly wrap the patient in a towel and support feet and spine. Ideally, these rabbits should be restrained on the floor to eliminate the possibility of a fall should the rabbit struggle during the injection. For SC injections, a preferred site is between the shoulder blades in the scruff of the neck. The lumbar muscle on either side of the spine just cranial to the pelvis is a preferred site for IM injections. When obtaining a blood sample for analysis, use the marginal ear, cephalic, or saphenous veins. Sedation may be required if there is a need to use the jugular vein.

Compile the information from the examination. Consider the ASA status of the patient presenting for anesthesia and surgery. Discuss with your attending veterinarian whether the patient needs any additional workup or stabilization

before anesthesia and surgery. Additional diagnostic testing and stabilization may need to be performed before the patient undergoes anesthesia. Tests include, but are not limited to, radiographs, ultrasound, echocardiogram, and complete blood count and chemistry profile, and stabilization may include fluid and electrolyte therapy and institution of analgesic and antibiotic treatment.

Anesthesia induction, care, and support

Before premedication ensure a complete setup. See setup for ferrets for a detailed list. The following are necessary tools and equipment for rabbit anesthesia:

- Endotracheal tubes, usually uncuffed, size 2–4 mm with a Murphy eye
- Otoscope

The anesthesia protocol needs to accomplish several goals: provide good sedation, decrease stress, allow facilitation of IV catheter placement, and provide analgesia and a smooth transition to anesthesia. Oxymorphone, an opioid, provides good sedation and analgesia. Ketamine, a dissociative anesthetic, provides chemical restraint and analgesia. The alpha-2 agonist, medetomidine may also provide useful sedation, chemical restraint and analgesia. Consider omitting ketamine and medetomidine from the premed for the critically ill rabbit. In sick rabbits, midazolam, a benzodiazepine tranquilizer, can replace the ketamine or medetomidine to provide good muscle relaxation. The drug combination, along with a quiet stress-free environment will provide facilitation of IV catheter placement. If the rabbit responds adversely to restraint or a needle stick, consider masking it with sevoflurane inhalant anesthetic in oxygen until the rabbit is more tolerant. This technique is best for reducing stress for the rabbit and anesthetist. The rabbit should be monitored during this procedure. Usually, a pulse oximeter will work on the ear. For induction to anesthesia, the use of ketamine and midazolam, as was detailed for ferret anesthesia, is preferred. If tiny volumes are difficult to titrate, the induction mixture can be diluted in saline to make titration easier. There are several techniques that can be used for intubation of the rabbit. The rabbit's long narrow oral cavity, inability to open the mouth wide, large tongue, and S-shaped neck all combine to make intubation challenging without sufficient training. Intubation of smaller pet rabbits is considered an advanced technique. Complications of intubation include damage to tongue and larynx (the latter can be fatal), hypoventilation, and hypoxemia. Pulse oximetry should be monitored closely. Time is an important factor when attempting intubation. In our hospital, we limit the total intubation attempt time to 10 minutes or less, after which time we proceed by mask maintenance unless an oral procedure is planned. The author's preferred method is to use an otoscope with a high-intensity light source to visualize the larynx. An expensive but worthy purchase would be a Storz® Otoscope, which is equipped with its own light source. Blind intubation, orotracheal or nasotracheal, can also be successful, but also requires training and experience. Before intubation preoxygenate for 5 minutes. It may take extra time for intubation, so draw up extra induction agent, roughly twice the amount calculated. The following discussion describes intubation of the rabbit with a Storz Otoscope. The intravenous induction agent is given to effect until the rabbit does not swallow or respond to stimulation, such as a toe pinch, or attempts to open its mouth. Continue to have someone provide oxygenation by mask over the nose. Scoop the tongue out of the mouth with a cotton swab, and hold it gently to the side of the lower jaw. Place the rabbit in sternal recumbency with head and nose in a straight line pointed toward the ceiling. Place the otoscope in the oral cavity ventrally and dorsally and advance until the larynx is visualized.

To see the larynx, elevate the soft palate with the endotracheal tube or stylet. The larynx will be extremely ventral. Use 0.1–0.2 mL of 2% lidocaine on the larynx to prevent laryngospasm. Intubation is not possible if the rabbit is at a light plane of anesthesia. If at any time the rabbit swallows, gags, or moves, give more induction

agent to effect. Place the endotracheal tube alongside the otoscope and advance until its tip is visualized.

Watch the tube move through the arytenoids into the trachea and remove the otoscope. The rabbit may cough or move at this time because intubation is very stimulating. Difficulty may arise when the proper angle or placement cannot be achieved. Manipulation of the head and neck to a different position may facilitate a better angle. Use the stylet through the endotracheal tube or otoscope. Watch as the stylet is passed through the arytenoids, and then pass the endotracheal tube over the stylet and advance into the trachea. Visualization must be maintained at all times to avoid esophageal intubation. Secure the endotracheal tube with Hy-Tape® or other available means. Place the endotracheal tube in the middle of the strip, crisscross over the tube and around the patient's head, sticking it to itself in a modified figure eight. The tape is extremely sticky and works well to prevent the tube from sliding out of place. Use good judgment to decide what is best for the patient and realize that intubation may not be necessary or advisable without a properly trained anesthetist. Mask placement and delivery of inhalant anesthetic is an acceptable technique. During masking, ensure that the head and neck remain extended for the best possible ventilation. Suctioning of the oral cavity may be necessary due to mucus accumulation.

Connect to the maintenance inhalant anesthesia either isoflurane or sevoflurane via a precision vaporizer in 100% oxygen. Administer the inhalant through a non-rebreathing delivery system, such as a Bain modified Mapleson D that is connected and pressure-checked before anesthesia begins. The ratio of abdominal size to thoracic size in the rabbit predisposes to hypoventilation under anesthesia; thus, ventilation may be necessary to ensure oxygenation of tissues and vital organs. Maintain atraumatic technique when ventilating a small patient through a non-rebreathing system or mechanical ventilator.

There are many variables that affect the fluid therapy plan. The fluid requirements are higher than most small-animal exotic patients. Rabbits under anesthesia require fluid rates averaging

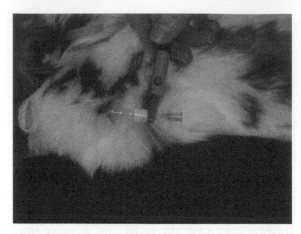

Figure 31.2. Placement of ECG clips in nontraumatic fashion with ECG clipped-on needle.

15 mL/kg/hr. See the ferret section for more information regarding fluids because products and administration are similar.

Effective monitoring can be achieved through a multiparameter monitor, individual monitors, and hands-on assessment (Fig. 31.2, 31.3).

See the ferret section for a detailed compilation of monitoring techniques and assessments. Arterial catheters may be placed in the ear; however, be advised that infection, sloughing, and necrosis can occur with any catheter placed in the ear. It is crucial to limit anesthesia time for rabbits and all exotic patients to achieve the

best outcome. Critically ill patients should undergo only quick procedures requiring anesthesia time of less than 1 hour for the best outcomes.

Anesthesia recovery

Place the patient in a quiet, well-ventilated and warmed environment. Give oxygen as needed if shivering or hypoventilation is observed. During the recovery period, continue to monitor until the rabbit is alert and able to hold its head up. Treat rabbits similarly to the treatment you would give a brachycephalic dog. Extubation should be performed only when appropriate alertness, chewing, and overall resentment of the endotracheal tube is observed. Activity level may inhibit the duration of time that the IV catheter can be kept in place. Compared to other exotic patients after anesthesia, rabbits have an increased amount of time before regaining normal activity. Be diligent about checking temperature, heart rate, and respiratory rate to ensure that they are within normal ranges. Monitor for pain, which may be difficult to assess in rabbits. Because they are a prey species, disguising their pain is a survival mechanism. Indicators of pain include decreased appetite, self trauma, and flinching during gentle palpation of incision. To control pain in the postoperative period, consider the use of multimodal analgesia. Assessment and evaluation after administration of analgesics is necessary to provide essential pain control in the rabbit patient.

Emergency Considerations

The anesthetic protocol is not complete until considerations are made for complications. Have emergency drug doses, epinephrine, atropine, lidocaine, and glycopyrrolate, calculated and drawn up ahead of time. Place in a location that is easily accessible and have means to administer them quickly in an emergent situation. When an IV or IO catheter is not in place, consider transtracheal administration of emergency drugs.

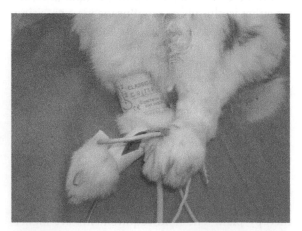

Figure 31.3. Rabbit instrumented with Doppler and blood pressure cuff.

References

Mayer, J. 2007. Use of behavior analysis to recognize pain in small mammals. Lab Anim (2007):43–48.

Quesenberry, KE, Carpenter, JW. 1997. Ferrets, Rabbits and Rodents, 2nd ed. St. Louis: WB Saunders, pp.136–147, 286–299.

Thurmon, J, Tranquilli, W, Benson, J. 1996. Anesthesia of wild, exotic and laboratory animals. In Lumb & Jones' Veterinary Anesthesia, 3rd ed. Philadelphia: Lippincott Williams & Wilkins, pp.712–727.

32

Basic Physiology of Pain

Lynette DeGouff

Evolution has played an important role in the development of an animal's response to pain. Survival may depend on an animal's ability to hide injury and pain from potential predators. Therefore, as animal advocates, we must be diligent in our observation of normal and abnormal behaviors—not only between individual species but also between individual patients because each patient has an individual response to pain. With recent advances in molecular neurophysiology our understanding of animal pain and how to treat it has advanced considerably. In the past, decisions regarding pain management were based primarily on behaviors, such as vocalizing, self-mutilation, writhing in the cage, and aggression in response to manipulation of a painful area.

Animals cannot tell us they are painful; we can only infer that they are experiencing pain by their behavioral response. We understand very little about the emotional aspect of pain that animals may experience. Therefore, to give our patients the best pain management we must anthropomorphize (attribute a human form or personality to an animal). That is, it is reasonable to assume that if the stimulus is painful to us, it is also painful to a veterinary patient receiving a similar stimulus. Armed with basic knowl-

edge of pain physiology and recognition, we can better understand pain in our patients.

Classification of Pain

Pain, as defined by the International Association for the Study of Pain, is the unpleasant sensory and emotional experience individuals have when they perceive actual or potential tissue damage to their body (IASP 2008).

Physiologic versus pathologic pain

Physiologic or adaptive pain is a warning pain that occurs after a noxious (physically harmful or destructive) stimulus. It is a protective response by the central nervous system to prevent tissue damage. Pathologic pain or clinical pain is a response to tissue damage and is typically characterized by sharp pain or dull burning pain, with exaggerated response to noxious stimulus (hyperalgesia) or a pain experience from a stimulus that is not normally painful (allodynia). "Pathologic pain may even take the form of neurogenic pain where there are no lesions to provide a noxious stimulus, but the perception of pain is still there, e.g., in phantom limb pain" (Livingston and Chambers 2000). This can be explained in part by the neurophysiologic processes of peripheral and central sensitization to pain.

Peripheral sensitization is a reduction in threshold and an increase in responsiveness of the peripheral ends of the pain fiber. Peripheral nociceptors are located in the skin, muscle, joints. and viscera (Woolf 2008). Inflammation and nerve injury are often the cause of pain, resulting in the release of a number of neuroactive substances to the site of tissue injury. The release of these substances increases the excitability of sensory and sympathetic nerve fibers and also activates inflammatory cells such as neutrophils. These cells begin expressing an enzyme known as cyclooxygenase 2 (Cox-2), which leads to the production and secretion of prostaglandin PGE2. Aspirinlike pain-killing drugs act by inhibiting Cox-2 and prostaglandin production (Woolf 2008). Whereas peripheral sensitization is localized at the site of the injury, central sensitization is a result of abnormal input at the level of the CNS.

Central sensitization is "an increase in the excitability of neurons within the central nervous system, so that normal inputs begin to produce abnormal responses" (Woolf 2008). With central sensitization, a light touch can cause pain and hypersensitivity that goes beyond the surgical site or the site of injury. The term *windup pain* is associated with central sensitization and often implies an increased pain response or a pain response to a nonpainful stimulus.

Acute versus chronic pain

Acute pain is a physiologic pain that is immediate and serves as a warning that tissue damage is occurring or is likely to occur unless action is taken. Due to reflex behavioral responses this should lead to a change in behavior or force an action, (i.e., flinching from a needle stick). As the problem begins to settle down, the pain subsides. Acute pain can be considered a protective pain, warning us about tissue injury. It is triggered by a chemical, thermal, or mechanical stimulus

linked to surgery, trauma, or acute illness. Acute pain is usually responsive to analgesic agents such as nonsteroidal antiinflammatory drugs (NSAIDs), local anesthetics, opioids, and heat or cold therapies. Based on origin, acute pain can be classified into two types, visceral and somatic (see below) (Morgan et al. 2002).

Acute pain that is not properly treated can lead to chronic pain. Chronic or maladaptive pain is defined as pain persisting beyond the normal period of healing in association with a particular type of injury or disease process. Depression and anxiety may be associated with chronic pain as well as decreased physical activity in fear of making the pain worse. It can be difficult to treat because it is often resistant to conventional medications. Chronic pain is typical of that associated with arthritis, cancer, neurologic injury, musculoskeletal injury, or sympathetic dystrophies.

Somatic versus visceral pain

Somatic pain is divided into superficial or deep pain. Superficial pain originates in the skin, subcutaneous tissues, and mucous membranes. It is typically well localized and associated with a sharp pricking, throbbing, or burning sensation (Morgan et al. 2002). Deep somatic pain comes from muscles, tendons, joints, or bones. It usually is less localized, and the degree of pain is affected by both duration and intensity of the stimulus. An example is a minor injury to your finger that is localized to the finger, but a more serious trauma to the finger (i.e., finger slammed in a car door) can cause pain in the whole hand. Deep pain typically has a dull, aching quality (Morgan et al. 2002).

Visceral pain is characterized as dull, diffuse, achy, spasmlike pain. It is caused by a disease process or abnormal function of an internal organ (Morgan et al. 2002). Visceral organs (intestine, liver, spleen, kidney, and bladder) transmit pain signals via Aδ and C fibers of the sympathetic and parasympathetic nervous system pathways. This difference means that most inputs coming from viscera are not perceived (Muir 2002). Therefore, clamping, cautery, and cutting generally produce no pain from the visceral structures (Thurmon and Tranquilli 1996). Conversely, inflammation, ischemia, and mesenteric stretching or dilation may produce severe unrelenting pain that activates numerous "silent nociceptors" in the gut and bladder. These silent nociceptors produce mechanosensitivity in response to normally innocuous smooth muscle contractile activity. It is believed that the viscera may contain more κ-opioid receptors than μ-opioid receptors; therefore, some visceral nociception may be more responsive to κ-opioid receptor agonists such as butorphanol (Muir 2002).

Referred versus neuropathic pain

Referred pain is a pain perceived at a site near to or at a distance from the site of injury. It is usually associated with visceral pain. Neuropathic pain is typically chronic in nature. It is a result of nerve damage, injury, or dysfunction resulting in abnormal signals being sent to the spinal cord and higher pain centers. Symptoms of neuropathic pain typically include burning and shooting pain, or tingling and numbness, or allodynia.

Pain Pathways

There are four physiologic processes of nociception (the detection of noxious stimulus). They are transduction, transmission, modulation and perception (Fig. 32.1). *Transduction* is the conversion of a chemical, thermal or mechanical noxious stimulus into an electrical signal that can be transmitted along a nerve. Transduction involves specialized encapsulated and bare (free) nerve endings (Muir 2002). These afferent (sensory) nerves send signals toward the central nervous system (CNS). *Transmission* occurs via the peripheral nerves that send signals to the dorsal horn and through the spinal cord to the brain. Both afferent (sensory) and efferent (motor) nerve fibers are found in the peripheral nerves. Transmission involves Aβ, Aδ, and C

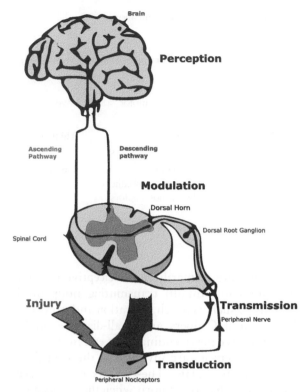

Figure 32.1. The four physiologic processes for the detection of a noxious stimulus are transduction, transmission, modulation, and perception. (Figure modified from artwork courtesy of Dr. Neil Castle.)

fibers. *Modulation* occurs in various regions of the spinal cord and brain. Signals pass through synapses within the CNS (spinal cord and brain) that are modified, either enhanced or inhibited by interneurons (neurons that communicate with other neurons). *Perception* is the process whereby the brain organizes the information that is transmitted and modulated. The information is then interpreted by an individual's unique psychology and physiology resulting in the experience of pain.

Afferent nerve fibers

The peripheral nervous system consists in part of Aβ, Aδ, and C fibers. These peripheral nerve fibers have a large degree of functional overlap, providing continuous sensation (Muir 2002). The Aβ fibers are large-diameter low-threshold

Table 32.1.   Nerve fibers classification.

Group	Sensory Receptor and Function	Myelination	Sensation	Velocity (m/sec)
Aβ	Mechanoreceptor, motor	Myelinated	Touch, pressure, vibration, limb movement	35–75
Aδ	Mechanoreceptors, thermareceptors, nociceptors	Thinly myelinated	Sharp, pricking, fast or 1st pain	12–30
C	Mechanoreceptors, thermoreceptors, sympathetic postganglionic nociceptors	Unmyelinated	Burning, aching, slow or 2nd pain	0.5–3

Sources: Muir 2002; Thurmon and Tranquilli 1996.

fibers that are primarily nonnociceptive (do not transmit pain stimuli) transmitting nonpainful sensations such as touch, vibration and pressure. The Aδ and C fibers are small-diameter high-threshold free nerve endings that end in the skin. Their nociceptors are involved in the transduction of pain signals. These fibers carry nerve impulses to the dorsal horn when the nociceptor threshold (minimum stimulus required to elicit a transmittable electrical signal) is exceeded. The dorsal horn contains a gating mechanism that determines whether a pain stimulus is transmitted to the CNS. Whether the "gate" is open or closed depends in part on the balance of input from the Aβ and Aδ/C fiber groups.

The *Aβ fibers* inhibit the input from Aδ and C fibers by closing the gate. This can explain why massaging and applying pressure, heat, or cold to a painful area can decrease the perception of pain.

The *Aδ fibers* are small-diameter, lightly myelinated, high-threshold "fast fibers." They signal first pain in response to an acute stimulus and are responsible for the sharp pricking sensation. They enable the animal to localize pain to the site of the stimulus. They cease after sensation is discontinued. Polymodal Aδ fibers respond to mechanical, chemical, and thermal stimuli. Other Aδ fibers respond only to specific stimuli, such as cold temperature or pressure.

C fibers are small, unmyelinated, mostly high-threshold nerves with polymodal neurons that are responsible for slow pain or chronic pain.

Slow pain has a burning, aching sensation, which indicates inflamed, damaged tissue. C fibers are abundant in the skin, skeletal muscle, joints, and viscera. Visceral nociception activity is primarily mediated by C fibers (Thurmon and Tranquilli 1996) (Table 32.1).

Silent nociceptors are Aδ and C fibers that are activated by tissue inflammation. Tissue damage and inflammation intensify the sensation of pain (activate silent receptors), producing hyperalgesia, allodynia, and hyperesthesia (Muir 2002).

Anatomy of the spinal cord dorsal horn

Interneurons are neurons that convey impulses from one neuron to another. They are typically inhibitory but can also be excitatory depending on which neurotransmitter is released. They serve as relays and participate in local processing. The dorsal horn is a collection of interneurons grouped into layers or laminae I to VI in the spinal cord. These laminae extend the full length of the spinal cord (Muir 2002). Nociceptive afferent fibers terminate on neurons within the dorsal horn of the spinal cord. Initial integration and modulation of nociceptive input occurs in the dorsal horn.

Most Aδ fibers terminate in the most superficial layer of lamina I, with a few projecting more deeply to lamina V. Lamina I is an important sensory relay junction for temperature and pain. Aδ and C fibers from the skin, skeletal muscle, joints, and viscera are responsible for most of the input. Nociceptive-specific neurons and projection neurons are contained within lamina I. Wide dynamic range (WDR) neurons are contained within laminae I, II, and V (Muir 2002).

It is thought that lamina II is important in the processing and modulating of nociceptive input from skin nociceptors due to its abundance of WDR neurons, which are mostly interneurons. It is also believed to be a major site of action for opioids (Morgan et al. 2002). In addition, lamina II is the end point for many C fibers (Fig. 32.2).

Laminae III and IV receive mostly nonnociceptive sensory input (Morgan et al. 2002). Lamina III combines descending information from the brain with sensory input (Muir 2002). Lamina V is where most visceral sensory fibers terminate, but lamina I may also be a termination point for these fibers. Sensory inputs received by wide dynamic range neurons (WDR) respond to both noxious and nonnoxious stimulus as well as pain sensations from visceral and somatic receptors. This unique quality can manifest clinically as referred pain (Hellyer et al. 2007; Morgan et al. 2002).

Second-order multireceptive neurons, WDR neurons have larger receptive fields than nociceptive-specific neurons. They respond to both noxious and nonnoxious stimuli (Hellyer et al. 2007) and receive afferent input from Aβ, Aδ, and C Fibers. WDR neurons are found throughout the dorsal horn; they are the most abundant in lamina V (Morgan et al. 2002). WDR neurons are also believed to be important in the occurrence of windup pain. C fibers are most likely the primary neuron facilitating windup pain, which occurs due to rapid and continuous firing of these fibers. It is important to recognize that general anesthesia does not prevent windup pain. Therefore preemptive analgesia becomes important and necessary for surgeries (i.e., orthopedic) likely to activate C fibers (Hellyer et al. 2007).

Projection neurons are excitatory neurons that participate in rostral transmission by extending axons beyond the spinal cord to the supraspinal centers such as the midbrain and the cortex.

Nociceptive specific neurons are concentrated in lamina I and are excited by noxious input from Aδ and C fibers. They have discrete, somatic receptive fields, are normally silent, and respond only to high-threshold noxious stimuli. It is believed that they are primarily involved in discriminative nociception (i.e., localization) (Hellyer et al. 2007).

Dorsal horn neurochemistry

Information from the dorsal horn is relayed to the brain by a number of neurotransmitters. Communication of nociceptive information between neurons occurs by chemical signaling mediated by excitatory and inhibitory amino acids and neuropeptides. These substances include peptides (substance P, calcitonin gene-related peptide [CGRP], somatostatin [SOM], neuropeptide Y, galanin [GAL]), excitatory (aspartate, glutamate) and inhibitory (gamma-aminobutyric acid [GABA], glycine) amino acids, nitric oxide (NO), prostaglandins, adenosine triphosphate (ATP), endogenous opioids, and monoamines (serotonin, norepinephrine) (Muir 2002). Glutamate and aspartate are neurotransmitters in fast excitatory synaptic response associated with Aδ fibers. Substance P, neurotensin, vasoactive intestinal peptide, calcitonin gene-

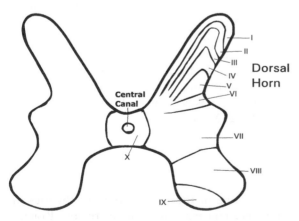

Figure 32.2. Cross section of the spinal cord. The dorsal horn of the spinal cord is composed of laminae I–VI. (Artwork modified from images courtesy of Wikipedia.com/Wikimedia.com.)

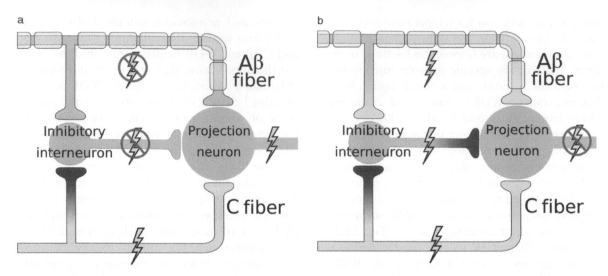

Figure 32.3 **a.** Inhibition is represented in blue, and excitation in yellow. A lightning bolt signifies increased neuron activation, while a crossed-out bolt signifies weakened or reduced activation. Increased input stimulates the C and/or Aβ fiber. This inhibits activation of the inhibitory interneuron and stimulates the projection neuron, therefore allowing a strong signal to be sent to the brain, which perceives the strong signal as pain. (Artwork courtesy of Wikipedia.com/Wikimedia.com.) **b.** A light touch will stimulate the Aβ fibers. If the stimulus is mild, the inhibitory interneurons prevent activation of the projection neuron, therefore preventing pain signals. (Artwork courtesy of Wikipedia.com/Wikimedia.com.)

related peptide, and cholecystokinin are neuropeptides capable of eliciting slow excitatory postsynaptic responses and are usually associated with C fibers.

Ascending spinal tracts

Ascending pathways are a series of neurons that transmit signals from receptors to the brain. The four ascending pathways of primary importance that carry information from the spinal cord to the brain are the spinothalamic, spinoreticular, spinomessencephalic, and spinohypothalamic tracts. These pathways have a large integrated degree of overlap in their function (Hellyer et al. 2007).

The spinothalamic pathway is considered the major pain pathway that originates from laminae I, IV, and VII (Morgan et al. 2002; Muir 2002). It transmits discriminative aspects of pain from the spinal cord to the thalamus, such as location, intensity, and duration. The sensations transmitted include superficial pain, temperature, itch, and touch. It is also responsible for mediating the

autonomic and unpleasant emotional perception of pain (Morgan et al. 2002). The spinoreticular pathway also originates from laminae I, IV, and VII (Muir 2002). It is believed to mediate arousal and more of the emotional aspect of pain (Morgan et al. 2002). The spinoreticular pathway is important in the transmission of deep pain and visceral sensations (Hellyer et al. 2007). The spinomesencephalic pathway is thought to be important in activation of antinociceptive, descending pathways and originates in laminae I and V (Morgan et al. 2002; Muir 2002). The spinohypothalamic tract originating from laminae III and IV participates in activating the motivational component of pain and evokes emotional behavior (Morgan et al. 2002; Muir 2002).

The Gate Control Theory of Pain

In 1965 one of the most important theories in pain mechanisms was put forth by Ronald Melzack and Patrick D. Wall, a theory they called the Gate Control Theory of Pain (Melzack and Wall 1965). Their theory proposed that pain phenomena are determined by interactions among three systems at the level of the spinal cord:

1. Gate control system: The substantia gelatinosa (now referred to as lamina II), functions as a *gate control system* that modulates the afferent patterns before they influence the T (central transmission cells now referred to as projection neurons) cells.
2. Central control trigger: The afferent patterns in the dorsal column system act, in part, as a *central control trigger*, which activates selective brain processes that influence the modulation properties of the gate control system.
3. Action system: The T cells activate neural mechanisms, which comprise the *action system* responsible for response and perception.

This theory was the basis for testing how noxious stimuli are transduced, transmitted, modulated, and perceived as pain. The theory continues to be important in our understanding of pain perception today.

Figure 32.3 (a and b) illustrates stimulation of the Aβ and Aδ and/or C fibers.

Pain physiology is a complex process. This chapter highlights some basic terminology that will allow you to understand the processes whereby pain occurs and how pain relief can be provided. Pain management is an ever-evolving specialty in the veterinary and human medical professions. It is coming to the forefront of veterinary care via drugs, procedures, diagnostics, and management therapies. Armed with this knowledge we can better design pain management protocols for each individual patient and strive for excellence in patient care.

Acknowledgments

I would like to give my sincere thanks to John W. Ludders DVM, Andrea L. Looney DVM, and William A. Horne DVM, PhD, for their encouragement and support in the development of this chapter.

References

Hellyer, PW, Robertson, SA, Fails, AD. 2007. Pain and its management. In Lumb & Jones' Veterinary Anesthesia and Analgesia, 4th ed., edited by Tranquilli, WJ, Thurmon, JC, Grimm, KA, editors. Ames, IA: Blackwell Publishing, pp.31–52.

Livingston, A, Chambers, P. 2000. The physiology of pain. In Pain Management in Animals, edited by Flecknell, PA, Waterman-Pearson, A. London: WB Saunders, pp.9–19.

Melzack, R, Wall, PD. 1965. Pain mechanisms: A new theory. Science 19;150(699):971–979.

Morgan, GE, Mikhail, MS, Murray, MJ. 2002. Pain management. In Clinical Anesthesiology, 4th ed., edited by Morgan, GE, Mikhail, MS, Murray, MJ. New York: McGraw-Hill, pp.359–373.

Muir, WW. 2002. Physiology and pathophysiology of pain. In Handbook of Veterinary Pain Management, edited by Gaynor, JS, Muir, WW. St. Louis: Mosby, pp.13–45.

Thurmon, JC, Tranquilli, WJ. 1996. Perioperative pain and distress. In Lumb & Jones' Veterinary Anesthesia, 3rd ed., Thurmon, JC, Tranquilli, WJ, Benson, GJ, Lumb, WV, edited by Thurmon, JC, Tranquilli, WJ. Baltimore: Williams & Wilkins, pp.40, 42.

Web Resources

International Association for the Study of Pain. IASP Pain Terminology. Available at http://www.iasppain.org/AM/Template.cfm?Section=General_Resource_Links&Template=/CM/HTMLDisplay.cfm&ContentID=3058#Pain. Accessed May 27, 2008.

Woolf, CJ. 2008. Pain Sensitization. Available at http://www.wellcome.ac.uk/en/pain/microsite/science4.html. Accessed May 15, 2008.

33 Pain Assessment

Kim Lockhead

Pain assessment in small animal practice has many challenges. One of these challenges is the lack of a standard, validated way of assessing pain in veterinary patients. Even in human medicine, accurate evaluation of pain is extremely difficult. Due to the fact that pain is always a subjective and individual experience, it is often difficult, even for humans, to accurately describe their level of discomfort and the quality of their pain. These challenges are magnified in veterinary medicine by the inability of veterinary patients to communicate verbally with their caretakers. Veterinarians and technicians are forced to make educated assumptions about the comfort level of their patients based on their own experiences, and they must draw parallels between human and veterinary patients. According to the AAHA/AAFP Pain Management Guidelines for Dogs and Cats, "It is now well established that animals and humans have similar neural pathways for the development, conduction, and modulation of pain. According to the principle of analogy, because cats and dogs have neural pathways and neurotransmitters that are similar, if not identical, to those of humans, it is highly likely that animals experience pain similarly" (Hellyer et al. 2007). This means that if a procedure or condition is thought to be painful in a human patient, it should be considered painful in a veterinary patient as well, based on the similarities in the nervous system of humans and many animals. This mind-set differs greatly from that of previous generations of veterinary professionals. Many used to believe that animals did not experience pain in the same manner as humans simply because they did not express pain in exactly the same ways. The 17th century French philosopher, René Descartes, expounded the belief that animals could not feel pain or experience suffering since they had no consciousness or rationality. This belief has been clung to by many in animal research and in the veterinary profession until somewhat recently. Because of this, painful conditions have not always been addressed appropriately. In fact, many believed that pain could be helpful to the patient. Pain has been used as a way of restricting activity in postsurgical patients. Some postsurgical animals were not given analgesics because it was thought that pain would restrict their activity and prevent them from injuring themselves. It was also believed that pain would be helpful in assessing the progression of a disease or condition. The current attitude is that pain should not be a tool used to restrict activity. Except in cases of complete sensory and motor blockade by a local anesthetic, analgesic therapy rarely completely eliminates pain, and some remaining sensation can limit activity that may be harmful. Withholding analgesics for the purpose of restraint is considered inhumane as well as unnecessary. Tranquilizers, e-collars, and cage confinement can be used to restrict movement and prevent injury as needed.

Attitudes toward animal pain and suffering have changed greatly since the days of Descartes, and the idea that animals experience pain differently from humans is now the minority view. Pain assessment and pain management techniques are now being treated as essential in the training of new veterinarians and veterinary technicians and as essential to the care and well-being of veterinary patients.

Role of the Technician in Pain Assessment

Pain recognition is a vital part of good nursing care. Minimizing pain is a very important aspect of overall patient care. It has been recognized by some veterinary clinicians that controlling pain in the perioperative period or during the acute painful phase of a medical condition helps patients begin to regain normal functions, such as eating and grooming, sooner (Carroll 1998). Unmanaged acute pain can lead to an activation of endocrine and cardiovascular responses that may play a role in perioperative immune suppression and act to impair recovery. The veterinary technician is so important in pain assessment because the technician is typically the individual that interacts with the patient most frequently and whose observations are most helpful in recognizing pain in veterinary patients. The technician and the veterinarian can work together to assess pain and anxiety and to develop an analgesic plan that will increase the quality of life of their patients and to help them return to normal function sooner.

Behavioral Signs of Pain

Behavioral assessment is the most common way of assessing pain in small animal patients. Pain in animals has been defined as "an aversive sensory experience that elicits protective motor actions, results in learned avoidance, and may modify species-specific traits of behavior, including social behavior" (Association 1986). Familiarizing oneself with normal behavior in a particular animal and species is the first step in learning to assess abnormal or painful behavior. A change from normal behavior is one of the most important signs of pain in veterinary species. These changes may be subtle and difficult to evaluate in some animals. The friendly, young cat that is postoperative and is now growling, biting, and trying to escape may be painful. The same could be true for the geriatric Golden Retriever that has begun having trouble getting out of bed and getting up and down the stairs. The rabbit that was previously friendly and enjoyed handling but is now reluctant to move and objects to handling may be painful as well. What about the dog that sits quietly in its cage and continually looks at its surgical incision? What about the one that paces in its cage and won't lie down? Are these dogs painful? It can be difficult to say for certain. Vocalization is often the first, overt sign that a patient is uncomfortable. Vocal patients are usually the first to be evaluated since they are the ones that are best at "telling" their caretakers that they are in pain. However, some patients do not vocalize when in pain, and attempt to hide it as a protective measure. The pain of these patients is more likely to go unrecognized. In fact, in the author's experience, the most painful patients are often not vocalizing at all.

Species differences

The signs of pain in veterinary patients can vary, but some commonalties are often observed. Figures 33.1 and 33.2 show some behaviors that are seen in acutely painful dogs and cats. There are some noticeable differences between these species but many behaviors are common.

- Abnormal sitting or lying posture
- Restlessness
- Splinting of abdomen
- Whining, groaning, crying
- Limping, unwilling to get up or move, unwilling to lie down
- Trembling, shivering
- Rapid, shallow breathing
- Lack of appetite
- Increased respiratory rate, heart rate, increased blood pressure
- Dilated pupils, bulging eyes
- Aggression, resents being touched
- Licking or biting the affected area
- Lack of grooming

Figure 33.1. Signs of acute pain in the dog.

- Crouching in the back of the cage
- Decreased grooming
- Decreased appetite
- Very likely to become aggressive when in pain
- Growling
- Increased heart rate, respiratory rate, and blood pressure
- Acting frantic, vocalizing
- Purring
- Squinting eyes
- Unwilling to use litter box
- Shivering, shuddering
- Biting at or trying to escape from the painful area
- Self-mutilation
- Hiding

Figure 33.2. Signs of acute pain in the cat.

Cats, rabbits, rodents, and other prey species often try to hide signs of pain or injury as part of a survival mechanism. In evolutionary terms, this behavior is a protective measure and would have given these animals a survival advantage. In the wild, predators single out injured or infirm animals from a group since they are easiest to capture and kill. By hiding an injury or illness, prey animals would be less likely to be singled out by predators. Though domestic animals are far less likely to have to worry about predation, some of these protective behaviors remain intact

→ **The Rabbit**
- Lack of grooming
- May appear hunched or droopy
- Lack of appetite
- Excessive scratching or licking
- Exaggerated responses to handling
- Teeth grinding
- Abdominal splinting
- May appear immobile, unwilling to move
- May hide or face the back of the cage
- Increased respiratory rate or effort

→ **The Rodent (Mouse, Rat)**
- Decreased exploring behavior
- Hunched appearance
- Porphyrin tearing
- Anorexia
- Decreased grooming, rough hair coat
- Self-mutilation
- Increased scratching, licking
- Increased aggression when handled

Figure 33.3. Signs of pain in small mammal species.

because they have been deeply ingrained as instinct.

Normal behaviors vary between species, and therefore abnormal behaviors will vary as well. It is often most difficult to evaluate species that are considered "exotic" because many people are unaware of the behaviors that are unique to these species. Figure 33.3 shows the signs of pain in some other small mammal species.

Breed differences

Responses to pain and distress are often breed related as well. Small-breed dogs, Nordic breeds (huskies, malamutes), and Labrador retrievers often have exaggerated responses to stress and pain. These animals are often considered less stoic than some other breeds when it comes to pain. However, it is important not to dismiss these responses without a proper evaluation of the individual patient. Occasionally, the behaviors seen in these patients are attributable to anxiety due to hospitalization, and administration of a sedative would be more appropriate than addition of an analgesic. However, if a proper assessment is done by a trained individual it may be found that the animal is painful and would benefit from administration of additional analgesics, a different type of analgesic, or an analgesic plus a sedative.

Age differences

Age can also complicate the evaluation process. Pediatrics and neonates tend to be very vocal and perhaps excessively communicative about their pain or discomfort. A proper assessment and adjustment of drug dosages is necessary in treating these patients effectively and safely. Adults or geriatric patients have a greater tendency toward stoicism. Though these older animals may be in an immense amount of pain due to a condition or procedure, they may tolerate it without complaint. This does not mean that analgesia is not needed and should not be provided.

Individual characteristics

Pain is always a very individual and unique experience. Every patient will have an individual response to a painful stimulus and stressful situation. There are several reasons for this. Every patient has different physiologic factors including different levels of endogenous opioids, individual drug receptor responses, and chronic pain states already present. Each patient must be assessed as an individual for these reasons. A procedure or condition that may not be painful for one patient may be quite painful for another due to individual characteristics. Flexibility is very important if treatment is to be successful.

Physiologic Signs of Pain

Some physiologic signs of severe pain include tachycardia, hypertension, cardiac arrhythmias, shallow or labored breathing, pale mucous membranes, increased body temperature, salivation, and dilated pupils. These physiologic signs can be used as part of the pain assessment plan but typically should not be used alone. Many signs of pain are also signs of other problems. Tachycardia is not always a reliable indicator of pain. High heart rate can be a sign of pain, but it may also signal other potential problems. These may include, but are not limited to, hypotension, shock, hypoxia, and hypercarbia. It is important to realize that painful animals will not always be tachycardic and/ or hypertensive. For example, animals on beta-blocker therapy for cardiac disease may not be able to become tachycardic in response to pain even though they may be painful.

Mucous membrane color can be an indicator of pain in some animals. Pale mucous membranes are sometimes seen due to vasoconstriction from release of catecholamines as part of a stress response. Of course, pale mucous membranes do not always signal pain. Anemia, shock, cardiac disease, and extreme stress should also be ruled out as causes.

Respiratory rate can be helpful as well. Often, a painful animal will have an elevated respiratory rate and/or an increase in respiratory effort. An increased respiratory rate and increased effort may also indicate pneumothorax, pleural effusion, pneumonia, hyperthermia, shock, etc. Animals with thoracic or cranial abdominal pain may have impaired ventilation because of their painful state. In some cases, the fear of opioid-induced respiratory depression leads to undertreatment of pain because opioid administration has the potential to worsen hypoxia by causing a degree of respiratory depression. However, administration of some kind of analgesic may enhance ventilation by allowing better expansion of the thoracic wall and diaphragm. Judicious use of opioid analgesics can be helpful. An analgesic with fewer proclivities for respiratory depression may also be used. Ketamine, gabapentin, NSAIDs, and local anesthetics are some possible options.

Neuroendocrine signs

Neuroendocrine values can occasionally be used as a part of pain assessment, but they really cannot be used as part of a cage-side evaluation. Parameters that can potentially be measured include cortisol levels, epinephrine, norepinephrine, blood glucose, stress leukogram, and endorphin levels. Generally, there are no blood tests that are considered practical pain measures for the clinical hospital setting. Blood tests are invasive, require processing, can be expensive, and can require days for results to be reported. For individual patients these tests may not be realistic, but they have been used in research settings and other controlled situations in which operated and unoperated controls are present for comparison. The other main problem with using neuroendocrine values is that they are not specific for pain and may indicate a generalized stress response. For these reasons, neuroendocrine values are of limited usefulness in the painful, hospitalized patient.

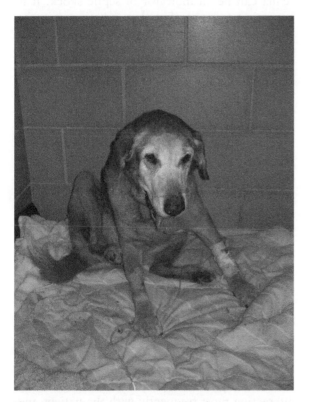

Figure 33.4. A splenectomy patient one day postop. Surgery went well and was uneventful. The dog was unwilling to lie down and held her hindleg up and away from her abdomen. She was currently on a fentanyl CRI for pain. The "rescue plan" included a dose of hydromorphone and the addition of a lidocaine CRI, which improved her comfort level immensely. Human beings report splenectomy surgery to be extremely painful.

Performing a General Acute Pain Assessment

It is difficult to say for sure in a given situation whether a patient is truly in pain. The best way to begin an assessment is by observation alone without interaction. Patients may change their behaviors if they know they are being observed, so it is important to simply watch from some distance at first. Note the patients' positions in the cage or run. Are they hiding in the rear of the cage and facing the back, or are they up at the front of the cage eager to interact? Are they sitting, lying down, or standing? A patient that is painful may try to lie down but be unable to. They may be observed trying to sleep while sitting or standing up (Fig. 33.4). They may tuck up or "splint" their abdomen if the area is uncomfortable (Fig. 33.5). They may be shivering, rigid, or thrashing in the cage. One should also note the respiratory rate and pattern and whether the patient is vocalizing.

The next step is to interact with the patient. When they are approached, is the patient willing

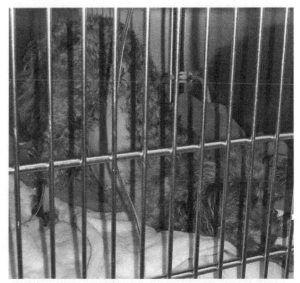

Figure 33.5. The classic "prayer position" in a miniature poodle 12 hours postoperatively for gallbladder removal surgery. Sadly, people in the room commented that they thought she was just being cute (which demonstrates the desperate need for education on pain assessment).

or able to stand or sit up? Do they acknowledge the presence of the caretaker, and do they appear more or less distressed when approached? The area on and around the suspected painful region should be gently palpated while the animal is lightly restrained. The patient should be watched closely to see whether they look over, whine, cry, yelp, bite, try to escape, scratch, grow tense, or growl. Be cautious during this part of the assessment because a painful animal is more likely to bite or scratch. Gentle restraint from an assistant may be helpful and can help to prevent injury to personnel.

It is important to assess additional sources of pain as well. Other parts of the body should be gently palpated. Some animals will also have pain from arthritis, poor positioning in surgery, or pressure points from inadequate bedding. Note the last time that the animal urinated and defecated. A source of stress and discomfort can be a full bladder. Is the patient hungry? An empty stomach can be painful and a small amount of food can improve the patient's overall level of comfort.

After a thorough evaluation it may still be unclear whether the patient is painful. It is impossible to say with complete certainty in every situation whether a patient is painful. A low, trial dose of an analgesic is usually a reasonable option, even in sick or debilitated patients. Opioid analgesics are generally considered the safest choices for these patients because they have limited effects on the cardiovascular system and they are reversible if undesirable side effects are seen. If an analgesic is administered and the patient's symptoms are diminished, it is reasonable to assume that pain was the cause. A sedative may be combined with an analgesic to cover anxiety that may contribute to worsening of the patient's discomfort. If the patient's behaviors improve, it may not be clear which drug was responsible for the change. However, this may not be important if the animal is improving. Generally, if pain is suspected, it should be treated.

For those working in emergency and critical care settings, distinguishing the painful patient from the patient in shock can be an especially large challenge. Both can be tachycardic. Both may be hypertensive, hypotensive, or normotensive depending on the stage of shock. Both may have pale mucous membranes. Both may have an elevated respiratory rate or increased respiratory effort. All of these factors can complicate assessment. A few procedures can be done to determine the difference. A blood lactate measurement may be helpful in these situations. An elevated lactate is indicative of anaerobic metabolism; this can occur due to hypoperfusion or hypoxemia, which is seen in states of shock. Typically, lactate will not be as elevated in painful states as it will be in shock, though some elevation may be seen due to stress. Typically, the elevation is much higher in severe states of shock. If sepsis is a possibility, it is important to screen for abdominal or other effusions. A blood glucose value may be obtained, because hypoglycemia can be an indicator of septic shock. It is important to remember that a patient may be very painful as well as in shock. In fact, this is often seen. Management of these patients should include normal treatments for shock as well as analgesic therapy where appropriate.

Frequency of assessment

Frequency of assessment is an important aspect of pain management to consider. Prevention of pain is usually much more effective than treatment of pain once it has already occurred. The goal for hospitalized patients should be to stay a step ahead of their pain. This goal can be difficult to achieve, so the frequency of assessment can vary according to the patient and the condition. One major limiting factor to identifying patients in pain at many hospitals is the inability of the staff to perform frequent, lengthy evaluations of each animal. Time limitations play a large role in the underrecognition of pain. Veterinary technicians play an essential role because they are the people who are generally interacting most frequently with the patient and can best assess changes in its behavior, demeanor, and physiologic parameters. Alerting the veterinarian to these changes is an important job of the technician. So the question remains: How often should the patient be assessed for pain? This depends on the health status of the patient, the extent of the injuries and/or the surgery, and the duration of the analgesic chosen.

A patient with severe disease may need to be assessed for pain more frequently than a patient that is generally healthy and having an elective procedure. A very ill patient may be in an unstable state and changes in its level of comfort could be indicative of changes in its disease process. This is also true of a patient suffering severe injuries or that has been through an extensive surgical procedure. A sudden increase in pain could signal the beginnings of infection or sepsis, so frequent assessment is essential in heading off these serious problems. The characteristics and duration of the analgesic that is already being administered can determine the frequency of assessment as well.

When monitoring analgesic therapy in the postoperative patient, hourly assessments should be done for the first 4–6 hours. These assessments may be brief if necessary. It is important to perform frequent evaluations during this period because the effects of anesthetics can alter normal behaviors and interfere with normal physiologic parameters. After 6 hours, the frequency of assessment can be reduced if the patient has stable vital signs, has recovered from anesthesia, and analgesia has been deemed adequate during the earlier period. The duration of analgesic therapy will vary, depending on many factors. Certain procedures or conditions will require long-term analgesic therapy. It can be challenging to predict a patient's analgesic needs, and therefore continuing evaluation is extremely important.

Painful Conditions and Procedures

Many hospitalized patients have painful conditions or undergo painful procedures. In assessing pain, it is helpful to have an expectation of how painful a certain condition or procedure is expected to be. This is usually subject to some bias based on the experiences of the veterinarian or technician. Most veterinary professionals will formulate an analgesic plan based on their preconceptions about the level of pain their patients will experience. The level of pain following a

surgery will depend on many factors. These include the type of surgery being performed, the type of tissue involved (bone, soft tissue), the amount of tissue manipulation by the surgeon, the length of the surgery, the skill and experience of the surgeon, whether preemptive analgesia was provided, and whether the patient already had a chronic pain state resulting in central sensitization. An ovariohysterectomy is a commonly performed surgical procedure. For some patients, limited analgesic therapy is needed because a skilled, experienced surgeon is performing the procedure in a healthy animal. Surgical skill and gentle handling of tissue may reduce, but not eliminate, the need for perioperative analgesia. For some patients, such as the arthritic Labrador with a severe pyometra, it can be quite painful. Additional analgesia may be required depending on the circumstances and the individual characteristics of the patient.

There is general agreement on the level of pain produced by certain procedures. Some procedures and conditions are considered more painful than others. Typically, anything involving bone, large amounts of tissue, nerve damage, or inflamed or infected tissue can be quite painful. Limb amputations, extensive burns, splenectomy, thoracotomy, bile peritonitis, pancreatitis, and anything involving extensive tissue trauma would generally be considered severely painful. Procedures causing moderate to severe pain would include enucleation, onychectomy (declawing), cranial abdominal procedures, and some fracture repairs. Procedures causing moderate pain would include caudal abdominal procedures, castrations, some fractures, and dental extractions. Mild pain can be caused by things like clipper burn and superficial lacerations (Carroll 1998). These are, of course, only a few of the potential procedures that can be performed and there are many factors that affect the amount of discomfort caused by each one.

Pain Scoring Systems

All pain scoring techniques in veterinary medicine have their drawbacks. No reliable scale has

| No pain | Mild pain | Moderate pain | Severe pain | V. severe pain |

Circle one

Figure 33.6. Example of the SDS.

been developed without differences between observers. Ultimately, each veterinary hospital needs to develop its own pain scoring system that works for the patients that are seen on a regular basis and that is easy for the veterinarians and technicians to apply quickly and reliably. No pain scale or worksheet will work for every patient in every circumstance, and no one scale has been approved for widespread use. Because pain is a very individual experience, it will manifest in different ways in different species and different individuals. Since veterinary patients cannot directly communicate with caretakers how they are feeling, assessment is completely reliant on the observations of an onlooker. Since these assessments are based on an observer's interpretations, they are therefore subject to bias. Pain assessment scales have been developed as tools to aid in the evaluation process and to decrease bias between observers. There are several different scales that can be used to assess pain. Each system has its advantages and its limitations.

The first and simplest pain scoring system described is the simple descriptive scale (SDS). This scale is a qualitative assessment of the level of an animal's pain made by an observer. The scale usually consists of four to five different descriptors varying from no pain to very severe pain. This system is the simplest pain scoring system and it is also the most subjective. Figure 33.6 shows an example of the simple descriptive scale.

The second commonly used pain scoring system is the numerical rating system (NRS). This scale is very similar to the SDS except that a numerical value is assigned to each pain descriptor. The NRS is not a quantitative scale. The scores are ordinal numbers that have no numerical relationship to each other. For example, a score of 4 is not twice as painful as a score of 2. The Categorized Numerical Rating System (CNRS) is an extension of the NRS that

takes a specific pain-associated behavior and assigns it a number based on the severity of the pain. A total score can be calculated and used to guide treatment. Intervention can then be applied accordingly. It is important to remember that animals that score low but appear painful to the observer may still require treatment. Figure 33.7 shows examples of the NRS and CNRS.

The third commonly used pain scoring system is the Visual Analog Scale (VAS). This scale has been used widely in human medicine. The scale consists of a continuous line of predetermined length, usually 100 mm long. The beginning of the line is assigned the value "0 to no pain" and the end is assigned the value "100 to very severe pain". The observer will assess the patient and mark the line where he/she believes the patient's pain level falls. The space can then be measured in millimeters from the zero mark to the mark of the observer to translate this mark into a numerical value. As with the other scales discussed, the VAS is subject to observer bias. However, since the VAS is not limited to defined categories, it may be more sensitive than the NRS or SDS (Firth and Haldane 1999). Some variations of the VAS may also be used. A modified VAS may consist of a continuous line with additional markings at predetermined lengths along the line. Figure 33.8 shows two examples of a VAS.

Each of the three main pain assessment scales discussed so far, while useful, has major limitations. In each system there is significant variability in scoring among observers. According to one paper, this variability was as high as 36% (Holton et al. 1998a). However, it has been suggested that the numerical rating scale may have the least variability of the three scales when observations are made by a trained observer (Holton et al. 1998b).

In addition to these three simple scales, more complex pain scoring systems have been developed. An extension of the visual analog scale

| 1 no pain | 2 mild pain | 3 moderate pain | 4 severe pain | 5 v. severe pain |

Circle one. Number chosen is the pain score. Higher pain score corresponds to higher level of pain.

Example of the CNRS

Vocalization	*Response to palpation*
None--0	None--0
Crying--1	Slight response--------------------------------1
Crying + escape behaviors------------------2	Strong response------------------------------2

Choose the appropriate value and total. The total is the pain score. Higher pain score corresponds to higher level of pain. Highest score is 4 according to this scale. A low score does not mean that intervention is not needed.

Figure 33.7.   (a) Example of the NRS. (b) Example of the CNRS.

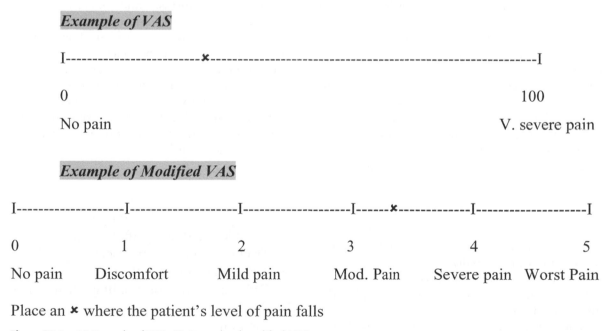

Example of VAS

I---------------------------**✗**---I

0   100

No pain   V. severe pain

Example of Modified VAS

I------------------I------------------I------------------I------**✗**------------I------------------I

0   1   2   3   4   5

No pain   Discomfort   Mild pain   Mod. Pain   Severe pain   Worst Pain

Place an **✗** where the patient's level of pain falls

Figure 33.8.   (a) Example of VAS. (B) Example of modified VAS.

called the Dynamic and Interactive Visual Analog Scale (DIVAS) may be used to do a more complete assessment of the patient (Lascelles et al. 1998). There are four main steps to performing this assessment. The first step is to simply observe the patient from a distance without disturbance and note its posture and behavior. The second step is to approach the animal and interact with it to see whether any of the behaviors that were seen previously change or whether new behaviors emerge. The third step is to palpate on and around the suspected painful area or surgical incision. The fourth step is an overall assessment of the patient's pain and level of sedation. These observations are used together to be translated into a VAS.

All the scales that have been discussed so far are one-dimensional scales. This means that they are used only to assess the suspected intensity of pain. A scale that is multidimensional can assess the intensity of pain as well as its sensory and emotional qualities. Multidimensional scales are infrequently used in veterinary medicine due to the difficulty of evaluating these qualities in veterinary patients. In humans, the McGill Pain Questionnaire has been used to perform more comprehensive assessments (Robertson 2007). This multidimensional scale requires the patient to assess its own pain. The patient must characterize its intensity and describe the specific qualities of the pain. The patient indicates whether the pain is dull, sharp, burning, stabbing, cramping, etc. It also requires the patient to assign an emotional quality to its pain, such as annoying, miserable, frightening, etc. Human patients will also be asked how much their pain "bothers" them and whether it interferes with their daily activities. Due to the inability of animal patients to communicate verbally with their caretakers, this type of assessment tool is more difficult to construct in veterinary medicine, despite the advantage it provides.

The Glasgow Composite Measures Pain Scale-Short form (CMPS-SF) was developed by the University of Glasgow and has been used to measure acute pain in dogs. The Glasgow Pain Scale can be considered a multidimensional pain assessment scale. It is possible to evaluate how patients' pain affects them by considering how their behaviors deviate from normal. If the patient is unable to catch a ball anymore or is unable to climb onto the couch with the family or other pets, it would seem that its pain is affecting its normal activity. One of the main advantages of this system is that it can be used reliably to assess acute postoperative pain in dogs and can be used quickly in routine clinical situations. There are six behavioral categories that are examined: vocalization, attention to painful area, mobility, response to touch, demeanor, and posture/activity (Reid et al. 2007). Pain intensity is scored and, based on the score, the clinician can determine whether or not the animal is in need of additional analgesia.

Assessment of Chronic Pain

Chronic pain states that are frequently seen in small animals include pain from cancer, dental disease, osteoarthritis, and musculoskeletal disease. Assessing these and other chronic pain states is different from assessment of acute pain in that it usually focuses on function and changes in function. Because of this, owner input can be extremely helpful since the owner is the person who is the most aware of what is normal behavior for that animal. Behaviors and signs that the owner may notice in the chronically painful animal are noted in Figure 33.9.

➢ Changes in exercise level
➢ Changes in general activity level
➢ Trouble standing up after rest periods
➢ Trouble ascending or descending stairs
➢ Tiring more quickly than usual
➢ Difficulty eating or drooling when eating
➢ Restlessness
➢ Limping
➢ Muscle wasting
➢ Decreased range of motion
➢ Alterations in voiding behaviors
➢ Decrease in grooming

Figure 33.9. Signs of chronic pain in the dog.

Owners should be asked to assess these behaviors in their pet to the best of their ability. This information combined with an exam performed by a veterinarian or veterinary technician can provide a basis for diagnosis and treatment of chronic pain states.

Conclusion

Recognition of pain in veterinary species has come a long way since the days of René Descartes; however, there are still many challenges to proper assessment and treatment. Veterinary technicians can play a huge role in increasing the comfort and welfare of animal patients by becoming familiar with normal species behavior and common signs of pain in those species that they treat. Becoming familiar with the expected level of pain from certain procedures is also important in providing preemptive analgesia and preventing pain. Finally, learning to use a pain assessment scale that is appropriate for the individual hospital and patients that are seen there can play a large role in decreasing bias between observers and more accurately evaluating patients so that they may receive the best treatment possible.

References

Association of Veterinary Teachers and Research Workers. 1986. Guidelines for the Recognition and Assessment of Pain in Animals. Vet Rec 118:334–338.

Carroll, GL. 1998. Small Animal Pain Management. AAHA Press, pp.21–25.

Firth, AM, Haldane, SL. 1999. Development of a scale to evaluate postoperative pain in dogs. JAVMA 214(5):651–659.

Hellyer, P, et al. 2007. AAHA/AAFP pain management guidelines for dogs and cats. JAAHA 43:235–248.

Holton, LL, et al. 1998a. Comparison of three methods used for assessment of pain in dogs. JAVMA 212(1):61–66.

Holton, LL, et al. 1998b. Relationship between physiological factors and clinical pain in dogs scored using a numerical rating scale. J Small Anim Pract 39:469–474.

Lascelles, B, et al. 1998. Efficacy and kinetics of carprofen, administered pre-operatively and post-operatively, for the prevention of pain in dogs undergoing ovariohysterectomy. Vet Surg 27(6):568–582.

Reid, J, et al. 2007. Development of the Short-Form Glasgow Composite Measure Pain Scale (CMPS-SF) and derivation of an analgesic intervention score. Anim Welfare 16(1): 97–104.

Robertson, SA. 2007. Acute Pain Evaluation. Proceedings of the Southern European Veterinary Conference and Congreso Nacional (AVEPA) 2007. Barcelona, Spain.

Pain Management Strategies

34

Kim Spelts and James Gaynor

"Pain management in dogs and cats has undergone a dramatic evolution in the past decade. Current approaches focus on anticipation and prevention of pain, as well as both pharmacologic and nonpharmacologic management techniques. The veterinary team plays an essential role in educating pet owners about recognizing and managing pain in their pets."

American Animal Hospital Association, 2007

Veterinary professionals are becoming increasingly proactive about identifying and treating pain in their patients. A multitude of strategies for managing pain are available, many of which were unheard of just a few years ago.

Designing an Optimal Pain Management Strategy

Designing an optimal pain management strategy for any patient requires a clear understanding of the following key definitions and concepts:

Multimodal analgesia

Normal pain sensation (nociception) occurs in four primary steps: transduction, transmission,

modulation, and perception (refer to Chapter 32 for more detail).

We have a variety of drugs available to us to address pain at each point along the nociceptive pathway. Providing such therapy to attack pain from different angles is known as *multimodal analgesia* and should be the primary strategy of any pain management plan. These drugs and their effects on the pain pathway are summarized in Table 34.1, and they are discussed in more detail later on and in other chapters of this book.

Central neuronal hypersensitization

Central neuronal hypersensitization, also referred to as *windup*, occurs when the dorsal horn of the spinal cord is bombarded with the transmission of noxious stimuli. N-methyl-D-aspartate (NMDA) receptors within the dorsal horn are activated and amplify the signal to the brain, much like turning up the volume on a stereo. Windup can result in exaggeration of painful impulses and the transmission and interpretation of an innocuous impulse as being painful. NMDA receptors act somewhat like light switches: once stimulated, they often require some intervention to turn them off. Likewise, once blocked,

Table 34.1.   Drug effects on the nociceptive pathway.

Pain Process	Mechanism	Anesthetic/Analgesic Agents
Transduction	Inhibit peripheral sensitization	Local anesthetics, opioids, NSAIDs, corticosteroids
Transmission	Inhibit impulse conduction	Local anesthetics, α_2 agonists
Modulation	Inhibit central sensitization	Local anesthetics, opioids, α_2 agonists, NSAIDs, NMDA antagonists, tricyclic antidepressants, anticonvulsants
Perception	Alter cerebral recognition of painful conditions	Inhalant anesthetics, opioids, α_2 agonists, benzodiazepines, phenothiazines

Adapted from Figure 1-3, Pain Management for the Small Animal Practitioner, 2004.

they can stay inactivated for extended periods of time.

Pain States

A newer understanding of the physiological processes of pain has led to definitions that accurately reflect microprocesses operating within the periphery and the CNS. Pain is a very complex process, and the way we define and treat pain in our patients must reflect this complexity.

Adaptive pain versus maladaptive pain

In an adaptive pain state, the body's central processes are operating normally. This type of pain serves a biological purpose—i.e., the body's pain response warns the individual of impending or actual tissue damage and helps to prevent further trauma. It also results in tissue healing. Pain related to surgery or acute traumatic injury and pain that results from inflammation are examples of adaptive pain.

In a maladaptive pain state, the body's central processing has gone awry. This is due to damage to the peripheral and/or central nervous system (neuropathic pain), or the CNS is not properly processing the pain. Spontaneous pain and hypersensitivity can occur. In this state, pain has actually become a disease process. Chronic pain, such as that related to osteoarthritis or cancer, is a good example of maladaptive pain.

Acute pain versus chronic pain

Acute pain is mild to severe pain that may be incapacitating. The degree of pain is related to the traumatic incident or procedure performed. Acute pain is relatively short-term (hours to days, up to a month) in duration and is generally adaptive in nature. Acute pain dissipates as the initial source of the pain (trauma, surgery, injury, etc.) resolves.

Chronic pain serves no biological purpose. Chronic pain may occur in the presence of a persistent stimulus (as with osteoarthritis), or there may be no stimulus at all (as happens when the pain has become maladaptive in nature).

Preemptive Analgesia

Although it is not always possible to achieve, *preemptive analgesia* should be one of the primary goals when creating a pain management plan, especially during the perioperative period. Lower doses of analgesics are required to prevent and keep pain under control than are required to "rescue" an animal that has become painful. Preemptive analgesia can also help prevent windup and can help prevent acute pain from developing into chronic pain, or adaptive pain into maladaptive pain.

Considerations

As in humans, pain in animals is an individual experience. Individuals may have very different responses to similar painful stimuli. Therefore, every pain management plan should be tailored to the individual, with periodic reassessments and modifications if necessary.

Providing preemptive and multimodal analgesia are goals in the management of both adaptive and maladaptive pain; however, the methods of doing so vary somewhat between the two.

Management of Adaptive Pain

Adaptive pain is the type most often associated with trauma and/or surgery. It is usually acute in nature, and it can be mild to severe. Most drugs administered for the management of this type of pain are administered on a relatively short-term basis, and the need for analgesic support should diminish as the initial source of pain resolves.

Nonsteroidal antiinflammatory drugs (NSAIDs)

NSAID administration is very common in small animal practices as a component of multimodal analgesia for the treatment of mild to moderate pain, both acute and chronic. Currently, six NSAIDs have FDA approval for use in dogs in the U.S.: etodolac, carprofen, deracoxib, tepoxalin, meloxicam, and firocoxib. Both carprofen and meloxicam are available in injectable formulations and can be given perioperatively. Deracoxib and carprofen are also approved for perioperative oral dosing for acute pain control. Injectable meloxicam is the only NSAID with FDA approval for use in cats.

The primary mechanism of action of NSAIDs is some preferential blockade of the cyclo-oxygenase-2 (COX-2) enzyme compared to the COX-1 enzyme (tepoxalin also inhibits the 5-lipoxygenase enzyme). The COX-2 enzyme converts arachadonic acid into prostaglandins. Some of these prostaglandins cause pain and inflammation, while others are crucial for the maintenance of GI mucosal integrity, renal blood flow, and proper platelet function during times of physiological stress (such as shock or dehydration). Because of the potential for blocking these beneficial prostaglandins, NSAID use should be avoided in patients with liver or kidney disease, those with a high likelihood of hemorrhage and/or low blood pressure, and those with GI ulcerative disease. Although carprofen and deracoxib are approved for preoperative dosing, these authors do not recommend their use for preemptive analgesia unless the patient will receive IV fluids as well as blood pressure monitoring and rapid and appropriate treatment of low blood pressure throughout the perianesthetic period.

NSAIDs may be prescribed for several days postoperatively; however, because of the increased risk of GI ulceration when multiple NSAIDs are administered (or an NSAID is administered concurrently with corticosteroids), it is important to remember to **never mix NSAIDs** without a 4–10 day washout period. It is also recommended to treat with a GI protectant such as omeprazole or misoprostal.

No data exists that shows that one NSAID provides better analgesia than any other. However, similar to humans, there does appear to be some individual variability in the response to NSAID therapy. If a patient has an adverse response to one NSAID, it doesn't mean that it will have an adverse effect from a different NSAID. Likewise, one NSAID may appear to provide better analgesia than another in the same patient.

Alpha-2 agonists

The alpha-2 agonists dexmedetomidine and xylazine provide excellent short-term (20 minutes–2 hours) visceral analgesia, and they also provide excellent sedation pre- and postoperatively. However, they drastically decrease cardiac output as well as tissue perfusion and oxygenation. They should be avoided, if possible, in patients with cardiopulmonary or renal compromise. The effects of these drugs are dose-dependent.

Effective sedation and analgesia can be achieved at doses significantly lower than those listed on the bottles. Microdoses (e.g., 0.5–1 mcg/kg of dexmedetomidine) can be used pre- and postoperatively for added analgesia and increased sedation in patients receiving concurrent opioids.

Opioids

Opioids, especially the mu agonists (morphine, methadone, hydromorphone, oxymorphone, fentanyl, and remifentanil) are the most efficacious analgesic drugs currently available. They are ideal as part of a presurgical protocol, providing outstanding preemptive analgesia. Opioids are discussed in detail in Chapter 14; however, some additional discussion is warranted.

The use of morphine in cats has recently come into question. Research has shown that it is the metabolite of morphine, morphine-6-glucuronide (M-6-G), that binds to the mu receptor and thereby produces analgesia. Since cats do not always metabolize drugs as effectively as dogs, it is unclear whether morphine produces the same level of analgesia in cats as it does in dogs. In research cats, M-6-G was detectable only after IV morphine dosing, and only in 50% of the cats studied. No M-6-G was detectable after IM morphine administration (Taylor et al. 2001).

Methadone, which has the same potency as morphine, has the lowest incidence of inducing vomiting in small animals. This makes methadone an excellent choice of premedication in patients where vomiting is contraindicated, such as those with gastric dilatation volvulus (GDV), laryngeal paralysis, or abdominal pain. Methadone also has NMDA receptor antagonist properties.

Remifentanil is an ultra–short-acting mu agonist. It requires no liver or kidney metabolism; rather, it is cleared by esterases that occur in blood and skeletal muscle (Gaynor and Muir 2009). It is best used as a constant rate infusion (CRI). There is only an 8–10 minute recovery time to normal after discontinuing the infusion, making it an ideal drug to use in trauma patients with a neurological component to their status and who require serial neurological exams. Remifentanil should be administered as a 4 mcg/kg IV bolus followed by 6–20 mcg/kg/hr.

Perianesthetic and postoperative opioids are best administered as CRIs. This ensures that a patient will have a steady state of plasma concentration of drug, decreasing the risk of the patient becoming painful. One study showed a clinically significant increase in the development of sepsis and DIC as well as death in infants who were treated with intermittent boluses of morphine for postoperative thoracotomy pain control as opposed to continuous fentanyl administration (Anand and Hickey 1992).

Intraoperative opioid CRIs can also reduce the amount of inhalant required to maintain an adequate plane of anesthesia.

Administering opioids continuously allows a practitioner to titrate the dose in order to effectively meet the patient's need for more or less analgesia. CRIs can be administered via a syringe pump (Fig. 34.1), or they can be diluted and dripped into an intravenous line. To calculate a CRI, utilize the formula found in Table 34.2.

Tramadol

Tramadol is a synthetic, centrally acting analgesic and is useful for moderate to severe pain. Although tramadol is not a true opioid, its metabolites bind to mu receptors, causing opioidlike effects. Dosing in dogs and cats is generally 2–5 mg/kg 2–4 times daily. Tramadol is an excellent oral analgesic for mild-moderate postsurgical or chronic pain, especially in combination with an NSAID.

NMDA receptor antagonists

Ketamine is commonly used as an anesthetic induction agent, but it also plays a role in perioperative pain management as a potent NMDA receptor antagonist, especially for orthopedic trauma/surgery and for limb amputation. Animals should be given a 0.5 mg/kg IV loading

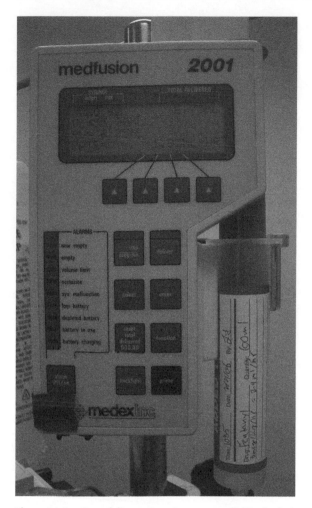

Figure 34.1. Drug delivery via syringe pump. (® Kim Spelts.)

Table 34.2. Drug infusion worksheet.

A	Desired dose (mcg/kg/min)
B	Body weight (kg)
C	Desired diluent volume (mL)
D	Drip set used (drops/mL)
E	Concentration of drug (mg/mL)
F	Desired drip rate (drops/min)

$$\text{mL of drug to add to diluent} = \frac{A \times B \times C \times D}{E \times F \times 1000}$$

Local anesthetics

Local and regional anesthetic blocks work by preventing painful signals from getting to the spinal cord. Patients are not only more comfortable, but it becomes easier to provide analgesia later since windup is unlikely to develop.

Lidocaine and bupivacaine are widely used for local and regional blocks in small animals. Lidocaine has a rapid onset and relatively short duration (~60 minutes). Bupivacaine has a slow onset, about 10–20 minutes but a long duration (~4 hours). Combining the two allows for a rapid onset and long duration of blockade. Both can be administered at 1.5 mg/kg alone or together for a block.

Bupivacaine may also be combined with epinephrine (1:200,000) to prolong a block by inducing peripheral vasoconstriction, slowing the uptake of the bupivacaine. Using this combination will extend the duration of the block for an additional 2–4 hours. Local anesthetics containing epinephrine **should not** be used for peripheral nerve blocks. Vasoconstriction from epinephrine may result in distal ischemia if there is not sufficient collateral circulation.

Local and regional blocks are valuable components of a balanced anesthesia plan. A detailed description of all nerve blocks is beyond the scope of this chapter; however, there are two simple blocks that warrant description because they can (and should) easily be incorporated into any small animal practice: the incisional block and the forepaw block for digit amputations.

dose followed by 10 mcg/kg/min during the perianesthetic period (initiating prior to surgery), and then 2 mcg/kg/min for the next 24–48 hours. It is unclear whether the higher dose of ketamine used for induction of anesthesia has the same NMDA receptor antagonist effects as a lower microdose administered as a constant rate infusion.

Although methadone is a potent mu agonist, it is also advantageous as an NMDA receptor antagonist, making it an ideal drug for trauma patients or for perioperative use during orthopedic procedures. IV methadone can be administered as a 0.05–0.1 mg/kg bolus followed by 0.05–0.1 mg/kg/hr.

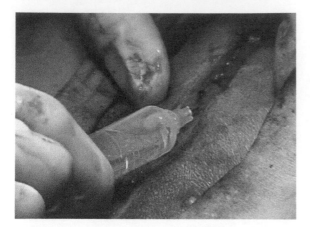

Figure 34.2.   Incisional block. (© Kim Spelts.)

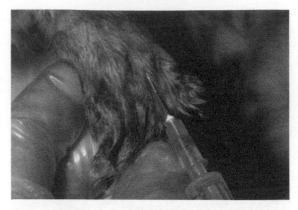

Figure 34.3.   Forepaw block. (© James Gaynor.)

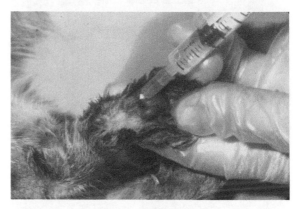

Figure 34.4.   Forepaw block. (© James Gaynor.)

Surgeons should perform an incisional block after body wall closure but before closure of the subcutaneous layer. A syringe and needle (25- or 22-gauge, at least 1 inch long) are passed to the surgeon aseptically, along with 1.5 mg/kg lidocaine mixed with 1.5 mg/kg bupivacaine. Insert the needle to the hub along one side of the incision, and if no blood is aspirated, inject local anesthetic in a fanlike manner as the needle is removed (Fig. 34.2). Repeat this procedure until the entire drug is distributed around the incision. For larger incisions, dilute the lidocaine/bupivacaine mixture 1:1 with sterile saline.

Forepaw blocks are effective for toe amputations, including declaw procedures in cats. The goal of this procedure is to block the radial nerve on the dorsal aspect and the median and ulnar nerves on the palmar aspect of the forepaw. As with the incisional block, combine 1.5 mg/kg lidocaine and 1.5 mg/kg bupivacaine. Begin by prepping both aspects of the paw using aseptic technique. Insert the needle (25-gauge) over the proximal-medial aspect of the metacarpus. If no blood is aspirated, inject local anesthetic until a small bleb appears. Repeat injections across the metacarpus to the lateral aspect until a line of local anesthetic is present (Fig. 34.3). Turn the paw over and inject a bleb of local anesthetic just distal to the accessory carpal pad (Fig. 34.4).

Despite the development of a strong pain management plan to deal with acute surgical pain, assessments and modifications must occur.

Figure 34.5 provides a good overview of developing and modifying a postsurgical pain management plan.

Management of Maladaptive Pain

Once a patient's pain has become maladaptive in nature, the analgesic strategy becomes more complex and requires ongoing reassessment and adjustment.

Pain related to osteoarthritis (OA) is the most common type of chronic, maladaptive pain in dogs and cats. Thankfully, the development of contemporary drugs, nutraceuticals, and other technologies has allowed more pets to live rea-

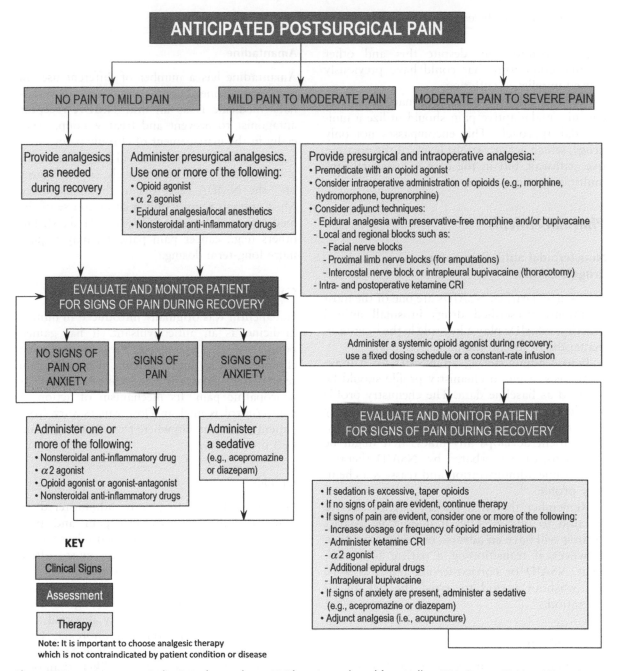

ANTICIPATED POSTSURGICAL PAIN

NO PAIN TO MILD PAIN

MILD PAIN TO MODERATE PAIN

MODERATE PAIN TO SEVERE PAIN

Provide analgesics as needed during recovery

Administer presurgical analgesics. Use one or more of the following:
- Opioid agonist
- α 2 agonist
- Epidural analgesia/local anesthetics
- Nonsteroidal anti-inflammatory drugs

Provide presurgical and intraoperative analgesia:
- Premedicate with an opioid agonist
- Consider intraoperative administration of opioids (e.g., morphine, hydromorphone, buprenorphine)
- Consider adjunct techniques:
  - Epidural analgesia with preservative-free morphine and/or bupivacaine
  - Local and regional blocks such as:
    - Facial nerve blocks
    - Proximal limb nerve blocks (for amputations)
    - Intercostal nerve block or intrapleural bupivacaine (thoracotomy)
  - Intra- and postoperative ketamine CRI

EVALUATE AND MONITOR PATIENT FOR SIGNS OF PAIN DURING RECOVERY

NO SIGNS OF PAIN OR ANXIETY

SIGNS OF PAIN

SIGNS OF ANXIETY

Administer one or more of the following:
- Nonsteroidal anti-inflammatory drug
- α 2 agonist
- Opioid agonist or agonist-antagonist
- Nonsteroidal anti-inflammatory drugs

Administer a sedative (e.g., acepromazine or diazepam)

Administer a systemic opioid agonist during recovery; use a fixed dosing schedule or a constant-rate infusion

EVALUATE AND MONITOR PATIENT FOR SIGNS OF PAIN DURING RECOVERY

- If sedation is excessive, taper opioids
- If no signs of pain are evident, continue therapy
- If signs of pain are evident, consider one or more of the following:
  - Increase dosage or frequency of opioid administration
  - Administer ketamine CRI
  - α 2 agonist
  - Additional epidural drugs
  - Intrapleural bupivacaine
- If signs of anxiety are present, administer a sedative (e.g., acepromazine or diazepam)
- Adjunct analgesia (i.e., acupuncture)

KEY

Clinical Signs

Assessment

Therapy

Note: It is important to choose analgesic therapy which is not contraindicated by patient condition or disease

Figure 34.5. Acute postsurgical pain in dogs and cats. (© Pfizer, Inc.; adapted from Hellyer PW, Gaynor JS: How I Treat Acute Surgical Pain in Dogs and Cats. Compend Contin Educ 1998;20:140.)

sonably comfortably despite this and other chronic conditions that could have previously caused unrelieved suffering.

As with adaptive pain, the management of chronic, maladaptive pain should utilize a multimodal approach. This encompasses not only drugs, which act at various levels of the nociceptive pathway, but in the case of osteoarthritis, multiple nondrug therapies also.

Pharmaceuticals

Nonsteroidal antiinflammatory drugs (NSAIDs)

As discussed earlier, NSAIDs are one of the most commonly prescribed drugs in small animal practice. NSAIDs play a key role in the long-term management of chronic pain.

Before administering an NSAID on a long-term basis, a blood chemistry profile should be assessed as baseline data. The chemistry profile should be reassessed at regular intervals (every 6–12 months) while continuing NSAID therapy. If a patient develops any illness that might be related to, or exacerbated by, NSAID therapy, discontinue administration and reassess a chemistry profile.

Remember that if a patient has an adverse reaction to one NSAID, it doesn't necessarily mean it will have an adverse reaction to another. However, if transitioning a patient to a different NSAID or corticosteroid, utilize a 4–10 day washout period to avoid the risk of GI ulceration.

Acetaminophen

Acetaminophen is a nonsteroidal analgesic drug that can be administered concurrently with other pain medications. In dogs, oral acetaminophen can be administered at 10–15 mg/kg BID for a maximum of 5 days so that pain medication is not completely withheld during NSAID washout periods. It is also beneficial in the long-term management of osteoarthritis in dogs as an adjunct to NSAID therapy to help manage breakthrough pain during the peaks of the osteoarthritis pain cycle.

Amantadine

Amantadine has a number of different uses in human medicine, but its primary use in veterinary medicine is as an oral NMDA receptor antagonist to prevent and treat windup, especially in the management of chronic pain.

A course of amantadine will help other analgesic drugs work more effectively, since it "turns off" the NMDA receptors in the spinal cord. Most animals require only a short course of the medication (3–5 mg/kg PO QD × 21 days), but others (e.g., cancer pain patients) may require more long-term dosing.

Gabapentin

Gabapentin was originally introduced in human medicine as an anticonvulsant. It has gained popularity as an integral part of managing chronic pain in dogs and cats, especially pain related to osteoarthritis and cancer, as well as neuropathic pain. Its mechanism of action in pain control is unclear. Dose ranges vary from patient to patient, anywhere from 2–40 mg/kg up to 3 times a day.

Opioids

Oral opioids are frequently administered to humans with refractory OA pain and pain related to cancer. Oral sustained-release morphine preparations are used most often. Anecdotally, oral morphine (regular or sustained-release formulations) seems to provide effective pain relief for OA (0.5 mg/kg PO TID-QID), with the most commonly reported side effect being constipation and anorexia. Oral oxycodone is also an effective drug for severe pain in dogs, and it may be less likely than oral morphine to produce dysphoria (Gaynor and Muir 2009). Oxycodone is effective in dogs at 0.3 mg/kg PO BID-TID.

Tramadol

As discussed earlier, tramadol is a centrally acting analgesic, useful for moderate-severe pain. It is particularly useful as an adjunct to NSAIDs and nutraceutical therapy in OA patients, for pain related to intervertebral disc disease, and for some types of cancer-related pain.

Joint/Cartilage Structure Modifiers and Other Nutraceuticals

A key component of managing chronic pain related to osteoarthritis is to provide not just analgesic drugs, but nutraceuticals and other products to prevent cartilage degradation and promote cartilage matrix synthesis.

A number of products are available that claim to provide joint and cartilage support in the presence of OA, and some claim to provide analgesia as well. Some products have apparent efficacy and varying degrees of research to support their use; however, most are nutraceuticals and have a number of problems with their claims, including the following:

- They are not classified as drugs and therefore have not undergone the scrutiny of the FDA approval process.
- Most have undergone very little to no product-specific research, and there is likely no scientific basis for their use. Any product can induce a placebo effect, and any company can choose to report only good testimonials and anecdotal information.
- Many do not contain what their labels say they do. A study from the University of Maryland showed that 80% of glucosamine-containing products do not contain the amounts indicated on the label (Adebowale 2000).

Glucosamine-containing supplements

In addition to many products not containing what they claim to, not all glucosamine formulations have the same in vivo effects. *Glucosamine HCl* is more efficacious than glucosamine sulfate. *Low molecular weight chondroitin sulfate* is absorbed from the GI tract of humans, dogs, and horses much better than high molecular weight chondroitin. Also, the addition of *manganese* significantly increases the bioactivity of glucosamine and chondroitin in cartilage.

Hyaluronic acid

Hyaluronic acid (HA) exists naturally in all living organisms, and it is the body's most abundant lubricant. It is found in greatest concentrations in the synovial fluid of joints, the vitreous humor of the eye, and in the skin. Hyaluronic acid plays an important role in tissue hydration and lubrication (especially in joints and muscle tissue).

In the presence of OA, HA concentration in the joint decreases. When present in a joint, even a joint with minimal or no cartilage, it can provide cushioning. High molecular weight (also known as long-chain) HA has been shown to provide better joint lubrication than low molecular weight (short-chain) HA.

Injectable hyaluronic acid is available as an FDA-approved drug for use in horses. There are no FDA-approved oral versions of HA. However, there is evidence that high molecular weight HA is absorbed through the GI tract in dogs and concentrated in joints (Balogh 2008). Clinical impressions of many veterinarians are that oral HA can act as a good adjunct to increasing pain control in dogs and cats with osteoarthritis.

Polysulfated glycosaminoglycans (PSGAGs)

PSGAGs have been investigated and approved for use in dogs and horses. Side effects are rare at a dosage of 5 mg/kg IM or SQ twice weekly. PSGAGs decrease cartilage catabolism and prevent adverse joint congruity changes.

Adjunct Therapies

Acupuncture

Ancient Chinese medical philosophy describes disease as an energy imbalance in the body.

Acupuncture is believed to balance this energy and thereby assist the body in healing disease. In modern physiologic terms, acupuncture can assist the body's efforts to heal itself by stimulating specific points on the body that have the ability to alter various physiological and biochemical conditions. Acupuncture stimulates nerves, increases blood circulation, relieves muscle spasms, and releases hormones such as endorphins and cortisol. Acupuncture can be very beneficial in pain alleviation in dogs and cats, with the duration of alleviation often being significant (days to months).

Therapeutic laser

Low-level laser is an FDA-approved treatment for arthritis in humans (Fig. 34.6). Therapeutic laser can have an antiinflammatory effect, optimize cell utilization of oxygen, and alter the transmission of painful impulses through the nervous system, all combining to provide pain relief. When used properly, low-level laser therapy is beneficial in treating OA and muscle pain, and helping to heal wounds as well as soft tissue injuries.

Weight loss

Weight reduction should be considered an integral part of the management of pain associated

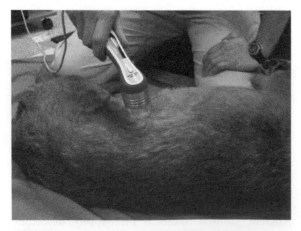

Figure 34.6.   Therapeutic laser treatment. (© Kim Spelts.)

with OA. All other interventions will work considerably better if the patient is not overweight. Weight loss can result in significant pain relief for arthritic patients. For patients who cannot lose weight with diet and exercise modifications, dirlotapide is an FDA-approved canine appetite suppressant.

A Purina study showed that dogs fed a more restricted diet over their lifetime exhibited a significantly lower prevalence of hip osteoarthritis, not to mention a longer life span, than dogs fed a higher-calorie diet (Kealy et al. 2000; Smith et al. 2006).

Physical Rehabilitation

Regular, *controlled exercise* is important for alleviating pain associated with OA. Patients are typically stiff after periods of inactivity but become more comfortable with mild regular exercise. Exercise is also important to maintain or build muscle mass to support joints.

Aquatic therapy provides an ideal low-impact exercise for dogs with chronic pain. The buoyancy of water reduces the load on painful joints and allows more comfortable exercise. Water pressure can reduce swelling and edema, and water resistance is useful for muscle strengthening (Millis et al. 2004).

Massage therapy enhances the circulatory, muscular, and nervous systems and their interdependent functioning. Massage increases blood flow to tissues, which improves oxygen delivery and the removal of metabolic waste products. Massage helps promote healing; it accelerates muscle recovery and breaks down adhesions that can result from acute and chronic inflammation. Massage also relieves pain by releasing endogenous endorphins (Millis et al. 2004).

Physical rehabilitation can play a vital role in both acute and chronic pain management, as well as in overall strengthening and conditioning (Fig. 34.7). Musculoskeletal pain, especially in the paraspinal musculature, often develops as a result of altered gait patterns. Animals benefit greatly from low-impact, low-intensity exercises, stretching, joint manipulation, localized heat and

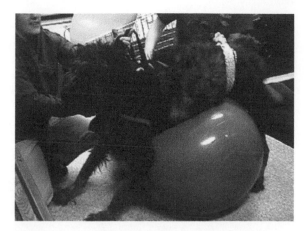

Figure 34.7. Therapeutic exercise on therapy ball. (© Kim Spelts.)

cold application, as well as modalities such as neuromuscular electrical stimulation and therapeutic ultrasound.

Regenerative Stem Cell Therapy (RSCT)

Regenerative stem cell therapy uses cells derived from an animal's own fat tissue to help regenerate cartilage and other tissues and to provide tremendous pain relief. RSCT is the gold standard for most cases of arthritis and multiple other musculoskeletal ailments.

Mesenchymal stem cells are part of the cell population utilized in RSCT. Mesenchymal stem cells (which are different from embryonic stem cells) are contained within each individual and are derived from the patient's own tissue. They have the potential of becoming cardiac cells, nerve cells, hepatocytes, chondrocytes, and vascular cells.

The process requires a short general anesthesia to extract a small amount of fat from the body wall. A cell therapy lab processes the fat and derives stem cells from the sample. Two to three days after the surgery, pets are sedated for injection of the regenerative cells directly into the joints and/or IV. Recently published data indicates tremendous improve-

ment in pain and function in dogs whose elbows, knees, or hips have been injected (Black et al. 2007).

References

Adebowale, A, Cox, D, Liang, Z, et al. 2000. Analysis of glucosamine and chondroitin sulfate content in marketed products and the Caco-2 permeability of chondroitin sulfate raw materials. JANA 3(1):37–44.

American Animal Hospital Association. 2007. AAHA/AAFP pain management guidelines for dogs and cats. JAAHA 43:235–248.

Anand, KJ, Hickey, PR. 1992. Halothane-morphine compared with high-dose sufentanil for anesthesia and postoperative analgesia in neonatal cardiac surgery. N Engl J Med 326(1):1–9.

Balogh, L, Polyak, A, Mathe, D, et al. 2008. Absorption, uptake and tissue affinity of high-molecular-weight hyaluronan after oral administration in rats and dogs. J Agric Food Chem 56(22):10582–10593.

Black, L, Gaynor, J, Gahring, D, et al. 2007. Effect of adipose-derived mesenchymal stem and regenerative cells on lameness in dogs with chronic osteoarthritis of the coxofemoral joints: A randomized, double-blinded, multi-center, controlled trial. Vet Therapeut 8(4): 272–284.

Gaynor, J, Muir, W. 2009. Handbook of Veterinary Pain Management, 2nd ed. St. Louis: Mosby, Inc.

Kealy, R, Lawler, D, Ballam, J, et al. 2000. Evaluation of the effect of limited food consumption on radiographic evidence of osteoarthritis in dogs. JAVMA 217(11):1678–1680.

Millis, DL, Levine, D, Taylor, RA, Adamson, CA. 2004. Canine Rehabilitation & Physical Therapy. St. Louis: WB Saunders.

Smith, G, Paster, E, Powers, M, et al. 2006. Lifelong diet restriction and radiographic evidence of osteoarthritis of the hip joint in dogs. JAVMA 229(5):690–693.

Taylor, PM, Robertson, SA, Dixon, MJ, et al. 2001. Morphine, pethidine and buprenorphine disposition in the cat. J Vet Pharmacol Therap 24(6):391–398.

Tranquilli, W, Grimm, K, Lamont, L. 2004. Pain Management for the Small Animal Practitioner, 2nd ed. Jackson: Teton NewMedia.

35

Equine Anesthesia

Lawrence E. Nann

Anesthesia is the use of drugs or drug combinations to depress the actions of central nervous system (CNS) tissues either locally, regionally, or generally. General anesthesia for horses is much like anesthesia for other animals, with some notable exceptions. For small and large animals alike, such as dogs, cats, horses and cattle, anesthesia will require the following in all cases:

1. "Sleep" (loss of awareness or sensation of surroundings)
2. Analgesia (loss of the sensation of pain)
3. Selective suppression of autonomic reflexes of the CNS
4. Muscle relaxation (which varies with the surgery)

To this list I would also add the following for horses and other large equids:

5. Immobility (lack of movement)

This latter quality has a special meaning to the large animal anesthetist who performs general anesthesia daily on horses. If a cat or dog were to wake up on the surgery table, it would typically take some fast work by the anesthetist to recover his/her dignity and get the patient back to sleep again. Movement of the small animal patient, even at 100 pounds, can be managed by an assistant or even the anesthetist's own quick hands. Movement of relatively small patients is easily controlled and the surgical team may be inconvenienced, but they will unlikely experience any harm to themselves. On the other hand, a horse waking up on the surgery table will put the safety of the patient, surgeon, and anesthetist at very serious risk. Twelve hundred pounds of horse moving on the table is not easily controlled, so it is a major consideration that the equine anesthetist be trained to provide an adequate margin of safety for all operating room personnel during the perioperative period. Ensuring that level of safety requires an understanding of the scale of equipment, the pharmacology of a significant number and class of drugs, and a concomitant level of comprehension about the cardiopulmonary physiology of the horse. At the same time, the risk to horses of an anesthetic-related death is significantly higher than with other species, about 1% (one death in a hundred anesthetics) (Johnston et al. 1995). Human risk of death related to anesthesia is significantly less, about one in a thousand (0.1%).

The Four Pillars

The safe equine anesthetist must first develop a comprehensive plan by which to avoid significant problems, especially the movement of a horse while under anesthesia. A four-part plan is helpful when teaching this to students. The "four pillars of equine anesthesia logistics" are assessment, readiness, familiarity, and planning.

Assessment

Adequate assessment of the patient's condition and readiness for surgery is paramount. The physical exam, evaluation of lab values, and heart auscultation (all mentioned later in detail) are needed for all patients. Personality evaluation of a horse is critically important (as is the breed and recent history) for understanding the selection and dose modulation of sedatives and other drugs that might be required to control each particular equine patient. The amount and type of restraint a particular horse might require will be determined by careful observation modulated by the experience of the anesthetist. A lead rope might be enough for a 15-year-old quarter horse mare, but a twitch and a chain shank over the gums might be needed for an Arab stallion that just unloaded from a 4-hour cross-country van ride. Placing an intravenous catheter (IV line) in the horse is a good opportunity for assessing a horse's personality quirks, as is flushing the patient's mouth with water to remove grass and straw that might otherwise be forced down the trachea during the intubation process (Fig. 35.1).

Sedatives might be needed to accomplish these tasks safely and this provides an opportunity to evaluate the effects of these drugs and perhaps even to infer what might be the effects of others to follow.

Readiness

It is crucial that the workspace and equipment are ready and organized to be available when needed. This includes both high-tech and low-

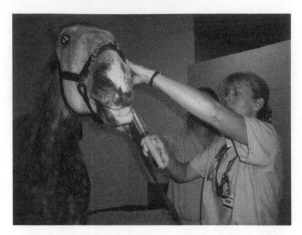

Figure 35.1. Flushing the horse's mouth prior to induction to rinse away debris that could potentially be carried into the trachea during intubation.

tech equipment. High-tech equipment, such as the anesthesia machine, cuffed endotracheal tubes, drugs, and monitors, should be tested and warmed up. Low-tech specialty equipment should be tested and ready as well. This includes 1-ton hoists, horse-sized surgery tables, heavy table padding, hobbles, and ropes (Fig. 35.2).

Pressure testing the anesthesia machine to detect leaks is an important task that should be done prior to each anesthetic event. Another might be checking that the hobbles are right where they are needed and that they are clean and not frayed. (Hobbles and ropes might be subject to a weight strain test every year or more frequently to certify that they will not fail under a known stress.)

Familiarity

Being familiar with the drugs that have useful properties in horses is critical. Sedatives, analgesics, induction drugs, and maintenance drugs are the general categories of drugs used in large animal anesthesia (see specific drug discussions later). Newer drugs have been found to have properties that can be used in special applications. Recently, for example, the use of medetomidine (or dexmedetomidine) CRIs during general anesthesia have been helpful in reducing MAC in "balanced anesthesia" cases. Newer,

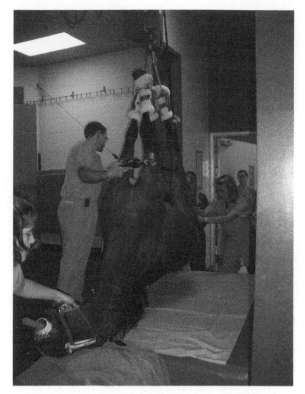

Figure 35.2. Hoisting and positioning the induced horse onto the surgery table.

fast-acting inhalants such as desflurane and sevoflurane may be useful as alternative inhalant anesthetics. Safe application of these newer drugs, however, requires adequate familiarity and regular use by the anesthetist in order to be used wisely. Familiarity breeds confidence and success.

Planning

Last, but not least, planning is what makes everything work. For example, the equine anesthetist must have a plan for a potentially dangerous excitement phase during the induction of anesthesia in the horse. Besides making good drug combination choices for induction of anesthesia, the anesthetist must be in full charge of everyone's safety. Besides the fully trained anesthetist, properly trained and experienced assistant personnel should be present to minimize risk

of potential injury to the patient or the caretakers. All participants present in an induction should know what they should and should not be doing during those very intense few moments of induction and early minutes of general anesthesia in the horse.

General Considerations Regarding Anesthesia Drugs

The anesthetist must develop and use finely honed skills of observation when giving a drug to an equine patient. The drug effects should be assessed in each individual horse and the anesthetist must have an alternative plan of action if the effects are not what is expected.

Individual differences

Equine patients may differ widely in their sensitivities to anesthetic drugs and to different noxious stimuli. Differences in breed, occupation, and environment can change how a drug can affect individual drug response in equine patients.

Dose range

A relatively broad range of doses may be used to produce a desired effect. These dose ranges may vary significantly even when giving the same drug to the same horse on different occasions. A drug may have "typical" effects on any one day and different, opposite effects on another. Variations in cardiac output, for example, may change how a drug is processed within the body, requiring either much more or much less drug for the same effect. (See "Uptake" and "Distribution.")

Circumstances

The dose providing an adequate effect in one set of circumstances (i.e., a castration) may be inadequate or excessive for another set of circumstances (compare a fracture repair versus taking radiographs). Environment is one of the keys to understanding why the "recommended dose" is not always the dose required to get the job done safely or effectively.

Cardiovascular effects

Virtually all inhalant anesthetics, induction agents, and sedatives alter cardiovascular function in some way or another, so it is imperative to monitor key indicators of these drug effects. This is why a watchful eye, good record-keeping habits, and concentration are essential during the entire perianesthetic period. Today's standards of equine monitoring now include invasive blood pressure, ECG, pulse oximetry, capnometry, and temperature. The addition of cardiac output and agent monitoring continue to gain popularity as cost of these modes of monitoring comes within reach of more veterinarians. (See "monitoring".)

The Five Phases

There are five phases of general anesthesia:

1. Preanesthetic Phase
    ■ Patient physical exam
    ■ Laboratory results
    ■ Emptying of the GI tract
    ■ Preanesthetic sedatives
2. Induction Phase
    ■ Muscle relaxants
    ■ General anesthetics
    ■ Analgesics
3. Maintenance Phase
    ■ Inhalants
    ■ TIVA
    ■ Balanced anesthesia
    ■ Padding
    ■ Monitoring
4. Recovery Phase
    ■ Sedatives
    ■ Sedative antagonists
    ■ Oxygenation

5. Postanesthetic Phase
    ■ Warming/cooling
    ■ Patient attitude/sedation

Preanesthetic Phase of General Anesthesia

Patient physical examination

Preparation of the equine patient for anesthesia requires a physical examination by the anesthetist, usually some laboratory testing, partial emptying of the gastrointestinal (GI) tract, and the use of preanesthetic medications.

The physical exam is important, in particular an exam of the cardiovascular and respiratory systems. However, other systems, such as the renal and hepatic functions, are of similar interest since they involve the metabolism and excretion of the anesthetic drugs. A systemic approach should be used to evaluate each patient.

History

Knowing the patient's health history is so important. The physical exam may never reveal as much as a thorough past history. Asking the owner key questions will likely reveal most serious predispositions including pneumonia, history of heaves, reaction to drugs, lameness problems, etc. Knowing the history may change the nature of the physical exam as well. If the horse has had previous anesthesia, knowing how it went and what the nature of the recovery was can be very helpful in planning subsequent anesthesia events.

Heart and pulse

Heart auscultation will allow the anesthetist to hear murmurs and other abnormal heart sounds if present. Abnormal rhythm disturbances may be noticed. Palpation of arterial pulses will similarly give the anesthetist an appreciation of heart strength and regularity.

Lungs and upper airway

Auscultation of healthy lungs should be difficult because air moving through normal lungs makes very little sound. Otherwise, the anesthetist is listening for sounds of fluid in each lung field, sounds that might indicate the presence of pulmonary edema. Lung sounds are checked bilaterally for indications of airway constriction, such as wheezes that might indicate pneumonia. The upper airway is also checked for signs of obstruction. The respiratory rate, respiratory pattern, and depth of chest excursions should be noted as well. The quantity of airflow being exhaled out of each nostril should be the same; otherwise, an obstruction might exist. Flaring nostrils while at rest may be an indication of excessive effort and likely represents some problem that should be addressed.

Skin

Skin is checked for normal sweating and skin turgor. In some places on a horse, "tenting" or skin turgor indicates the degree of dehydration of the patient. A healthy coat is also an indicator of general good health.

Mucous membranes

Dryness of mucous membranes (MM) may indicate another reason to suspect dehydration in a patient whereas moist membranes tend to indicate adequate hydration. Pink color of MM indicates good peripheral perfusion, indirectly giving the anesthetist a rough idea of oxygen saturation and cardiac output.

Laboratory results

After the physical exam, the decision about what laboratory testing should be performed needs to be made. The minimum lab testing that should be done for each patient is packed cell volume (PCV) or hematocrit, total plasma solids (TS), and white blood cell count (WBC) with fibrinogen (Muir and Hubbell, 2009). Horses with inflammatory, traumatic, or neoplastic disorders may have an elevated fibrinogen. Blood should be drawn once the horse is calm because PCV may be elevated in the excited horse (contraction of the spleen).

If the physical exam sheds light on other possible problems, other tests might be added, including electrolytes (sodium, potassium, or calcium), creatinine, hepatic enzymes, and others. Electrolyte imbalances may contribute to postoperative muscle weakness, cardiac dysrhythmias, and acid-base imbalance. Elevated creatinine may indicate possible urinary dysfunction, while elevated hepatic enzymes may predict potential problems with anesthetic drug clearance (Muir and Hubbell 2009).

The PCV is a measure (%) of the cellular portion of the blood after being centrifuged in a microhematocrit device. High values indicate possible dehydration; low values indicate anemia. Total solids (TS) is a measure of the refractive index of plasma proteins, which indicates either hemodilution (low value) or hemoconcentration (high value).

A dehydrated patient would have a high PCV and high TS. A patient with hemolytic anemia would have a low PCV and normal TS. The presence of a "left shift" in white cell count (lots of immature emerging new white cells) and a high fibrinogen might indicate a festering pulmonary infection such as pneumonia. In the presence of a fever, these three things might be enough for a surgeon to consider postponing general anesthesia.

Emptying of the GI tract

A horse can rupture its stomach on induction of general anesthesia. This is almost always a fatal complication and can happen if the stomach is full of ingesta or fluids. Horses are normally kept off feed for several hours before induction of general anesthesia, some for as long as 6 to 12 hours and others much less. Free access to water is allowed. If horses have not been muzzled for some reason and ate only hay, the surgery is not cancelled. However, if the patient ate grain in any quantity, gas formation in the stomach is possible, and elective surgery should be postponed 24 hours to allow for gas reabsorption.

Preanesthetic sedatives

The anesthetist relies upon these drugs to decrease fear and anxiety in horse patients, making them safer and easier to work with. Preanesthetics facilitate smooth inductions and recoveries from anesthesia. They constitute an integral part of the anesthesia sequence of induction. By controlling the excited or painful or violent patient we can help protect the people who handle the patient. Preanesthetics can have the following effects:

- Reducing the amount of general anesthetic used
- Calming the patient and reducing pain
- Providing muscle relaxation
- MAC reduction
- Blocking the vasovagal reflex (although considered controversial, anticholinergics such as atropine have been used to treat bradycardias resulting from vagal stimulation or alpha-2 agonist effects).
- Smooth recovery

The more debilitated or ill the patient is, in general, the less preanesthetic medication required. Conversely, the more excited, painful, or active the patient, the lower is the effect of the preanesthetic, and preanesthetic drug requirements go up. In every individual patient, the preanesthetic should be tailored to the patient and not just given routinely. The following is a list of commonly used preanesthetic drugs used in horses.

Xylazine

Xylazine is an alpha-2 adrenergic agonist drug that is used for sedation and analgesia. Its commercial name is Rompun®. Xylazine is not an ideal drug for sick or debilitated animals because of its negative cardiopulmonary effects, which include potent peripheral vasoconstriction and bradycardia with possible 2nd degree AV block. Xylazine can also cause relaxation of the equine airways and occasional upper airway obstruction (both vagal and alpha-2 effects) (Muir and Hubbell 2009).

- Equine Dose: 0.5–1.1 mg/kg IV/IM
- Time to peak effect: 5–10 minutes
- Length of sedation: 15–30 minutes (typical)
- Length of analgesia (visceral): 45–60 minutes (typical)
- Antagonists: Yohimbine, atipamizole, tolazoline

This widely used drug causes sedation, ataxia, and analgesia, especially visceral analgesia. It will initially cause a transient increase in blood pressure due to vasoconstriction, commonly resulting in compensatory atrioventricular block and bradycardia. This initial hypertension is followed by hypotension. Xylazine can occasionally cause personality changes manifested as ear pinning, tail switching, biting, and kicking, thought to be due to a decrease in inhibition. Arousal is possible in response to loud noises or touch. Although the horse appears well sedated, it may be stimulated and awakened enough to deliver a powerful kick if startled.

Xylazine is supplied as either 20 mg/mL (small animal) or as 100 mg/mL (large animal).

Detomidine

- Category: alpha-2 adrenergic agonist
- Major uses: sedation and analgesia
- Cardiopulmonary effects: similar to xylazine
- Equine dose: 0.01–0.02 mg/kg IV/IM, 0.02 mg/kg sublingual (Taylor and Clarke 2007); CRI 0.01–0.02 µg/kg/min following initial IV dose of 0.01–0.02 mg/kg
- Length of sedation: 20–40 minutes (typical)
- Length of analgesia (visceral): 120–180 minutes (typical)
- Antagonists: same as xylazine
- Supplied as 1.0 mg/mL

This drug, although more expensive than xylazine, is being used widely for both equine sedation and pain control because its analgesic effect (and other side effects) lasts longer and sedation is slightly more potent.

Medetomidine (Dexmedetomidine)

- Category: alpha-2 adrenergic agonist
- Major uses: sedation, analgesia, and balanced anesthesia (MAC reduction)
- Cardiopulmonary effects: similar to xylazine, potent peripheral vasoconstriction
- Equine dose: 5–20 µg/kg IV/IM (0.0005–0.0020 mg/kg); CRI 3.5 µg/kg/min (Muir and Hubbell 2009)
- Antagonists: same as xylazine

Acepromazine

- Category: phenothiazine derivative
- Major use: tranquilizer, preoperative sedative
- Cardiopulmonary: potent peripheral vasodilation, lowering blood pressure. Clinical doses can lower blood pressure 15–20 mm Hg (Muir and Hubbell 2009) and so should not be used in patients that are anemic, hypotensive, shocky, or seizuring. Vasodilation effects can abolish thermoregulation and heat loss can be significant. Ace can cause penile retractor muscle paralysis (paraphymosis), and for this reason it is not recommended for use in breeding stallions.
- Equine dose: 0.03–0.10 mg/kg IV/IM (Muir and Hubbell 2009)
- IV tranquilization onset is about 20–30 minutes, lasting an hour or more for sedation; vasodilation effects may last from 6 to 12 hours. Ace can also be given orally. Acepromazine can be used to reduce the excitement effects seen with opioids such as morphine in the horse (Muir and Hubbell, 2009).

Atropine

- Category: anticholinergic
- Major use: decreasing sympathetic tone, increasing heart rate (for treating bradycardia—horses have high vagal tone at rest, and drugs [alpha-2] and surgical manipulations [pulling on an optic nerve, for example] may lead to bradyarrhythmias or even cardiac arrest), bronchial dilation, decreasing salivation.

- Cardiopulmonary: see earlier in this chapter.
- Equine dose: 7–10 µg/lb IV/IM (0.007–0.010 mg/lb)

Pretreatment of a horse with atropine may not eliminate bradycardia, but it may prevent cardiac arrest (Taylor and Clarke 2007). Presurgical treatment of sinus bradycardia may include reduction/reversal of the anesthetic drug, administration of atropine, and administration of catecholamine such as dobutamine or epinephrine (Muir and Hubbell 2009). Atropine may take as long as 5 minutes to take effect and may cause an initial bradycardia before heart rate increases. Atropine can cause decreased gut motility, resulting in postoperative colic, and so routine use remains controversial.

Diazepam

- Category: benzodiazepine
- Major use: sedation, muscle relaxant, anticonvulsant
- Used as a premedicant mainly only in foals because it does not provide adequate sedation in healthy adult equines
- Can be combined with ketamine to provide muscle relaxation for induction (in place of guaifenesin)
- Cardiopulmonary: little effect
- Equine dose: 0.10–0.25 mg/kg
- Antagonist: flumazenil

Diazepam increases cough reflexes and laryngospasm; it is inexpensive and is dissolved in propylene glycol, which can cause it to sting on administration.

Another popular benzodiazepine is midazolam, commercial name, Versed®. Midazolam is dissolved in water (faster IM/SQ dosing) and has 1/2 the half life of diazepam and 1/2 the dose (0.0045–0.01 mg/kg), but it is also more expensive per dose (Adams 2001).

Butorphanol

- Category: synthetic opioid agonist antagonist

- Major use: used synergistically with alpha-2 sedatives for sedation and visceral analgesia
- Equine dose: 0.01–0.02 mg/kg IV/IM

Butorphanol has fewer negative side effects as with morphine but provides good analgesia in horses as compared to canines. Butorphanol can cause ataxia and "twitching" or head jerking. It is a kappa agonist mu antagonist with a duration of about 60 minutes (IV).

Morphine

- Category: opioid agonist
- Major use: analgesia
- Cardiopulmonary: may increase heart rate, cardiac output, and blood pressure at clinical doses (Muir and Hubbell 2009)
- Equine dose: 0.1–0.3 mg/kg IV/IM (NOTE: Give IV morphine very slowly after a tranquilizer. Duration of effects is 3–5 hours. Convulsions are possible.)
- Antagonist: naloxone (0.05 mg/lb)

Besides potent analgesia, morphine can produce excitement in the horse in the absence of a tranquilizer, although using the drug IM can minimize this effect. Morphine can be a potent respiratory depressant and can increase GI sphincter tone (constipating effect) (Muir and Hubbell 2009).

Induction Phase

Induction agents for horses

Guaifenesin

- Category: centrally acting skeletal muscle relaxant
- Known as "GG" or "GGE," for its old name (glyceryl guaiacolate ether), it is a mild sedative with little or no analgesic properties.
- Cardiopulmonary: little cardiopulmonary depression in the dose range below
- Equine dose: 25–50 mg/kg to effect (duration 20 minutes, longer in stallion ponies)

- Supplied most often as 5% guaifenesin in 5% dextrose and typically given under pressure (pressure infusor) to effect until signs of ataxia are seen, at which time IV bolus of general anesthetic (thiopental or ketamine) is given. Halves the induction dose of thiopental necessary, and masks the seizurelike excitement of typical ketamine inductions. Smoother inductions and recoveries than without GG. Some common problems include:
  - Residual muscle weakness in recovery
  - Tissue irritant if GG goes perivascularly (sloughing)
  - Hemolysis if concentration is over 5%
  - Mild cardiovascular depressant at higher doses

Thiopental

- Category: ultra–short-acting thiobarbiturate
- Major use: general anesthetic, causes loss of conscience.
- Equine dose: 4–6 mg/kg IV
- Duration: 4–10 minutes

Thiopental is a potent dose-dependent cardiovascular and respiratory depressant. Problems include the following:

- Apnea
- Excitement during induction and recovery
- Little analgesia or muscle relaxation
- Narrow margin of safety
- Tissue irritant if injected perivascularly
- Highly protein-bound (reduce dose in hypoproteinemia)

Caution: Do not use for patients in shock, dehydrated, or otherwise hypovolemic. Geriatrics are more sensitive to its effects.

Ketamine

- Category: cyclohexlamine, dissociative anesthetic
- Major use: general anesthetic, analgesic
- Commercial name: Ketaset, Vetalar

- Equine dose: 1.5–2.2 mg/kg IV, duration 5–10 minutes
- Cardiopulmonary: minimal cardiovascular and respiratory depression

Allows for very brisk reflexes, muscle rigidity, and myotonic contractions. Used without preanesthetic muscle relaxants (not recommended), rigidity is pronounced. May cause an increase in blood pressure and heart rate. Inductions (in well-sedated horses) and recoveries are smooth, but repeated doses tend to increase the incidence of rough recoveries. Poor surgical conditions when used alone. Muscle rigidity and swallowing may make intubation difficult. Use with diazepam, midazolam, or guaifenesin for good muscle relaxation. Good choice for anesthesia for shocky patients and those with hypovolemia.

Tolazoline-Zolazepam

- Category: paired drugs—a dissociative anesthetic and a benzodiazepine
- Major use: general anesthesia (imitation of ketamine-valium mixture)
- Commercial name: Telazol®
- Cardiopulmonary: similar to ketamine
- Equine dose: 0.7–1.0 mg/kg IV
  - Dried powder mixed with water is good for 2 weeks.

Maintenance Phase

Inhalant anesthetics

Induction and maintenance of anesthesia is often performed using inhalational agents delivered by an anesthesia machine of some kind. These agents are potent and rapid acting. In addition, they allow rapid adjustment of the depth of anesthesia during the perioperative period. Recovery from these inhalants involves "blowing off" the anesthetic agent into the environment. Induction and recovery can be rapid, even in neonatal foals with immature liver function. All of the inhalants below are potent vasodilators,

profound respiratory depressants, nonexplosive and nonflammable.

Halothane

No longer in production

Isoflurane

- Vapor pressure 240 mm Hg
- Equine MAC 1.31–1.64%
- Cost per mL $0.08
- Saturation in oxygen 32%
- Percent metabolized 1.7%
- Good analgesia; peripheral vasodilation and hypotension
- Potent respiratory depressant (usually requiring a ventilator); short cases recover relatively smoothly, longer cases can be rougher.

Sevoflurane (Ultane®)

- Vapor pressure 160 mm Hg
- Equine MAC 2.31–2.84%
- Cost per mL $0.48
- Saturation in oxygen 21%
- Percent metabolized 3%
- Good analgesia, rapid change in depth
- Compound "A" can produce nephrotoxins in absorbent, but no clinical evidence of kidney damage has been seen.
- Reaction with dry KOH can produce CO.
- Quick recoveries, requires aid of sedatives

Desflurane

- Vapor pressure 664 mm Hg
- Equine MAC 7.02–8.06%
- Cost per mL $0.60
- Saturation in oxygen 87%
- Percent metabolized 0.02%
- Good analgesia, very rapid change in depth
- Quick recoveries; may require aid of postoperative sedatives to avoid too rapid recovery (Muir and Hubbell 2009)

TIVA

Total Intravenous Anesthesia (TIVA) is popular for short surgical procedures. Most recommendations limit TIVA to under 2 hours due to the cumulative effects of IV drug metabolism. This involves the use of "triple drip," which is most commonly made with 1 L 5% guaifenesin, 500 mg xylazine, and 1.5–2.0 g of ketamine all mixed together. Sedation and induction are accomplished in the usual manner, and triple drip may be used for maintenance of anesthesia at a rate of about 2 mL/kg/hr to effect. Horses will maintain a brisk palpebral reflex and may blink spontaneously under a surgical (minor) plane of anesthesia.

Balanced anesthesia

Balanced anesthesia refers to the combination of multiple drugs to reduce the amount of any one particular drug to produce general anesthesia. In the horse, we may balance the effects of a number of drugs, such as isoflurane plus lidocaine infusion, with a medetomidine CRI and induction with ketamine/diazepam.

Padding/Positioning

One of the most important differences between small animals and horses is that there is a significant potential for developing neuropathy and myopathy with a horse on the surgical table while under anesthesia.

Simply stated, the horse's weight combined with hypotensive effects of general anesthetics could reduce the flow of blood to large portions of the musculature. This could result in serious nerve and muscle damage unless the anesthetist takes appropriate preventative measures, such as maintaining adequate blood pressure and proper positioning and padding. Most surgical tables for horses use some form of foam padding to spread the weight of the horse over a larger area (Fig. 35.3).

Others may use water-filled mattresses and inflated air bladders to accomplish the same result. Attention to the details of positioning is required to prevent a number of classic neuropathies such as radial nerve paresis/paralysis. In this case, the horse in lateral recumbency can develop radial nerve damage unless the lower leg

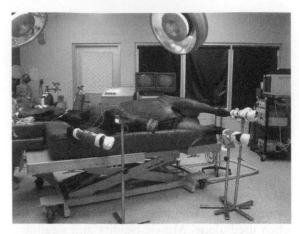

Figure 35.3 A horse well padded and positioned on the surgery table. Note the use of stands to support the legs and joints. The front down leg is pulled well forward.

is properly pulled forward, either on the table or in the recovery stall.

Monitoring

Proper monitoring of the anesthetized horse is crucial. Besides the basic physiologic parameters, the depth of anesthesia must be monitored so that the horse may be kept at the appropriate anesthetic level for the specific surgery or procedure at hand. As mentioned above, the depth of anesthesia in the horse is critical. A horse that is too lightly anesthetized may physically respond to surgical stimulus, risking contamination of the surgical site or injury to personnel. A horse that is too deeply anesthetized may suffer from respiratory or cardiovascular depression, leading to serious complications.

Heart rate, strength, and rhythm

Note that the relatively small changes seen in heart rate (HR) during anesthesia makes HR an unreliable indicator of anesthetic depth in the horse.

Physical signs and reflexes

The assessment of depth of anesthesia in the horse involves physical signs such as muscular movement, eye position, and eye reflexes (palpebral and corneal). In addition, the rate and depth of respiration, swallow reflex, and response to surgical stimulation can contribute to the evaluation of anesthetic depth. Use the following physical signs to assess the depth of anesthesia in the horse:

- Lateral nystagmus—moving laterally back and forth signifies a lightening plane of anesthesia.
- Palpebral reflex (blink)—progressive depression as plane deepens, and reflex may disappear.
- Heart rate does not normally change with anesthetic depth except in excessively deep planes.
- Arterial blood pressure can be a good indicator of anesthetic depth if trends are monitored. Mean arterial blood pressures should be maintained above 70 mm Hg in horses.
- Corneal reflex (wink) may be absent during deep surgical planes and during the use of neuromuscular blocking drugs.
- Anal tone—absence of anal tone indicates deeper planes of anesthesia.
- Ocular position—the globe will roll ventral/medial with the lateral canthus visible. Moderate to rapid movement (nystagmus) indicates a lightening plane.
- Lacrimation—tearing indicates a lighter plane of anesthesia.
- Muscular relaxation—absence of purposeful muscular movement indicates adequate depth.

ECG (Electrocardiogram)

Detection of dysrhythmias is the goal. Set leads in base apex configuration, lead I or II, and chart recorder to 25 mm/sec. Note rate, rhythm, and normal/abnormal complexes.

Treatment of hypotension in horses

Hypotension resulting in poor tissue perfusion can be a problem after IV injections of anesthetic drugs or by inhalants delivered by anesthesia machines. Symptoms are poor peripheral pulse quality, blanched mucous membranes, and an increased capillary refill time greater than 3 seconds. These clinical signs can be caused by poor cardiac contractility, vasodilation, or both, and also possibly caused by bradycardia. Alpha-2 agonists are known to produce atrioventricular block at times, and acepromazine may cause vasodilation, for example. Myopathy, shock, and ultimately death will result if hypotension is allowed to continue for an extended period. For a horse to survive, pressures must be returned to a mean arterial value of greater than 70 mm Hg using fluids, vasopressors, and cardiac stimulants, and by turning down the anesthetic to some degree. The following five drugs can be used to combat hypotension.

Dobutamine

Dose: 1–5 µg/kg/min.

Dobutamine is a beta-1 adrenergic agonist. The beta-1 receptors are located in the muscular walls of the heart, which, when stimulated, cause an increase in the force of contraction of each beat of the heart (improved contractility). Each stroke of the heart then ejects a greater volume (increased stroke volume) into the aorta and therefore results in an increase in cardiac output (CO); that in turn results in higher blood pressure. Used as a CRI starting at low dose rates, dobutamine is the drug of choice for increasing blood pressure in horses. However, at higher dose rates it may cause sinus tachycardia, especially in the face of hypovolemia.

Phenylephrine

Dose: 0.01 mg/kg or CRI to effect.

Phenylephrine is an alpha-1 adrenergic agonist, and it stimulates alpha-1 receptors in the peripheral circulation to cause vasoconstriction. It, in effect, causes increased vasomotor tone, increasing diastolic pressure and improving the volume of blood returning to the heart (preload). It is not without problems because if given too rapidly, phenylephrine can result in a reflex vagal bradycardia. If used too long as a constant rate infusion (CRI), there is the possibility that it may decrease blood flow (and oxygen supply) to tissues, especially in the periphery. Judicious, short-term use is recommended.

Ephedrine

Dose: 0.03–0.06 mg/kg bolus.

Ephedrine is a sympathomimetic drug that increases blood pressure from stimulating both alpha-1 receptors (causing vasoconstriction) and beta-1 receptors (increased contractility). It is used as a bolus dose only because a CRI will cause tachycardia. Ephedrine is also a CNS stimulant and may possibly cause movement or arousal in lightly anesthetized patients. The beta-1 effect of ephedrine is both direct (working directly on the beta-1 receptors) and indirect. It indirectly amplifies the direct beta-1 effect by stimulating the release of adrenaline (norepinephrine) from the adrenal glands (another beta-1 agonist).

Epinephrine

Dose: 1–3 µg/kg/min.

Epinephrine is an endogenous catecholamine that is both a positive inotrope (contractility) and a chronotrope (increasing heart rate). Its primary effect on the cardiovascular system is its potent vasoconstriction. Its use in cardiac resuscitation is primarily in constricting peripheral vessels so that blood volume is forced to the body core where it can be circulated to the major organs.

Beta-1 activity of epinephrine increases the strength of the beating heart. There is also beta-2 receptor activity causing bronchodilation (better breathing and gas exchange) as well as some selective vasodilation (depending on the tissue). On the negative side, epinephrine can cause tachyarrhythmias, even ventricular fibrillation, especially with higher dose rates. It remains one of the primary drugs for treating cardiac arrest as a bolus, and it can be used as a CRI for stubborn hypotension in the horse.

Vasopressin

Dose: 0.4–0.6 µ/kg (Muir and Hubbell, 2009)

Vasopressin is a nonadrenergic endogenous stress hormone and the most potent vasocon-strictor known. It also enhances cardiac contractile function, elevates blood pressure and improves tissue perfusion. Repeat doses are not necessary. It works to stimulate the release of catecholemines from the adrenal medulla and is currently the drug of last choice for serious cases of hypotension in our clinic.

Respiration

Note rate, depth, and rhythm, and whether it is spontaneous or CMV (continuous mechanical ventilation); if it is CMV, the peak airway pressure, breaths per minute, and tidal volume should be noted. Further evaluation of ventilation should be done through blood gas analysis.

End-Tidal CO_2 (and inspired CO_2)

Capnography can help monitor the effectiveness of lung ventilation. The CO_2 waveform (capnograph) is useful for monitoring ventilator and anesthesia machine functions. The goal for $ETCO_2$ is 35–45 mm Hg; the goal for inspired CO_2 is less than 5 mm Hg (Taylor and Clarke 2007).

Blood gases and electrolytes

Include evaluation of acid-base balance and electrolyte abnormalities. Blood gas analysis is the ideal method of assessing ventilation.

Pulse oximetry (SpO_2)

Noninvasive measurement of % saturation of hemoglobin should be done. Adult human finger probes work well on equine tongues; large C-clamps are commercially available.

Mucous membrane color and CRT (in seconds)

Make a quick assessment of oxygenation, blood flow, and hydration.

End-Tidal agent monitoring

Monitor the dose response effects to ensure adequate depth and compare to the physical signs of anesthetic depth listed above.

Ventilation

Ventilation, oxygenation, and CO_2

Before the discussion of general anesthesia by use of the above inhalants, an understanding of oxygen uptake and carbon dioxide elimination is needed. The regulation of these two gases, O_2 and CO_2, in the horse or foal undergoing general anesthesia is usually provided by the anesthesia machine. This device usually provides the inhalant general anesthetic via oxygen as a carrier gas and removes CO_2 either by dilution, out the APL valve (also called the pop-off valve), or by chemical means via absorption through sodalime.

Regulation of ventilation

Ventilation regulates the oxygen and carbon dioxide environment of the cells in the body. When awake, the respiratory functions are controlled by the respiratory center in the hypothalamus, and normal awake horses (as well as humans) will breathe to keep the level of CO_2 in the blood close to a partial pressure of 40 mm Hg. In disease, the horse may also have to work harder to breathe to keep the level of oxygen in the blood above a partial pressure of 80 mm Hg (normal oxygen is 90–100 mm Hg on room air) (Muir and Hubbell 2009).

During anesthesia, the respiratory drive of the patient is ablated or even eliminated through the CNS depression provided by the inhalant and other drugs. Without the anesthesia machine to provide oxygen, remove CO_2, and perhaps ventilate the patient, if necessary, the patient can become hypoxemic, and CO_2 will accumulate in the blood producing a respiratory acidosis.

Ventilation and inhalational anesthesia

Delivery of the general anesthetic via the lungs rather than by IV (as during induction) requires not only an understanding of the inhalants, but an understanding of ventilation, the uptake of inhalants in the lungs, distribution of inhalants via the circulation, and redistribution of those inhalants during the different periods of gas anesthesia. The brain "sees" the blood levels of inhalant that rise, are maintained, and fall, keeping those portions of the CNS responsible for the perception of pain quiescent.

The concentration of inhalant that the brain sees is affected by a number of things:

- Inhalant amount delivered to the circuit: This is controlled by setting the % dial on the vaporizer and setting the total flow of the carrier gas (O_2). Together they provide the amount of anesthetic vapor that is being transported to the circulating blood volume. The brain and the CNS will "see" the amount of inhalant that is in the blood.
- Cardiac output (CO): The anesthetic gas can be carried to the CNS (brain) only via the circulatory system. Without CO there will be no transport of inhalant from the lungs to the brain. Blood from the pulmonary circulation picks up inhalant from the alveoli in the lungs as it passes through the capillaries surrounding the alveoli. The blood transfers the agent to the brain and other tissues.
- Ventilation: Lungs receive the inhalant when the horse is ventilated. Respiration rate (breaths per minute) and tidal volume (volume of each breath) control the exposure to the pulmonary bronchioles and alveoli.
- Agent: The anesthetic agent (inhalant) of choice possesses the ability to become soluble in both blood and tissues. This degree of solubility is key to the delivery and uptake of inhalant to the CNS.
- Uptake: The transfer of anesthetic agent from the anesthesia machine fresh gas to the lungs and alveoli and then from the alveoli to the blood are the first two steps. The rate at which this takes place is based upon how soluble the agent is in the blood.
- Distribution: This is the transportation of agent throughout the body via the blood circulation. Transfer of anesthetic from blood to tissues (CNS, muscle, fat, etc.) is dependent upon this issue of solubility.

■ Redistribution: This is the reshuffling of the inhalant between blood and initial tissue locations to locations where the new levels are desired. Increased cardiac output will mobilize the agent in some tissues into a larger tissue bed, lowering the blood level and causing a "wake-up" event. The vaporizer is turned up to reload the CNS with more inhalant so the patient goes back to sleep. As another example, when the patient needs to wake up, the anesthetic is redistributed out of tissues by decreasing inhalant settings. Ventilation is continued to remove inhalant from the patient to the circuit. Inhalant is either metabolized (small amount) or diluted by oxygen and moves back into the anesthesia machine where it is finally eliminated out the scavenging system or as the patient exhales during recovery.

Induction flows of oxygen range from 10 to 15 mL/kg/min or more. It is intended to wash out both nitrogen and CO_2. It saturates the circle rubber and plastic, including hoses and bag, with inhalant agent, while supplying oxygen for metabolism and ventilation. At the same time it rapidly supplies the volume of the anesthesia machine with enough anesthetic gas to safely keep the patient asleep.

Maintenance flows of oxygen range (low flow) from 4 to 8 mL/kg/min. Low flow is the most economical flow setting, conserving both agent and oxygen. There is also less environmental contamination because less anesthetic gas is allowed to escape into the scavenger. There is only a need to supply the metabolic oxygen needs of the tissues. Uptake of the agent decreases with time due to redistribution. The use of low flow comes with a price: FiO2 must be monitored. This can be by monitoring blood gases, pulse oximeter, or oxygen monitor. High oxygen flows must be run long enough and at high enough flow settings that nitrogen washout is significantly accomplished. If the inspired oxygen is allowed to stay closer to room air gas levels (21%), hypoxemia is a possibility. An FiO2 monitor dedicated to each individual circuit is the safest way to know the actual inspiratory oxygen level.

Recovery Phase

Elimination of anesthetic agents

A similar process takes place during recovery as took place during induction, only in reverse: A washout of inhalant (agent elimination) occurs, depending upon the same factors above required for uptake:

■ Ventilation (minute volume)
■ Cardiac output
■ Agent selection (potency and solubility)
■ Tissue blood flow (systemic vascular resistance, SVR)
■ Alveolar to mixed venous partial pressure difference

Sedation

Depending on the inhalant chosen for the anesthesia, a horse may spend between 10 minutes (rarely) and several hours in recovery before standing. At least 45 minutes is required for washout of inhalant in the case of most healthy horses. If the horse tries to struggle to rise too soon, while it still has nystagmus, a sedative dose of xylazine is typically administered to smooth out the recovery. This recovery sedative is hardly ever needed when halothane is used, is frequently used for isoflurane, and is almost always needed for sevoflurane and desflurane anesthetics.

Antagonists

When recovery times are extended well beyond expected periods, reversal (antagonism) of the alpha-2 agonists may be considered. The antagonists for alpha-2 agonist reversal in horses are atipamazole (0.05–0.1 mg/kg) and yohimbine (0.04–0.15 mg/kg). Recovery is often seen in just a few minutes if this is effective. Reversal of the analgesia provided by the alpha-2 agonist is to also be expected and may need to be replaced by another analgesic.

Patent airway

During the recovery phase of anesthesia there is a chance of a horse developing an airway obstruction or displacement. To maintain a patent airway, a nasal tracheal tube can be placed. When the horse is in recovery and is breathing spontaneously, the cuffed oral endotracheal tube is removed and a lubricated uncuffed nasal tracheal tube (NTT) is placed. This maintains a minimal open airway of about 16–18 mm diameter providing airflow until the horse is standing. In certain cases the NTT may be lubricated with a gel mixed with phenylephrine to provide a degree of vasoconstriction and thus minimizing the potential of epistaxis. Others may secure the orotracheal tube (OTT) in place instead of a nasal tube or place and secure a shorter nasopharyngeal tube for recovery. In these cases, the ETT is strapped with tape so it is firmly in place through the interdental space so the patient does not occlude the tube by clamping its teeth on it or risk aspiration of the tube.

Oxygenation

Oxygen supplementation in recovery is provided by running a Levin tube through the NTT with oxygen by insufflation at a typical flow of 5 liters per minute. The NTT can be made from a length of Tygon tubing with a collared attachment to prevent it from being sucked into the trachea. Alternatively, the ETT can be used in recovery to ventilate the patient by demand valve until the horse is ready to breathe on its own.

Conversion to the NTT is accomplished by extubating the oral tube and intubating with the NTT. Oxygen is run from a bubble-jet humidifier located outside the recovery stall. It is imperative that the O_2 flow be confirmed to be in the trachea, not the esophagus.

Postanesthetic Phase

Warming and cooling

Heat loss on the surgery table is often unavoidable, although there are several methods to minimize losses and to replace lost heat energy. In lateral recumbency, blankets are effective in reducing heat loss as are forced warm air units like the Bair Hugger® and the Warm Touch®. When heat loss is unavoidable, as in dorsal positioning of colic cases, the use of active fluid warming systems can warm IV fluids to 37°C as they are flowing during the surgery. In these cases heat loss is reduced, and shivering during recovery is minimized. Oxygenation of the horse in the recovery stall will likely be improved if shivering is kept to a minimum because oxygen may otherwise be depleted by the extraordinary amount of energy required to maintain shivering muscle activity.

References

Adams, HR. 2001. Veterinary Pharmacology and Therapeutics, 8th ed. Ames, IA: Iowa State University Press.

Johnston, GM, Taylor, PM, Holmes, MA, Wood, JLN. 1995. Confidential Enquiry of Perioperative Equine Fatalities (CEPEF=1) Survival Curves. Vet Surg 25:171–182.

Muir, WW, Hubbell, JAE, eds. 2009. Equine Anesthesia, 2nd ed., Monitoring and Emergency Therapy. St. Louis: Saunders-Elsevier.

Taylor, PM, Clarke, KW. 2007. Handbook of Equine Anesthesia, 2nd ed. Philadelphia: Saunders-Elsevier.

Ruminant Anesthesia

Sharon Kaiser-Klinger

Ruminants such as cattle, sheep, and goats are not good candidates for heavy sedation or general anesthesia, although anesthetic management can be accomplished if the anesthetist takes into consideration complications that can occur due to these animals' physiology. Cattle, sheep, and goats are animals with four stomachs: the rumen, the reticulum, the omasum, and the abomasum. These animals regurgitate and remasticate their food, which then is digested through a fermentation process. During the anesthetic and recovery periods, ruminants are predisposed to regurgitation, which can lead to aspiration of rumen contents. Bloating and increased salivation are also common among ruminant patients under anesthesia. When a ruminant is placed in dorsal or lateral recumbency, normal eructation is impaired and gas is formed. If the patient has a large volume of ingesta in its stomach and a large amount of gas is produced by the fermentation process, bloating can become significant, particularly if the anesthetic period is prolonged. Regurgitation results if the rumen becomes overly distended. In cattle, the weight of the enlarged rumen can impair free movement of the diaphragm and cause shallow rapid respirations and poor ventilation and gas exchange.

Dose rates of some drugs are very different in ruminants than in other species. This difference needs to be considered when determining anesthetic protocols. Also to be considered is the prey animal behavior of ruminants to disguise signs of illness or pain. Therefore, a seemingly healthy ruminant may have masked conditions and require decreased doses of anesthetic drugs due to its health status. This chapter offers both local and general anesthetic protocols to use to anesthetize cattle, sheep, and goats. Some anesthetic techniques for use in the small camelids, llamas, and alpacas will also be included.

In general, much of ruminant surgery is carried out in the standing animal, especially in cattle, under local anesthetics. Surgery is made easier by both physical and chemical restraints. In cattle, the use of chutes and ropes is common, and the bovine technician is usually very skilled in tying numerous types of knots and quickly applying restraints for the purpose of casting a patient. Goats and sheep can also be restrained by the use of ropes, but they are more commonly sedated and manually restrained.

There are very serious risks to heavy sedation and general anesthesia in the ruminants. Recumbency can compound the adverse side effects of regurgitation and salivation associated with general anesthesia. Regurgitation can occur in both light and deep planes of anesthesia. The risk of death is unusually high in recumbent bovine patients following regurgitation. Salivation is increased tremendously by anesthesia also and aspiration or inhalation of either fluid should be prevented. Precautions should be taken to help decrease the probability of regurgitation and inspiration of ingesta.

Withholding food for 24 hours tends to produce rumen contents that are less likely to be regurgitated; 2–4 hours is sufficient in calves, kids, and lambs less than 1 month of age. Longer periods of fasting tend to make the ingesta watery and easily regurgitated. Water should be withheld 6–12 hours. Fasting can also decrease pressure on the diaphragm minimizing lung collapse and decrease in PaO_2, although hypoxemia and respiratory acidosis occur in most anesthetized ruminants in varying degrees. Fasting for lengths of time greater than 48 hours has been shown to cause decreased heart rates, especially in cattle. Therefore, it is important for the anesthetist to be familiar with normal values in the unsedated healthy cow. Heart Rate: 60–90 bpm. MAP: 120–180 mm Hg (Hall et al. 2001)

In lateral recumbency, the patient's head should be placed over a towel or pillow so that the poll is elevated to a position higher than the nose to allow saliva and regurgitated matter to flow out of the mouth (Fig. 36.1).

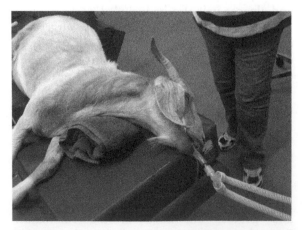

Figure 36.1. Goat positioned with a towel under the neck to facilitate drainage of salivation and regurgitation.

Local Analgesia and Nerve Blocks

Local analgesia and nerve blocks are used extensively in ruminants in an attempt to avoid general anesthesia.

Auriculopalpebral nerve block

An auriculopalpebral nerve block is used to aid in examination and surgery of the eye by preventing the eyelid from closing. There is no analgesia associated with this block. For painful procedures, topical or injectable analgesia should be added. Insert the needle in front of the ear at its base at the end of the zygomatic arch until the point reaches the dorsal border of the arch; 10–15 mL of 2% lidocaine can then be injected underneath the fascia in this location (Hall et al. 2001).

Cornual nerve block

A cornual nerve block is used for dehorning. The horns receive sensory innervation from the corneal branches of the lachrymal and infratrochlear nerves. The cornual nerve has several branches, but the lateral and caudal parts of the horn are supplied by only a couple of them. For this block to be effective, the corneal branches of both the lachrymal and infratrochlear nerves must be blocked. To produce blockade of the corneal branch of the lachrymal nerve, the needle insertion site is as close as possible to the caudal ridge of the root of the supraorbital process. The needle should be inserted to a depth of 1.0–1.5 cm in the adult goat (Fig. 36.2).

The anesthetist should be aware that there is a large blood vessel at this site, and care should be taken that the needle is not in this vein. The dorsomedial margin of the orbit is the site to block the corneal branch of the infratrochlear nerve. Applying pressure and manipulating the skin over this area can allow for palpation of this nerve. The needle is inserted under the muscle and close to the margin of the orbit approximately 1/2 cm deep. Local analgesic such as lidocaine is injected at each site with a maximum

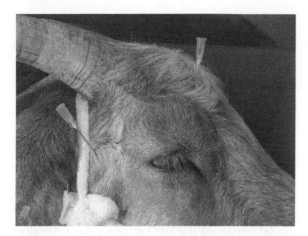

Figure 36.2. Needle placement for a cornual block in a goat.

total dose of 6 mg/kg per animal. Caution should be exercised not to exceed the toxic dose of lidocaine, particularly in kids and calves, and not to inject the local anesthetic intravenously. Other options for dehorning are sedation with xylazine, general anesthesia with diazepam and ketamine, propofol, or inhalant anesthesia. If inhalant anesthesia is used, the oxygen must be turned off when a hot iron is being used (Muir et al. 2000).

Caudal block

For obstetric procedures of the vagina and/or vulva and for tail docking, the caudal block is very effective. The hair is clipped over the sacrum and base of tail. By moving the tail up and down, the injection site can be found. The anesthetist palpates for the most cranial point of articulation, the first intercoccygeal space, and inserts a 20-gauge needle at the midline at a 45° angle to the body where the needle enters the vertebral column; 2% lidocaine (1–4 mL) is then injected into the epidural space (Hall et al. 2001). If continuous caudal block is desired, an epidural catheter can be placed using a Tuohy needle whose curved end is helpful in directing the advancement of the catheter. The catheter is advanced 3–5 inches, the needle removed, and the catheter capped and secured to the animal in position so that repeated doses of local analgesic can be given (Hall et al. 2001).

Epidural blocks

Epidural anesthesia is used for many procedures from the diaphragm caudally, providing anesthesia of the abdominal wall, the flank, and the inguinal and perineal regions. In calves, sheep, and goats, the epidural is usually administered at the lumbosacral space because it is easily palpable. In adult cattle, the epidural is administered at the sacrococcygeal or first intercoccygeal space (Muir et al. 2000). The effects of the epidural in regard to the blocked area are dose-dependent. Epidural injections should be given slowly to minimize patient discomfort and vascular absorption. If vascular absorption is not minimized, reduced neural uptake results and anesthesia may be incomplete. Epidurals are contraindicated in patients with cardiovascular disease, coagulopathies, or signs of shock or toxemia. Improper injection in the subarachnoid space or overdose can cause side effects, including unconsciousness, muscular spasm or contractions, seizures, paralysis of the respiratory system, hypotension, and/or hypothermia. In the small ruminants, the injection is placed at the lumbosacral space between L6 and S1, and the landmarks are similar to those of the dog. The dose of 2% lidocaine is 1 mL/10 lb of body weight. Onset of action is 2–5 minutes with a duration of 1–2 hours. Paralysis is achieved 3/4 of the distance from pubis to umbilicus (Hall et al. 2001). If the subarachnoid space is infiltrated upon insertion of the needle, only half of the dose of lidocaine should be injected. Onset of anesthesia with similar effects as the epidural injection will occur in 1–3 minutes. Preservative-free morphine (0.05 mg/lb) can be diluted with saline to a volume of 0.06 mL/lb and used epidurally for analgesia and sedation (Hall et al. 2001). In adult cattle, the spinal cord ends at the last lumbar vertebra. The epidural needle is placed between the 1st and 2nd coccygeal vertebra past the end of the spinal cord and meninges. This space is larger and more readily found than the sacrococcygeal space. In the cow, the anesthetist grips the tail, and raising and lowering it determines the first articulation behind the sacrum that is the first intercoccygeal space. The spinal needle is applied between the 1st and 2nd coccygeal spines on the midline. The needle is advanced at a 15° angle to vertical until it reaches the floor of the canal. The anesthetist needs to be aware that the patient may make sudden movements if a caudal nerve is disturbed. If there is resistance to the injection of lidocaine, the needle may be penetrating the intervertebral disc and needs to be repositioned by retracting it slightly. If the needle is positioned correctly, there should be no resistance to injection; 2% lidocaine or, for prolonged effect, 5% bupivicaine is used and injected over 10–15 seconds. The dose of lidocaine is 5–10 mL based on the size of the patient (Hall et al. 2001) The analgesia will be provided in the tail, croup, anus, vulva, perineum, and posterior region of the thighs. Maximum effect lasts for 5–10 minutes and then diminishes over 2 hours until it's gone. Xylazine can be used to provide epidural analgesia at a dose of 0.05 mg/kg diluted to 5 mL in 0.9% saline (Hall et al. 2001). Analgesic onset is 20 minutes with a duration of 2 hours (Blaze and Glowaski 2004). The xylazine is absorbed and can cause sedation, decreased motility of the rumen (possibly causing bloat), bradycardia, and decreased MAP. These side effects may have adverse effects in sick patients.

In cattle, because general anesthesia is associated with numerous complications such as bloating, excessive salivation, myelopathy regurgitation, and aspiration associated with recumbency, many surgeries are performed in the standing position. The small ruminants are at a slightly decreased risk of these complications, but some surgical procedures are performed standing in these patients. Infiltration anesthesia is a set of common procedures that have minor disadvantages and several advantages. One of these procedures, the line block, is the easiest of the blocks. A 20-gauge or smaller needle is used to block the skin and 18-gauge, 1-1/2–3-inch needles are used for the muscle layers and peritoneum; 50 mL of 2% lidocaine are used for numerous subcutaneous injections of 0.5–1 mL volumes 1/2–1 inch apart along the proposed incision line (Muir et al. 2000). Then the muscle layer is injected through the already blocked skin. Disadvantages and compli-

cations of this block include the necessity for large volumes of anesthetic and possible lidocaine toxicity, particularly if the anesthetic is injected into the peritoneal cavity. There can be minimal to no block in the deeper layers of the abdominal wall. Lidocaine can inhibit healing. Despite these possible complications, the line block is easily and commonly used successfully for many standing procedures. Another widely used infiltration anesthetic procedure is the inverted L block. This block is achieved by injecting with an 18-gauge 3-inch needle up to 100 mL of 2% lidocaine in a line down the caudal border of the last rib and a line ventrally between the last rib and the 4th lumbar vertebra (Muir et al. 2000); thus, the inverted L. This procedure blocks the flank caudally and ventrally from the injection lines, eliminating anesthetic agent at the incision line, therefore limiting complications of incisional edema and interrupted healing.

Intravenous Regional Anesthesia

Intravenous regional anesthesia (IRA) can be used for surgery of the limbs. In sheep and goats, a tourniquet or sphygmomanometer cuff is used by placement on the foreleg above the elbow or hindleg above the hock. Care must be taken to allow enough of the saphenous vein to be visible to facilitate injection. A tourniquet must be tightened just enough to block arterial flow. The sphygmomanometer cuff should be inflated to above systolic blood pressure. A 25-gauge needle is inserted into the vein, directed toward the foot, and secured to prevent movement from the vein while injection is performed. Lidocaine at a dose of 4 mg/kg without epinephrine is injected slowly with an onset of action of 15–20 minutes (Hall et al. 2001). The tourniquet should remain for at least 10 minutes to allow for thorough diffusion of lidocaine into the tissues. The tourniquet can be released at any time after the initial 10–15 minutes with no decrease in effect. No residual effect has been seen in goats or sheep when the tourniquet has remained tightened for up to 2 hours.

Peroneal and tibial nerve blocks

Peroneal and tibial nerve blocks provide excellent analgesia to the hindlimb below the hock. The peroneal nerve is blocked by injecting 5 mL of 2% lidocaine over the nerve that runs across the lateral side of the leg caudodorsally to cranioventrally 1 inch below the condyle of the tibia (Hall et al. 2001). Applying pressure and moving the skin and tissues covering it can facilitate palpation of the nerve. The tibial nerve block is achieved by injecting 4 mL of 2% lidocaine at the hock between the flexor tendons and the gastrocnemius tendon on the medial side of the leg. An additional 1 mL should be injected on the lateral side of the leg in the same general area because there is a small superficial nerve that is a branch of the peroneal nerve that originates in the middle of the thigh (Hall et al. 2001). When the combination of the peroneal and tibial nerve blocks are used successfully, the hock will straighten and the animal will stand on the dorsum of the fetlock. Onset of action for each of these blocks is 15 minutes or less.

Digital blocks in cattle

Besides intravenous regional anesthesia used in all ruminants, in cattle local anesthesia can be achieved by the use of a ring block or local regional anesthesia of specific nerves. The ring block, of course, is the easiest to perform but with the least reliable results. Local anesthetic is injected, infiltrating the tissues around the limb. Success of this block is variable because specific nerves are not targeted. Because the nerve supply to the digits in cattle is complex, local regional anesthesia is complicated. Location of the nerves is hindered by tense skin and subcutaneous fibrous tissue in the distal limb. There are five separate injection sites in the forelimb to block the whole digit:

1. Dorsal metacarpal nerve: middle of the metacarpus medial to the extensor tendon
2. Dorsal branch of ulnar nerve on lateral aspect of leg, 2 inches above the fetlock in the groove running between the metacarpal bone and suspensory ligament
3. Palmar branch of ulnar nerve behind the suspensory ligament
4. An injection in the midline just above the fetlock blocks the lateral branch of the median nerve and may block both branches.
5. The medial branch of the median nerve is reliably blocked in the groove between the suspensory ligament and the flexor tendons about 2 inches above the fetlock on the medial side of the limb.

Blocking the peroneal nerve behind the caudal edge of the lateral condyle of the tibia over the fibula blocks the hindlimb below the hock. The tibial nerve can be blocked about 5 inches above the top of the calcaneous in front of the gastrocnemius tendon on the medial aspect of the leg. (Hall, 2001)

Sedatives and Sedation Agents

Sedatives and tranquilizers are not to be used in food animals. Acepromazine may be used for mild sedation in ruminants (0.05–0.1 mg/kg IV, IM, SQ) (Blaze and Glowaski 2004). The onset of action is 10–20 minutes with a duration of sedation being 2–4 hours (Hall et al. 2001). It is infrequently used due to prolonged elimination and recovery.

The alpha-2 agonists and antagonists are more commonly used. Xylazine, detomidine, medetomidine, and romifidine induce dose-dependent mild to heavy sedation. These drugs can be used alone to sedate patients for restraint or combined for premedication before induction of anesthesia. Xylazine (0.02–0.2 mg/kg) is the most commonly used of the alpha-2 class of drugs (Blaze and Glowaski 2004). When using xylazine in ruminants, it is recommended that the 20 mg/mL concentration preparation be used. The ruminants and goats in particular are quite sensitive to xylazine. A 0.2 mg/kg dose will provide profound prolonged sedation. Young or sick patients should be given only the lowest of doses if at all. The dose of detomidine or medetomidine is 10–20 mcg/kg (Hall et al. 2001). The side effects of the alpha-2 agonists are dose-dependent and can include cardiovascular and respiratory depression, bloat, hyperglycemia, decreased plasma insulin, diuresis, decreased hematocrit, and premature delivery in late pregnancy. Cardiovascular changes that occur differ between the alpha-2 drugs. Xylazine causes a transient mild bradycardia and hypertension and then a decrease in MAP. Detomidine, medetomidine, and romifidine all cause profound bradycardia and increased MAP. The effects of the alpha-2 agonists can be reversed by the specific antagonists atipamazole (25–50 mcg/kg IV), yohimbine (0.1 mg/kg IV slowly), or tolazoline (2 mg/kg IV slowly) (Hall et al. 2001).

Sedation achieved in the ruminants by use of the benzodiazepines is unreliable and of short duration (15–30 minutes). The dose of both diazepam and midazolam is 0.2–0.3 mg/kg, with the higher dose prolonging but not deepening sedation. Flumazenil (0.1–1.0 mg/kg) antagonizes the effects of the benzodiazepines (Blaze and Glowaski 2004).

Meperidine, butorphanol, and buprenorphine are the opioids most commonly used in the ruminants. Butorphanol (0.02–0.03 mg/kg) can provide sedation in sick cattle and intensify xylazine sedation in healthy cattle (Hall et al. 2001). In sheep and goats, butorphanol (0.05–0.2 mg/kg) is used as an adjunct to xylazine, acepromazine, and diazepam (Hall et al. 2001). It has a rapid onset of action and can also be used 5–10 minutes prior to induction of anesthesia to provide analgesia and a smoother induction. The duration of action is 1–2 hours. Meperidine has been used in sheep and goats as a premedication for many years. Buprenorphine (0.006–0.01 mg/kg IM) can be given to sheep or goats 30 minutes before induction of anesthesia to decrease the concentration of inhalant needed during the anesthetic period and to provide analgesia peri- and postoperatively and can be redosed every 4–6 hours (Hall et al. 2001).

Anticholinergics such as atropine and glycopyrrolate are not generally used or recommended in ruminants. Anticholinergics tend to increase viscosity of the saliva without decreasing the amount, making it harder to drain from the pharynx. The anticholinergics cause a decrease in intestinal motility, predisposing the patient to bloat. A dose of atropine at 2 mg/50 kg IM or SQ is useful in treating severe bradycardia and hypotension during anesthesia (Muir et al. 2000).

Preanesthetic Preparation

Preanesthetic preparation should include a physical exam and various laboratory tests, the minimum of which should be a PCV and total protein. In addition, if the patient is geriatric or sick, a complete blood count, serum chemistry, and urinalysis may also be warranted. Not only do the health concerns of the ruminant need to be considered, but the type of ruminant must also be factored in (Tables 36.1, 36.2). For instance, if the patient is a food animal the choice of anesthetics may be limited based on the legislation in effect. Dairy breeds of cattle tend to be more tolerant of anesthetics than are some of the beef breeds. Beefmaster, Santa Gertrudis, and Brahman purebred or crosses appear to have lower anesthetic requirements (Hall et al. 2001). It is not imperative that the ruminant patient be premedicated prior to general anesthesia, because excitement is not common during induction, particularly in the small ruminants. In cattle, an acepromazine or xylazine premedication will reduce the dose of induction drugs needed and may prolong recovery. It is recommended that premedication is used prior to ketamine induction. In adult cattle, alpha-2 drugs are commonly used preoperatively. In sheep and goats, adding butorphanol or buprenorphine enhances muscle relaxation and provides analgesia for prolonged or painful procedures. Commonly, a diazepam/ketamine combination is used for induction in the small ruminants (1 mL of 50/50 mix per 20 lbs).

Placement of an indwelling catheter is recommended for all anesthetic events whether all injectable or injectable and inhalant anesthetics are to be used. The catheter not only allows for ongoing fluid therapy and safe injection of drugs that cause irritation if injected perivascularly, but it also provides reliable venous access for

Table 36.1. Anesthetic drugs in goats, sheep, and calves.

Drugs	Dosage (mg/kg)	Duration	Notes
Diazepam Ketamine	0.2–0.3 mg/kg IV 6–7.5 mg/kg IV	10–15 min	Can add butorphanol 0.1 mg/kg for analgesia
Xylazine Ketamine	0.1 mg/kg IM 6 mg/kg IV or 10 mg/kg IM	30 minutes	Xylazine 0.1 mg/kg can be added for increased anesthetic depth
Thiopental	7–20 mg/kg IV	10 minutes	Not in animals <30 months of age Inject 1/3 dose IV; then titrate remaining dose to effect
Xylazine Telazol	0.1 mg/kg IM 4 mg/kg IM	45–60 minutes	May cause transient apnea
Butorphanol Telazol	0.1 mg/kg IV 4–6 mg/kg	Variable	Unreliable duration of action
Propofol	4 mg/kg IV	Short–can be prolonged by bolus injections or CRI	Works better following premedication

Dosages used by Anesthesia Department, University of Georgia.

adjunct drugs perioperatively. In cattle, a 14-gauge 5.25-inch catheter is generally placed through a small incision in the skin into the jugular vein. The incision is made necessary by the thickness of the skin, especially in adult bulls. In sheep and goats, catheter placement is deter-mined by the procedure performed and anesthe-tist preference. Both the cephalic vein in the forelimb and the saphenous vein in the hindlimb are accessible with restraint assistance and after wool or hair is clipped away. The cephalic vein of goats is relatively short and lies obliquely

Table 36.2. Anesthesia in adult cattle.

Drugs		Dosage (mg/kg)	Duration	Notes
Calves 200–350 kg Xylazine Ketamine		0.1 mg/kg IM 4 mg/kg IV or 6 mg/kg IM	20 minutes	Can be prolonged with "triple drip"
Thiopental		11 mg/kg IV	10 minutes	Can be prolonged with bolus doses or CRI Premedication decreases dose rate
"Triple Drip" Xylazine Guaiphenesin 5% Ketamine	Guaiphenesin 5% Thiopental	50–100 mg/kg IV 3–4 mg/kg IV	15 minutes	Dose can be decreased by premedication or in cattle weighing >600 kg Endotracheal intubation recommended
	Xylazine Ketamine	0.1 mg/kg IM 2.2 mg/kg IV	15–20 minutes	Can be prolonged with "triple drip"

Dosages used by Anesthesia Department, University of Georgia.

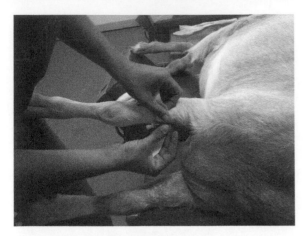

Figure 36.3. Cephalic catheter in a goat.

across the leg. An 18-gauge 2 inch catheter is commonly used in the limbs, capped and secured to the leg with tape much like in the dog (Fig. 36.3).

Because of their long necks and prominent jugular veins, catheterization at this site is easily achieved with a 14-gauge 3 inch catheter (Fig. 36.4).

Sheep by contrast have shorter thicker necks, making jugular catheterization harder although possible. The ear vein is very superficial and easily used for blood collection and intravenous injection.

Small-gauge catheters can also be placed and secured in the ear. The auricular artery is also very prominent, so be sure to identify which is

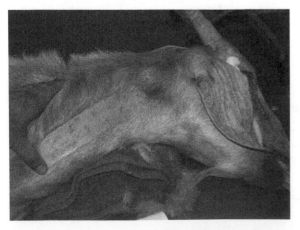

Figure 36.4. The jugular groove in a goat. Notice also the prominent auricular veins and arteries in this goat.

the vein and which is the artery prior to injecting any drugs.

Injectable drugs can be used alone for both induction and maintenance of short anesthetic events or as premedication and induction of anesthesia followed by maintenance with inhalants. In the small ruminants, most surgeries and diagnostics that require extended length of anesthesia are best done with inhalants, after induction and endotracheal intubation. This affords the anesthetist the opportunity to secure a patent airway to protect against aspiration and provide the ventilation necessary to counteract respiratory depression and hypoxia created by the injectable premedication and induction drugs. Additionally, recovery is prolonged following anesthetic maintenance with injectable drugs, with the exception of propofol.

Endotracheal intubation should be considered vital for all ruminants undergoing general anesthesia. In the small ruminants and cattle under 300 kg, endotracheal intubation can be challenging because of the size of the oral opening (small) and the length of the incisors from the larynx (long). With practice and the correct technique, it becomes easier. The patient is placed in sternal recumbency with nose pointed upward until the endotracheal tube has been placed and the cuff inflated. In the event that the patient regurgitates during this procedure, it should be turned to lateral recumbency with its head tilted downward allowing the rumen material to drain out. Solid rumen matter should be flushed or wiped out of the animal's mouth prior to endotracheal intubation. A laryngoscope will help visualize the pharynx and trachea and facilitate intubation. Extending the head and neck in a straight line will also be of assistance. Strips of gauze positioned around the animal's jaws will help the assistant hold the mouth open wider, keeping the fingers out of the way of the anesthetist's view of the trachea. The assistant must also grip the tongue and pull it out of the mouth. A stylet is often of benefit to help keep the endotracheal tube stiff and bent at the correct angle to facilitate intubation. In small ruminants particularly, the use of a guide wire is helpful because the endotracheal tube can completely occlude the anesthetist's view of the arytenoids. The laryngoscope blade is used to depress the base of the tongue and allow the anesthetist to see the opening of the larynx. The tip of the endotracheal tube is used to flatten the epiglottis as it is inserted into the trachea. There may be slight resistance at the vocal chords. Once the endotracheal tube is placed, it can be secured to the patient's head with a strip of gauze tied around the tube and then tied behind the ears or around the lower jaw. The cuff is then inflated just enough for an airtight seal. In large bovines, palpation by the anesthetist is often used for intubation. A gag is placed in the patient's mouth. The anesthetist holds the end of the tube and places an arm in the cow's mouth staying in the middle so that the cow's teeth will not tear the tube's cuff. A finger is used to lower the epiglottis and the tube is advanced slightly. The anesthetist then opens the arytenoids and larynx with the hand holding the tube and uses her free hand to feed the tube into the trachea. Once the endotracheal tube is placed, the cuff is inflated and the tube secured to the cow's head or the mouth speculum with tape or gauze. This "blind" method can also be used in small ruminants but is sometimes difficult due to the narrowness of the mouth of goats and sheep.

Thiopental can be used in adult cattle, sheep, and goats for induction alone or anesthetic maintenance also. The onset of anesthesia is rapid and the duration is short (5–10 minutes). Therefore, it is suitable for only very short procedures or for endotracheal intubation prior to inhalant anesthesia. Young calves less than 3 months of age should not be anesthetized with thiopental. Thiopental is generally safe in healthy ruminants, and recovery is usually uneventful. If injected perivascularly, it will cause irritation and tissue damage; therefore, the injection site should be infiltrated with 2% lidocaine and a large volume of 0.9% sodium chloride. In cattle, 5% guaiphenesin(GG) alone can be used at a dose of 80–100 mg/kg to sedate an adult into recumbency (Hall et al. 2001). If deeper anesthesia is needed for a painful procedure, thiopental can be combined with the GG at a dilution of 50 g GG with 2 g thiopental. This combination, when used at a dose rate of 2 mL/kg/hr causes an increase in respiration and heart rate with a

decrease in blood pressure (Hall et al. 2001). Xylazine prior to induction will reduce the dose of thiopental/GG needed.

Although ketamine can be used alone for induction, using it in combination with xylazine smoothes induction, produces good muscle relaxation, and provides for quiet recovery. In calves and the small ruminants, diazepam or midazolam is combined with ketamine for induction with or without the addition of butorphanol. Muscle relaxation is improved when butorphanol is added. It should be noted that the dose requirement for ketamine in calves is higher than in adults. In the small ruminants, ketamine and diazepam administered together in low doses have been used to produce profound sedation and analgesia with minimal loss of swallowing and cough reflexes. When xylazine and ketamine are used together, the xylazine can be given intramuscularly 5 minutes prior to injection of the ketamine. This may result in recumbency prior to IV or IM injection of the ketamine. The xylazine combination will result in 15–30 minutes of anesthesia dependent on the route of administration of the ketamine. Intramuscular injection of ketamine creates longer duration of anesthesia. Prolonging anesthesia further can be achieved by CRI of GG/ketamine (1 g ketamine in a 1 L bottle of 5% GG) or by inhalant anesthesia. This mixture is given at a dose rate of 1–2 mL/kg/hr (Blaze and Glowaski 2004). Oxygen supplementation is advisable with this protocol. In calves, which depend on heart rate for cardiac output, diazepam-ketamine is used to avoid the bradycardia side effect of xylazine. The anesthesia can be prolonged with intermittent bolus doses of the combination or by inhalation anesthesia. Medetomidine (0.02 mg/kg) and ketamine (0.5–2 mg/kg) can be combined and administered intravenously to provide 30 minutes of strong sedation that, with local analgesia, is adequate for surgery (Hall et al. 2001). Tiletamine-zolazepam (12 mg/kg IV) provides similar but extended anesthesia to diazepam-ketamine in small ruminants (Hall et al. 2001). It is recommended that butorphanol be added for procedures requiring analgesia because unlike ketamine, tiletamine does not provide adequate analgesia. In calves and cattle under 500 lb, the dose of tiletamine-zolazepam is 4 mg/kg and is generally combined with 0.1 mg/kg of xylazine (Hall et al. 2001). The duration of action of this combination is 60–90 minutes. Due to hypoxia associated with this protocol, the anesthetist should be prepared for oxygen supplementation, especially in patients in dorsal recumbency.

Propofol can be used in sheep and goats (5–7 mg/kg IV) for induction and intubation (Hall et al. 2001). Premedication can cause a reduction in this dose. Due to the rapid elimination of propofol it can be given either as multiple bolus doses or in a constant rate infusion for anesthetic maintenance without causing a prolonged recovery. The CRI dose of propofol is 0.3–0.6 mg/kg/min and can be adjusted based on premedication given and extent of painful stimulus (Hall et al. 2001). Oxygen supplementation is imperative during anesthesia maintained on propofol CRI because hypotension and hypercarbia can result.

Inhalation anesthesia can safely produce a reliable anesthetic plane for both surgery and medical procedures. Isoflurane is the most commonly used inhalant in cattle, sheep, and goats. Generally, injectable agents are used for induction in lieu of the "masking" technique so that a protected patent airway can be established quickly. Adult animals are also hard to restrain for mask induction. A disadvantage of inhalants is the cardiovascular and respiratory depression that develops and intermittent positive pressure ventilation (IPPV), and inotropic drugs may be required. Sheep, goats, and small calves can be maintained on small-animal equipment. Breathing systems are chosen by size and weight similar to dog and cat parameters. In general, a vaporizer setting of 1–2% isoflurane is adequate in the premedicated patient. Sevoflurane can also be utilized, remembering that higher percentages need to be used due to its lower potency. Nitrous oxide should not be used in ruminants.

When placing the patient on the table, great attention should be paid to positioning. The patient should be placed with his head positioned so that the poll is higher than the nose to facilitate draining of saliva from the mouth. Additionally, the horns should be padded to protect them from breakage. In cattle, myopathy and radial nerve damage are a risk in extended anesthetic events of 20 or more minutes. Because of the anatomy of the shoulders, it is difficult to pull the lower foreleg forward as in horses. Therefore, the upper limbs should be positioned horizontally and elevated to remove the weight from the lower limbs. Any portion of the limbs resting on the table, floor, or supports should be well padded. Fluid therapy can be continued throughout the recovery period if a prolonged recovery or patient postoperative need is anticipated.

Monitoring during anesthesia can be accomplished either manually or mechanically or both. Often, a combination of manual and electronic monitoring is required for optimal observation of the patient. In anesthetized goats and sheep, the eye position is rostroventral during light to medium anesthetic depths and becomes centrally positioned when a deep anesthetic plane is achieved. "Star gazing," where the eye rolls dorsally, can occur with light anesthesia. In cattle, eye position changes from light to deep anesthesia differently than in the small ruminants. During light- and medium-depth anesthesia, the eye is in a ventral position where only the sclera can be seen, and in deep anesthetic planes the eye returns to a central position. Although ketamine can cause the pupil to dilate and the eye to remain central, generally in all ruminants the pupil constricts to a horizontal slit. Palpebral reflex is lost in all but light anesthesia or when ketamine is used for general anesthesia. Respiratory rates in anesthetized ruminants is generally quick and shallow, with goats and sheep being 15–30 bpm and cattle 20–40 bpm (Hall et al. 2001). Higher rates may indicate hypoventilation, hypoxemia, or hypercapnia, which is especially common in adult cattle. IPPV at a rate of 10 bpm and a tidal volume of 10 mL/kg will generally maintain a $PaCO_2$ of approximately 40 mm Hg. In small ruminants, the IPPV values are about 12 bpm and tidal volume 15 mL/kg (Hall et al. 2001). Inspiratory pressure should be adequate at 20–25 cm H_2O. Calves should be ventilated with small-ruminant values. Pulse oximetry and capnography can be used to measure oxygenation and ventilation. Monitoring both oxygenation and ventilation are important when the ruminant is in dorsal recumbency, which causes impairment of respiration. Rumen bloat, which can produce pressure on the diaphragm, can also cause reduced ventilation. This is more common in the small ruminants. A tube can be passed into the rumen to release the gas and pressure, but care must be taken to ensure that the tube remains unblocked by rumen contents. Tachycardia and hypertension are also side effects of hypercapnia and generally return to normal after IPPV is instituted.

Heart rate and blood pressure can easily be monitored in the ruminant. Heart rates for the small ruminants are generally 60–120 bpm, with <55 beats/min considered bradycardia and >140 bpm considered tachycardia where any underlying cause should be determined and treated. In adult cattle, HR should be 60–80 bpm under anesthesia (Hall et al. 2001). Adult cattle commonly develop hypertension, sometimes with systolic pressure >200 mmHg. Indirect blood pressure measurement has a large margin of error, and arterial direct blood pressure measurement is recommended with either a manometer or electrical transducer connected to a catheter in the auricular artery. In calves and the small ruminants, a mean arterial pressure (MAP) less than 65 mmHg should be considered hypotension and the cause determined and treated. Indirect blood pressure measurement is accurate in small ruminants and can be easily obtained by oscillometric monitor on either the fore- or hindlimbs. Treatment of hypotension in all ruminants can include IV boluses of crystalloid fluids at a rate of 10–20 mL/kg and decrease in anesthetic depth (Muir et al. 2000). Inotropic drugs may be required to stimulate cardiac output and increase blood pressure. Ephedrine (0.03–0.06 mg/kg) can be given IV, or a positive inotrope, dopamine, or dobutamine (5–7 mcg/kg/min) can be administered as a CRI in 0.9% NaCl (Blaze and Glowaski 2004). For hypotension associated with minimal blood loss, crystalloid fluids can be infused at a volume three times the volume of blood lost.

In calves, kids, and lambs, blood glucose levels should be monitored. Pediatric patients less than 3 months of age should be given 5% dextrose in water at 2–5 mL/kg/hr (Hall et al. 2001).

When the anesthetic period is complete, the ruminant should be moved to recovery and placed in sternal recumbency, propped up so that eructation and gas release can occur. The endotracheal tube should be left in the patient with the cuff inflated to protect its airway from regurgitation until the patient can chew, swallow, and move its tongue. The tube should be removed with a partially inflated cuff. Ruminants tend to be content to remain sternal in recovery until they can stand with little effort. Food and water can be offered 2–3 hours after standing.

Local anesthesia and epidural analgesia are commonly used in llamas and alpacas. Physical restraint includes placing the camelid into submissive sternal recumbency. It is best not to tie the patient, especially if 1 year old or less, because struggling could cause cervical vertebra injury. For caudal epidural analgesia, a 20-gauge 1–1-1/2-inch needle is placed in the sacrococcygeal space angled toward the base of the tail. An injection of lidocaine and xylazine or lidocaine alone is administered. Doses are those used for ruminants. The camelid usually will cush but have minimal signs of ataxia. The combination of lidocaine and xylazine will, of course, provide prolonged duration of analgesia. For standing castration, a combination of intramuscular butorphanol (0.1 mg/kg) and 2–5 mL of 2% lidocaine injected into each testicle, 10–15 minutes after the butorphanol injection works well (Hall et al. 2001). Additionally, 1–2 mL of lidocaine can be administered subcutaneously at the incision site.

Preanesthetic considerations for llamas and alpacas are the same as in the small ruminants. These camelids are susceptible to bloat, regurgitation, and aspiration and therefore should be fasted for 24 hours and water deprived for 8 hours (Fig. 36.5) (Muir et al. 2000). In young patients, no fasting is necessary.

In emergency cases, a protected airway needs to be established immediately upon induction of anesthesia.

Endotracheal intubation is achieved in much the same way as in sheep and goats. A laryngoscope with a long blade and a stylet placed in the

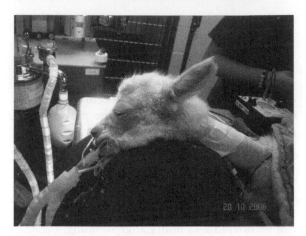

Figure 36.5 Alpaca cria anesthetized for enucleation surgery.

tube make intubation simpler. Intubation is important in llamas because they are obligate nasal breathers and are susceptible to airway obstruction due to displaced soft palate and nasal edema.

Xylazine (0.4–0.6 mg/kg IV) can be used for sedation. This dose will cause recumbency of 30-minute duration. Medetomidine (0.005–0.03 mg /kg IM) can also be used with high end dose causing sedation for 1–2 hours. Atipamazole (0.125 mg/kg IV) can be used for reversal (Hall et al. 2001).

To induce general anesthesia prior to inhalant anesthesia maintenance or to provide 30 minutes of anesthesia, one of two drug combinations can be used: Xylazine (0.25 mg/kg IV) with or without butorphanol (0.05 mg/kg IV or 0.1 mg/kg IM), wait 10–15 minutes, and then ketamine (2.5 mg/ kg IV or 5 mg/kg IM). The same combination can be used with the addition of diazepam or midazolam (0.1–0.2 mg/kg IV) to the ketamine (Hall

et al. 2001). In patients with urethral obstruction, xylazine should be avoided. Diazepam (0.1 mg/kg) and butorphanol (0.1 mg/kg) can be combined with 5% guaiphenesin (up to 0.5 mL/ kg), given to effect (sternal recumbency), and ketamine (2.5 mg/kg) in sick patients (Hall et al. 2001). In small llamas and alpacas, propofol (2.0–3.5 mg/kg IV) can be used for induction (Muir et al. 2000). Anesthetic maintenance can then be accomplished with inhalants or a constant rate infusion of propofol (0.4 mg/kg/min) (Hall et al. 2001).

Analgesia will need to be provided additionally. MAP and cardiac output are generally not depressed by propofol CRI; however, this protocol can be expensive. Inhalant anesthesia should be considered for prolonged procedures. Most llamas will breathe spontaneously 10–30 bpm and ventilate well. IPPV would be necessary in the face of hypoventilation.

Camelids should be recovered with the procedure outlined under ruminant recovery, with a plan for potential upper airway obstruction in place.

References

Blaze, CA, Glowaski, MM. 2004. Veterinary Anesthesia Drug Quick Reference. St. Louis: Elsevier Saunders, pp.1–99, 105–108, 156–167.

Hall, LW, Clarke, KW, Trim, CM. 2001. Veterinary Anaesthesia, 10th ed. London: WB Saunders, pp.315–365.

Muir, WW, Hubbell, JAE, Skarda, RT, Bednarski RM. 2000. Handbook of Veterinary Anesthesia, 3rd ed. St. Louis: Mosby, Inc., pp.57–81, 343–358.

Index

Printed and bound by CPI Group (UK) Ltd, Croydon, CR0 4YY

27/10/2024

14580250-0003